Bowel Imaging

Editor

PERRY J. PICKHARDT

RADIOLOGIC CLINICS OF NORTH AMERICA

www.radiologic.theclinics.com

Consulting Editor
FRANK H. MILLER

January 2013 • Volume 51 • Number 1

ELSEVIER

1600 John F. Kennedy Boulevard • Suite 1800 • Philadelphia, Pennsylvania 19103-2899

http://www.theclinics.com

RADIOLOGIC CLINICS OF NORTH AMERICA Volume 51, Number 1
January 2013 ISSN 0033-8389, ISBN 13: 978-1-4557-7326-8

Editor: Adrianne Brigido

Radiologic Clinics of North America (ISSN 0033-8389) is published bimonthly by Elsevier Inc., 360 Park Avenue South, New York, NY 10010-1710. Months of issue are January, March, May, July, September, and November. Periodicals postage paid at New York, NY and additional mailing offices. Subscription prices are USD 421 per year for US individuals, USD 659 per year for US institutions, USD 202 per year for US students and residents, USD 491 per year for Canadian individuals, USD 827 per year for Canadian institutions, USD 606 per year for international individuals, USD 827 per year for international institutions, and USD 290 per year for Canadian and foreign students/residents. To receive student and resident rate, orders must be accompanied by name of affiliated institution, date of term and the signature of program/residency coordinatior on institution letterhead. Orders will be billed at individual rate until proof of status is received. Foreign air speed delivery is included in all *Clinics* subscription prices. All prices are subject to change without notice. **POSTMASTER:** Send address changes to *Radiologic Clinics of North America*, Elsevier Health Sciences Division, Subscription Customer Service, 3251 Riverport Lane, Maryland Heights, MO63043. **Customer Service: Telephone: 1-800-654-2452** (U.S. and Canada); **1-314-447-8871** (outside U.S. and Canada). **Fax: 1-314-447-8029. E-mail: journalscustomerservice-usa@ elsevier.com** (for print support); **journalsonlinesupport-usa@elsevier.com** (for online support).

Reprints. For copies of 100 or more of articles in this publication, please contact the Commercial Reprints Department, Elsevier Inc., 360 Park Avenue South, New York, New York 10010-1710. Tel.: (+1) 212-633-3812; Fax: (+1) 212-462-1935; E-mail: reprints@elsevier.com.

Radiologic Clinics of North America also published in Greek Paschalidis Medical Publications, Athens, Greece.

Radiologic Clinics of North America is covered in *MEDLINE/PubMed (Index Medicus), EMBASE/Excerpta Medica, Current Contents/Life Sciences, Current Contents/Clinical Medicine, RSNA Index to Imaging Literature, BIOSIS, Science Citation Index,* and *ISI/BIOMED*.

Printed in the United States of America.

Contributors

CONSULTING EDITOR

FRANK H. MILLER, MD
Professor of Radiology; Chief, Body Imaging
Section and Fellowship Program and GI
Radiology; Medical Director MRI, Department
of Radiology, Feinberg School of Medicine,
Northwestern University, Chicago, Illinois

EDITOR

PERRY J. PICKHARDT, MD
Professor of Radiology and Chief,
Gastrointestinal Imaging, University of
Wisconsin, School of Medicine and Public
Health, Madison, Wisconsin

AUTHORS

MAHMOUD M. AL-HAWARY, MD
Diagnostic Radiology, Abdominal Imaging
Division, University of Michigan, Ann Arbor,
Michigan

MICHAEL BELAND, MD
Assistant Professor, Diagnostic Imaging;
Director of Ultrasound, Warren Alpert School
of Medicine, Brown University, Providence,
Rhode Island

RITU BORDIA, MBBS
Fourth Year Radiology Resident, Department
of Radiology, Winthrop-University Hospital,
Mineola, New York

**CATHERINE E. DEWHURST, MB, BCh,
BAO, BMedSc**
Fellow, Divisions of Abdominal Imaging and
Body MRI, Department of Radiology, Beth
Israel Deaconess Medical Center, Boston,
Massachusetts

DAVID J. GRAND, MD
Assistant Professor, Diagnostic Imaging;
Director, Body MRI, Warren Alpert School
of Medicine, Brown University, Providence,
Rhode Island

ANNO GRASER, MD
Associate Professor of Radiology and Head
of Oncologic Imaging, Department of Clinical
Radiology, University of Munich, Munich,
Germany

ADAM HARRIS, MD
Assistant Professor of Medicine, Department
of Gastroenterology, Warren Alpert School of
Medicine, Brown University, Providence,
Rhode Island

CESARE HASSAN, MD
Digestive Endoscopy Unit, Nuovo Regina
Margherita Hospital, Roma, Italy

JOHN J. HINES, MD
Assistant Radiology Residency Director, Long
Island Jewish Medical Center, New Hyde Park,
New York; Assistant Professor of Radiology,
Department of Radiology, Hofstra University
School of Medicine, New York

BRUCE R. JAVORS, MD, FACR
Director of Abdominal Imaging, Department
of Radiology, Winthrop-University Hospital,
Mineola, New York

DOUGLAS S. KATZ, MD, FACR
Director of Body CT and Vice Chair of Clinical
Research and Education, Department of
Radiology, Winthrop-University Hospital,
Mineola, New York; Professor of Clinical
Radiology, State University of New York,
Stony Brook School of Medicine, Stony Brook,
New York

RAVI K. KAZA, MD
Diagnostic Radiology, Abdominal Imaging
Division, University of Michigan, Ann Arbor,
Michigan

DAVID H. KIM, MD
Department of Radiology, University of
Wisconsin School of Medicine and Public
Health, Madison, Wisconsin

SEUNG SOO LEE, MD
Associate Professor, Department of Radiology
and Research Institute of Radiology, Asan
Medical Center, University of Ulsan College of
Medicine, Songpa-Gu, Seoul, South Korea

JONATHAN A. LEIGHTON, MD
Professor of Medicine, Division of
Gastroenterology, Department of Internal
Medicine, Mayo Clinic Arizona, Arizona

DEAN D.T. MAGLINTE, MD
Distinguished Professor of Radiology and
Imaging Sciences, Indiana University School of
Medicine, IU Health – University Hospital,
Indianapolis, Indiana

KOENRAAD J. MORTELE, MD
Director, Division of Clinical MRI; Staff
Radiologist, Divisions of Abdominal Imaging
and Body MRI, Beth Israel Deaconess Medical
Center; Associate Professor of Radiology,
Harvard Medical School, Boston,
Massachusetts

SEONG HO PARK, MD
Associate Professor, Department of Radiology
and Research Institute of Radiology, Asan
Medical Center, University of Ulsan College of
Medicine, Songpa-Gu, Seoul, South Korea

SHABANA F. PASHA, MD
Assistant Professor of Medicine, Division
of Gastroenterology, Department of Internal
Medicine, Mayo Clinic College of Medicine,
Arizona

PERRY J. PICKHARDT, MD
Professor of Radiology and Chief,
Gastrointestinal Imaging, University of
Wisconsin, School of Medicine and Public
Health, Madison, Wisconsin

JOEL F. PLATT, MD
Diagnostic Radiology, Abdominal Imaging
Division, University of Michigan, Ann Arbor,
Michigan

PETER M. RODGERS, FRCR
Consultant Radiologist, Radiology
Department, Leicester Royal Infirmary,
University Hospitals of Leicester, Leicester,
United Kingdom

CYNTHIA S. SANTILLAN, MD
Associate Professor of Radiology;
Vice-Chief of Body Imaging Section and
Chief of Body CT, Department of Radiology,
University of California San Diego, San Diego,
California

CHRISTOPHER D. SCHEIREY, MD
Assistant Professor of Radiology, Tufts
University School of Medicine, Boston,
Massachusetts; Radiology Residency Director,
Department of Radiology, Lahey Clinic,
Burlington, Massachusetts

FRANCIS J. SCHOLZ, MD, FACR
Professor of Radiology, Tufts University School
of Medicine, Boston, Massachusetts

RATAN VERMA, FRCR
Consultant Radiologist, Radiology
Department, Leicester General Hospital,
University Hospitals of Leicester, Leicester,
United Kingdom

Contents

> Crohn's disease represents a heterogeneous group of patients who have different clinical phenotypes. Computed tomography enterography (CTE) has been validated and optimized over the recent years since its introduction in the past decade and now has a clear established role as one of the primary diagnostic tools in the evaluation of patients with Crohn's disease. This article describes the current clinical concepts in Crohn's disease activity assessment and the use of imaging as well as the typical imaging findings in different subtypes of Crohn's disease using CTE.

> Multidetector computed tomography (CT) is a powerful tool for the assessment of patients with small bowel obstruction (SBO). CT can provide important information about the cause and site of obstruction and the presence of a closed-loop obstruction or ischemia. Under investigation is the ability of CT to accurately identify patients without clear indications for urgent surgery who may benefit from earlier intervention. This article reviews the appropriate CT technique for assessment of SBO, common causes for obstruction, imaging findings in SBO, and the significance of those findings for determining whether a patient is likely to require surgical management for SBO.

> Gastrointestinal bleeding and acute mesenteric ischemia are conditions that generally require an urgent and accurate diagnosis. In this setting, multidetector computed tomography (MDCT) can play an important role. This article discusses current techniques, the findings in correlation with pathophysiology, and the proper use of MDCT in the diagnostic evaluation and management of these patients.

> This article reviews the computed tomography (CT) findings of miscellaneous regional and diffuse small bowel disorders. CT technique and potential pitfalls are discussed. Several categories of regional and diffuse small bowel conditions are reviewed, with representative CT images. These disorders often have relatively nonspecific CT appearances, and correlation with the history, clinical, and laboratory findings in each specific case is critical. In selected conditions, the CT findings are highly specific. The imaging literature of some of the common as well as some of the less common entities is reviewed, and clues to narrowing the differential diagnosis are provided.

As with any radiologic imaging test, there are several potential interpretive pitfalls at CT colonography that need to be recognized and handled appropriately. Perhaps the single most important step in learning to avoid most of these diagnostic traps is simply to be aware of their existence. With a little experience, most of these potential pitfalls are easily recognized. This article systematically covers the key pitfalls confronting the radiologist at CT colonography interpretation, primarily dividing them into those related to technique and those related to underlying anatomy. Tips and pointers for how to effectively handle these potential pitfalls are included.

Simulation modeling is extensively applied to CT colonography (CTC) to define its long-term efficacy and cost-effectiveness for colorectal cancer (CRC) screening. CTC is effective in reducing CRC incidence and mortality (40%–77% and 58%–84%, respectively). Several factors may explain this variability. CTC is cost-effective compared with no screening, indicating that it represents an attractive test noncompliance with the available options. CTC needs to achieve a higher attendance rate or cost less than colonoscopy to be cost-effective relative to colonoscopy. Fortunately, both conditions appear to be achievable if CTC becomes a widely utilized and reimbursed screening tool.

Magnetic resonance (MR) enterography is a targeted examination of the gastrointestinal tract, particularly the small intestine, without nasojejunal intubation (in which case it is referred to as MR enteroclysis). Until recently, MR imaging of the small bowel could not reliably compete with the high-quality small bowel images generated by computed tomography (CT). Now, however, MR enterography is not only a feasible alternative to CT, but may provide superior diagnostic information, specifically with regard to differentiating active, inflammatory disease from chronic, fibrostenotic disease. MR enterography is no longer merely adequate and radiation-free; it is an essential part of the imaging armamentarium.

Magnetic resonance colonography (MRC) is performed on a whole body scanner after laxative-based purgation and distension of the large bowel with water. To achieve good image quality, acquisition of sequences within a comfortable breath-hold time is essential. Frequently, fast 3D fat-saturated T1-weighted techniques with parallel imaging are used to meet this demand, providing "dark lumen" contrast of the bowel with high signal intensity of the bowel wall after intravenous injection of contrast agent. This article sheds light on MRC technique, image acquisition, post processing, and normal findings, relevant pathologies, and differential diagnoses of the most frequent pathologies encountered at MRC.

This article aims to discuss the anatomy of the anorectum, the MRI protocol parameters required to optimize diagnosis of rectal cancer, and the diagnostic MRI criteria essential to stage rectal cancer accurately, using the TNM staging classification. A brief review of more emerging important aspects of rectal cancer staging, such as the circumferential resection margin, extramural vascular invasion, and the staging of low rectal cancers, will also be provided. Finally, the authors will touch upon the evaluation of tumor response to neoadjuvant chemoradiation therapy in the setting of locally advanced rectal cancer.

PROGRAM OBJECTIVE:

The objective of the Radiologic Clinics of North America is to keep practicing radiologists and radiology residents up to date with current clinical practice in radiology by providing timely articles reviewing the state of the art in patient care.

TARGET AUDIENCE

Practicing radiologists, radiology residents, and other health care professionals who provide patient care utilizing radiologic findings.

ACCREDITATION

The Elsevier Office of Continuing Medical Education (EOCME) is accredited by the Accreditation Council for Continuing Medical Education (ACCME) to provide continuing medical education for physicians.

The EOCME designates this journal-based CME activity for a maximum of 12 *AMA PRA Category 1 Credit*(s)™. Physicians should claim only the credit commensurate with the extent of their participation in the activity.

All other health care professionals completing continuing education credit for this activity will be issued a certificate of participation.

DISCLOSURE OF CONFLICTS OF INTEREST

The EOCME assesses conflict of interest with its instructors, faculty, planners, and other individuals who are in a position to control the content of CME activities. All relevant conflicts of interest that are identified are thoroughly vetted by EOCME for fair balance, scientific objectivity, and patient care recommendations. EOCME is committed to providing its learners with CME activities that promote improvements or quality in healthcare and not a specific proprietary business or a commercial interest.

The planning committee, staff, authors and editors listed below have identified no financial relationships or relationships to products or devices they or their spouse/life partner have with commercial interest related to the content of this CME activity:
Mahmoud M. Al-Hawary, MD; Michael Beland, MD; Ritu Bordia, MBBS; Nicole Congleton; Catherine E. Dewhurst, MB, BCh, BAO, BMedSc; David J. Grand, MD; Adam Harris, MD; Cesare Hassan, MD; John J. Hines, MD; Bruce R. Javors, MD; Douglas S. Katz, MD; Ravi K. Kaza, MD; Seung Soo Lee, MD; Jill McNair; Frank H. Miller, MD; Koenraad J. Mortele, MD; Nagaraj Paramasivam; Seong Ho Park, MD; Joel F. Platt, MD; Peter M. Rodgers, FRCR; Christopher D. Scheirey, MD; Francis J. Scholz, MD; Katelynn Steck; and Ratan Verma, FRCR.

The planning committee, staff, authors and editors listed below have identified financial relationships or relationships to products or devices they or their spouse/life partner have with commercial interest related to the content of this CME activity:
Anno Graser, MD is on the speakers bureau for Siemens AG Healthcare Sector, Bayer AG Healthcare, Pfizer Pharma and is a consultant for Siemens AG Healthcare Sector.
David H. Kim, MD is a consultant/advisor for Viatronix and owns stock in VirtuoCTC.
Jonathan A. Leighton, MD is a consultant/advisor for Given Imaging and Olympus and received a research grant from Given Imaging and Capsovision.
Dean D.T. Maglinte, MD received royalties/patents from Cook Inc.
Shabana F. Pasha, MD received a research grant from Capsovision.
Perry J. Pickhardt, MD is a consultant/advisor for Virtuo CTC, Viatronix, iCAD, Bracco, and Check-Cap.
Cynthia S. Santillan, MD is a consultant for Robarts Clinical Research.

UNAPPROVED/OFF-LABEL USE DISCLOSURE

The EOCME requires CME faculty to disclose to the participants:

1. When products or procedures being discussed are off-label, unlabelled, experimental, and/or investigational (not US Food and Drug Administration (FDA) approved; and
2. Any limitations on the information presented, such as data that are preliminary or that represent ongoing research, interim analyses, and/or unsupported opinions. Faculty may discuss information about pharmaceutical agents that is outside of DA-approved labelling. This information is intended solely for CME and is not intended to promote off-label use of these medications. If you have any questions, contact the medical affairs department of the manufacturer for the most recent prescribing information.

TO ENROLL

To enroll in the *Radiologic Clinics of North America* Continuing Medical Education program, call customer service at 1-800-654-2452 or sign up online at http://www.theclinics.com/home/cme. The CME program is available to subscribers for an additional annual fee of $288 USD.

METHOD OF PARTICIPATION

In order to claim credit, participants must complete the following:

1. Complete enrolment as indicated above.
2. Read the activity.
3. Complete the CME Test and Evaluation. Participants must achieve a score of 70% on the test. All CME Tests and Evaluations must be completed online.

CME INQUIRIES/SPECIAL NEEDS

For all CME inquiries or special needs, please contact elsevierCME@elsevier.com.

RADIOLOGIC CLINICS OF NORTH AMERICA

DOWNLOAD Free App!

Review Articles
THE CLINICS

NOW AVAILABLE FOR YOUR iPhone and iPad

Preface

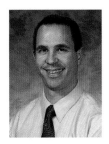

Perry J. Pickhardt, MD
Guest Editor

This issue of the *Radiologic Clinics of North America* is devoted to imaging of the small and large intestine. Of the 12 articles in total, 8 are focused primarily on diseases of the small bowel and 4 are focused on colorectal imaging. The contents are also organized by modality, with 6 articles devoted to CT imaging, 3 articles devoted to MR imaging, and the remainder primarily covering ultrasound, fluoroscopy, and endoscopy.

The small bowel has often been regarded as a "final frontier" of sorts, largely due to its relative inaccessibility to conventional diagnostic means. Although fluoroscopic evaluation certainly remains relevant for small bowel evaluation, cross-sectional and endoscopic imaging have largely revolutionized the field. From the diagnostic standpoint, CT enterography, MR enterography, and capsule endoscopy have each made an enormous impact on clinical practice, whereas techniques such as double-balloon enteroscopy are now shifting the therapeutic paradigm. Perhaps the greatest collective strength of these studies lies in their complementary nature, ranging from exquisite mucosal assessment to transmural and extraintestinal evaluation. Specific small bowel topics covered herein include Crohn's disease, mechanical obstruction, ischemia, and a host of other miscellaneous conditions.

As with the small intestine, imaging evaluation of the large intestine has also undergone remarkable advances over the past decade. The general shift toward less-invasive diagnostic evaluation through the use of cross-sectional imaging is allowing the more invasive endoscopic techniques to focus more appropriately on their therapeutic role. Prior validation of CT colonography as an accurate diagnostic technique should now logically give way to expanding clinical utilization. Rather than regurgitate past performance results from CT colonography trials herein, this issue instead tackles the more practical and current issues of interpretive pitfalls and cost-effectiveness. The use of MR for rectal cancer staging has also rapidly matured in recent years and is now an invaluable component for patient care. Finally, the current status of MR colonography is also covered in this issue.

I am deeply indebted to all of the contributing authors for generously sharing their cutting-edge expertise and insights in such an illustrative and understandable fashion. I am confident that this installment of the *Radiologic Clinics of North America* will be a valuable and unique resource for both practicing radiologists and allied clinicians for years to come.

I would like to dedicate this issue to the memory of Dr Michael Macari, a dear friend and colleague, who contributed so much to the field of gastrointestinal imaging over a regrettably short period of time—and who will be greatly missed on both the professional and the personal level.

Perry J. Pickhardt, MD
Gastrointestinal Imaging
University of Wisconsin
School of Medicine and Public Health
Madison, WI 53792-3252, USA

E-mail address:
ppickhardt2@uwhealth.org

CT Enterography: Concepts and Advances in Crohn's Disease Imaging

Mahmoud M. Al-Hawary, MD*, Ravi K. Kaza, MD,
Joel F. Platt, MD

KEYWORDS

- Computed tomography • CTE • Crohn's disease • Small bowel • CT radiation dose

KEY POINTS

- Crohn's disease represents a heterogeneous group of patients who have different clinical phenotypes.
- Cross-sectional imaging evaluation can alter patient management in a significant number of patients detecting clinically unsuspected disease.
- Computed tomography enterography can assess the extent and location of bowel involvement with Crohn's disease and can help detect complications, such as fistula, abscess, stricture, and obstruction.

INTRODUCTION

Computed tomography enterography (CTE) has been validated and optimized over the recent years since its introduction in the past decade and now has a clear established role as one of the primary diagnostic tools in the evaluation of patients with Crohn's disease. CTE is a noninvasive examination that offers important and relevant information in the diagnosis and management of patients with proven or suspected Crohn's disease and is supplemental to clinical and endoscopic findings. Recent advances in radiation dose reduction from CT examinations will likely help in maintaining the role of CTE in the follow-up of patients with Crohn's disease to assess disease complication as well as treatment response. This article describes the current clinical concepts in Crohn's disease activity assessment and the use of imaging as well as the typical imaging findings in different subtypes of Crohn's disease using CTE.

Background and Current Concepts in Crohn's Disease Activity Assessment

Crohn's disease is a chronic inflammatory condition that represents 1 of 2 major clinically recognized phenotypic types of inflammatory bowel diseases: Crohn's disease and ulcerative colitis. Crohn's disease can affect any part of the gastrointestinal tract extending from the mouth to the anus. There is more recognition recently with improved understanding of the genetic and environmental basis of inflammatory bowel diseases that patients affected with Crohn's disease represent a heterogeneous group, which appears to vary in observed disease location, behavior, severity, and responsiveness to therapies.[1] Clinical classifications of the disease, such as the proposed Vienna classification and the later modification in the Montreal classification, can help in defining recognized subgroups of patients with different disease phenotypes that may be suitable for studying the influence of specific genetic or environmental factors.[2,3] Based on these classification systems, some patients have long-standing and stable inflammatory disease, whereas others have a more complicated form of the disease that can arise at any time point in the disease course, developing fistulizing or stricturing complications.[4] The Vienna and Montreal classification systems categorize patients with Crohn's disease into distinct subgroups that reflect the characteristic disease involvement based on age, location, and

Diagnostic Radiology, Abdominal Imaging Division, University of Michigan, University Hospital, 1500 East Medical Center Drive, Room B1 D502, Ann Arbor, MI 48109, USA
* Corresponding author.
E-mail address: alhawary@med.umich.edu

Radiol Clin N Am 51 (2013) 1–16
http://dx.doi.org/10.1016/j.rcl.2012.09.001

predominant phenotype or behavior of the disease (**Table 1**).

A study of the behavior of Crohn's disease according to the Vienna classification by Louis and colleagues[4] showed that the location of the disease remained stable over the course of the disease except in a small proportion of patients (15.9%) who had a change in location over 10 years (**Fig. 1**). However, they also observed significant change in the disease behavior in 45.9% of patients over a 10-year period, with the most prominent change seen from nonstricturing, nonpenetrating B1 disease to either stricturing B2 (27.1%) or penetrating B3 (29.4%) disease. The importance of recognizing the different patterns of disease behavior, especially early in the disease course, may help in tailoring specific therapies, predicting future complications, and possibly offer better timing of surgical interventions. Ongoing investigations studying a variety of clinical, endoscopic, genetic, serum, and stool biomarkers are underway to help better predict disease behavior.[5–7] An important emerging concept in assessing disease activity, in particular based on imaging evaluation, is to understand the interplay of inflammation and fibrosis in patients with Crohn's disease. Traditionally, Crohn's disease is classified as active or inflammatory versus fibrotic based on CTE findings, suggesting that both forms are mutually exclusive. However, a recently published study by Adler and colleagues[8] showed that strictures identified on CTE with the most active disease activity also had the most fibrosis on histology. Their results suggest that both active inflammation and fibrosis appear to coexist in the same bowel segment and possibly that inflammation progresses to fibrosis over time. This concept bears important implications on correlating the clinical disease assessment with the imaging findings detected by CTE.

Use of CTE in Crohn's Disease

Cross-sectional evaluation of bowel pathology with CT has come a long way since the concept of optimized small bowel imaging or CTE was first introduced by Raptopoulos and colleagues[9] in 1997. Several validation studies have been published since then in the radiology literature correlating cross-sectional evaluation of patients with Crohn's disease to clinical, pathologic, endoscopic, and other established imaging modalities that validate the use of CTE as one of the primary imaging modalities in the evaluation of patients with known or suspected Crohn's disease.[10–19] This validation has led to progressive increase in the use of CTE in recent years, with significant shift from predominant fluoroscopy-based imaging to cross-sectional imaging evaluation. In addition, recent evidence has also shown that cross-sectional evaluation has significant impact on patient management, helping better characterize disease activity and involvement, especially with frequent nonspecific nature of the patient symptoms and clinical presentation, leading to detection of clinically unsuspected disease. A study by Higgins and colleagues[20] showed that CTE findings are not equivalent to clinical assessment, demonstrating either unsuspected strictures in up to 16% of patients or absence of a radiologically significant stricture in more than half the subjects with clinically suspected strictures. CTE findings also changed the perceived likelihood of steroid benefit in a significant proportion of patients (61%) in their study population. These investigators concluded that CTE altered the management plans in more than 50% of patients with established or suspected Crohn's disease. Another recent study by Bruining and colleagues[21] showed that CTE altered management plans in up to 51% of patients with established or suspected Crohn's disease, with

Table 1
The vienna and montreal crohn's disease clinical classification

	Vienna Classification	Montreal Classification
Age at Diagnosis:	A1: below 40 y A2: equal to or above 40 y	A1: below 17 y A2: 17–40 y A3: Above 40 y
Location:	L1: terminal ileum L2: colon L3: ileocolon L4: upper gastrointestinal	L1: TI+-limited cecal disease L2: colon L3: ileocolonic L4: isolated upper gastrointestinal
Behavior:	B1: nonstricturing nonpenetrating B2: stricturing B3: penetrating	B1: nonstricturing nonpenetrating B2: stricturing B3: penetrating p: perianal disease modifier

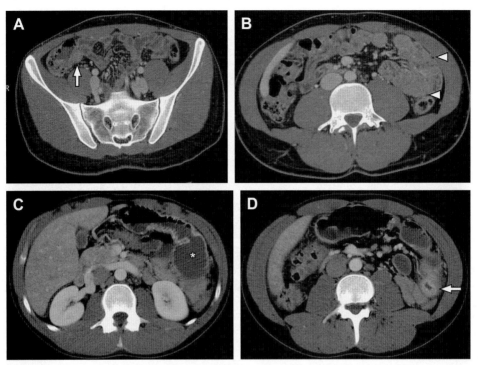

Fig. 1. (*A, B*) Axial images from CTE examination in a patient with isolated terminal ileum Crohn's disease (*arrow*). Note normal appearance of the jejunum (*arrowheads*). (*C, D*) Follow-up examination show unsuspected proximal bowel obstruction (*asterisk*) due to new site of disease in the proximal ileum (*arrow*) showing signs of active inflammation and luminal narrowing leading to the bowel obstruction.

the most frequent changes being the exclusion of small intestinal inflammation and medication alterations. A second important finding in the same study was the effect of CTE on the physician's level of confidence for the findings of active small bowel disease, fistula, abscess, or stricture formation, which was altered in more than 90% of cases, with clinically significant changes in up to 77.6% (**Fig. 2**A, B). Booya and colleagues[22] also reported detection of clinically unsuspected penetrating disease on CTE examinations, leading to alteration in therapy in up to 61% of patients with Crohn's disease. One of the major limitation of clinically unsuspected stricture is the potential for capsule endoscopy retention if a small bowel stricture is not excluded before the capsule administration (see **Fig. 2**C, D). In conclusion, these studies show the limited sensitivity for detecting disease distribution and complications based on clinical impression alone, emphasize the clinical benefit of CTE in assessing small bowel disease activity and complications, and help in altering the patient management.

CTE
Imaging Protocol

Historical sensitivity of CT imaging for small bowel disorders has been suboptimal because of compounding limiting factors including the lack of appropriate or adequate bowel distension, which limits the assessment for bowel wall thickening and lack of visual contrast between the bowel lumen and the adjacent mucosa to detect inflammatory changes in the bowel wall. Recent advances in CT imaging include the introduction of newer oral contrast agents, the currently widely available multidetector CT scanners, and availability of newer CT radiation dose reduction techniques.[23–28]

Oral contrast preparation

The use of routine high attenuation or positive, barium- or iodine-based, enteric oral contrast can mask the visualization of the bowel wall enhancement pattern, especially along the mucosal side (**Fig. 3**). The ideal oral enteric contrast for optimization of the bowel wall evaluation should provide 2 tasks. The first task is to appropriately distend the bowel lumen in a more or less uniform pattern throughout the small bowel to better assess the presence of bowel wall thickening, which is present in most affected bowel segments with Crohn's disease, and decrease the incidence of false-positive results (**Fig. 4**). Ideally, the oral agent should be nonabsorbable to achieve more uniform distension in particular toward the distal small

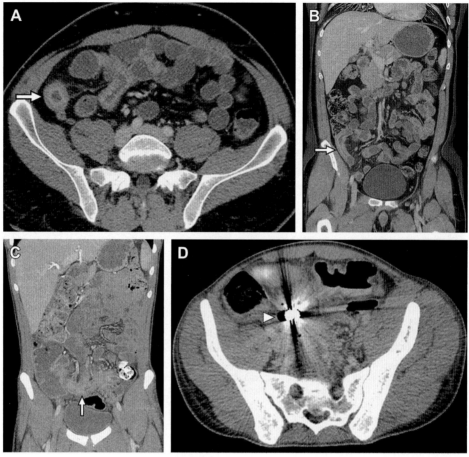

Fig. 2. Axial (*A*) and coronal reformatted (*B*) CTE images in a patient with unsuspected distal ileal stricture demonstrating bowel wall thickening and luminal narrowing (*arrow*). No proximal bowel dilatation noted to suggest significant obstruction. (*C*) Coronal reformatted image from CTE examination in a different patient with terminal ileum Crohn's disease (*arrow*). There is luminal narrowing without proximal dilatation. Endoscopic capsule was administered before the CTE examination to investigate suspected Crohn's disease. (*D*) The axial CT image demonstrates the retention of the capsule (*arrowhead*) proximal to the site of the ileal stricture.

bowel or terminal ileum, which is affected in a significant proportion of patients. The second task is to provide adequate difference in the visual contrast between the bowel lumen and the bowel wall.

Because the intended evaluation in patients with Crohn's disease is the enhancement pattern of the bowel wall, especially the mucosal side, which is bright on CT examinations, these ideal oral agents

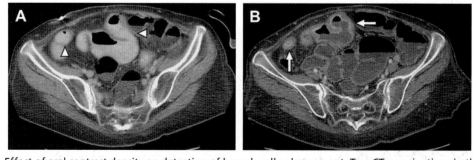

Fig. 3. Effect of oral contrast density on detection of bowel wall enhancement. Two CT examinations in the same patient with ileal Crohn's disease (*A*) obtained with positive oral contrast and (*B*) with neutral oral contrast. The mural enhancement pattern and bowel wall stratification are only appreciated on the examination performed with the neutral oral contrast (*arrows*) and not on the scan with the positive oral contrast (*arrowheads*).

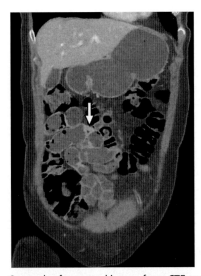

Fig. 4. Coronal reformatted image from CTE examination in a patient with nonspecific abdominal pain. Collapsed bowel segment in the proximal ileum (*arrow*) shows apparent increased bowel wall enhancement compared with the adjacent well-distended bowel segments, which is likely secondary to bowel peristalsis and contraction with lack of appreciable bowel wall thickening, adjacent engorged mesenteric vascularity, or mesenteric fat haziness.

should be of sufficient low density to contrast the bowel wall and are most commonly referred to as neutral (or low Hounsfield units) oral contrast. One limitation of the similar density between the neutral oral contrast and fluid-containing structures, such as abscesses, is the potential risk of missing a small interloop abscess (**Fig. 5**). This limitation can be avoided by carefully following the bowel lumen and confirming lack of continuity and correlation with multiplanar projections in suspected extraluminal fluid collections. Several oral contrast agents have been used as neutral oral contrast agents, such as milk, Mucofalk, mannitol, methylcellulose solution, lactulose, polyethylene glycol electrolyte solution, and low-concentration barium oral suspension.[29–33] The neutral oral contrast agent most commonly used for peroral CTE is dilute 0.1% barium sulfate mixed with sorbitol (VoLumen; Bracco Diagnostics, Inc, Princeton, NJ, USA). The dilute barium sulfate suspension contains sorbitol to reduce water absorption and gum to increase viscosity.[34] This oral contrast suspension is nonabsorbable and demonstrates low attenuation that would fit the profile of intended oral contrast for CTE. Several different oral contrast administration regimens have been used, but the most common protocol involves the administration of high volume of the oral contrast (usually between 900 and 1350 mL) to achieve adequate distension. Average range

of oral contrast timing varies between 30 minutes and 90 minutes. In the authors' department, 1350 mL of the oral contrast is administered over a course of 1 hour before the examination, starting with 450 mL administered at 1 hour, 450 mL at 40 minutes, and splitting the last dose into 225 mL at 20 minutes and the other 225 mL immediately before the scan. Water can be substituted for the last dose, depending on patients' tolerance, because absorption is not a significant issue for distending the stomach and duodenum.

Intravenous contrast
The enteric system can be imaged at multiple phases of enhancement depending on the clinical scenario. The enhancement phases are divided into the arterial, enteric, portal venous, and delayed phases. In patients with Crohn's disease, most commonly a single phase of scanning is obtained, which includes either the enteric phase, obtained at maximal bowel enhancement, or the portal venous phase, which provides acceptable enhancement pattern of the bowel wall and surrounding structures including the mesenteric fat and terminal mesenteric vessels that allows appropriate evaluation of the disease activity and detection of extraintestinal complications.[23,24] The authors' CTE protocol includes the administration of 125 cc of high iodine concentration contrast (Isovue-370; Bracco Diagnostics, Inc, Princeton, NJ, USA) at an injection rate of 4 cc/s followed by 50 cc saline flush injected at a rate of 4 cc/s, with scan acquisition at 65 seconds from the start of the injection to obtain nearly portal venous images.

CT technique
The introduction of multidetector CT technology (MDCT) allowed for the acquisition of multiple imaging slices through the patient during each gantry rotation, with resultant improvement in both the spatial and temporal resolutions of image acquisition. The multi-slice acquisition results in a longer area of coverage during a shorter time, allowing for a more homogeneous acquisition in a single phase of enhancement without appreciable bowel motion effect, which in turn leads to improved imaging of the enteric system. The thin slices also allows better depiction of the mucosal edge and transmural changes noted in inflammatory bowel disease with better visualization of the terminal mesenteric vessels. Because thin slices offer the possibility of obtaining isotropic or near-isotropic resolution voxels with 16-detector or higher CT scanners, the acquired slices can then be reconstructed in any thickness perservering the quality of the examination while decreasing

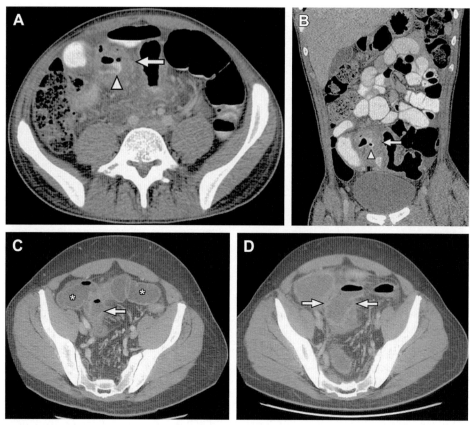

Fig. 5. (*A*) Axial and (*B*) coronal reformatted images from CT examination performed with positive oral contrast in a patient with ileal Crohn's disease. An interloop abscess is present in the right lower quadrant (*arrows*) containing extraluminal high-density oral contrast (*arrowheads*). (*C*) Axial CT examination performed with neutral oral contrast in a patient with ileal Crohn's disease show a small gas containing interloop fluid collection (*arrow*), which was confused with a fluid-filled bowel segment due to the similar density with the surrounding bowel (*asterisks*). (*D*) Follow-up CT in the same patient following the start of immunosuppressive therapy shows increase in the size of the fluid collection (*arrow*) confirming a worsening interloop abscess.

the number of images for easier review while the sub-millimeter slices are used to generate the 3-dimensional (3D) and multiplanar images.[26,34] Our imaging display includes the source 0.625 mm images, which are reconstructed at 2.5 mm thickness, coronal reformat at 2 mm thickness, and 3D volumetric thick section in the coronal and both oblique projections.

CT dose reduction

Although the true biologic effects from low-level radiation exposure of CT scan are not well established, the increased cumulative effective dose (CED) in patients with inflammatory bowel disease who require multiple imaging studies has become a growing concern.[35,36] Chatu and colleagues,[37] in their meta-analysis of diagnostic medical radiation exposure in patients with inflammatory bowel disease, reported that about 1 in 10 patients may be exposed to potentially harmful levels of radiation

(defined as ≥50 mSv). Peloquin and colleagues[38] reported that CT scans accounted for 51% of the CED in patients with Crohn's disease. Desmond and colleagues,[39] in their 15-year study period of patients with inflammatory bowel disease, noted that the portion of CT scans contributing to CED increased from 46.3% during the first 5 years to 84.7% during the final 5 years. This increase in part is likely due to the increased reliance on CT as a primary diagnostic tool in the follow-up of patients because it can detect clinically unsuspected complications of the disease in a significant proportion of patients, which can alter their management.[20] Recent improvement and validation of magnetic resonance enterography (MRE) as a radiation-free alternative to CTE with diagnostic efficiency equivalent to CTE in evaluating patients with Crohn's disease has led to increased use of MRE in the imaging follow-up, in particular when evaluating younger patients with inflammatory bowel disease or as the primary imaging modality in the pediatric population.[18,40] Although MRE offers additional advantages to CT, including higher signal to noise ratio; repeated multiphase postcontrast imaging without added risk; assessment of the biophysical characteristics of the tissue; and potential ability to at least semiquantitatively quantify edema and fibrosis and cine imaging, several factors limit the widespread use of MRE. These factors include scanner availability, higher cost of examination, variability in examination quality, need for expertize in MR imaging because of more complex technical demand of this imaging modality, longer acquisition time needed, and lower spatial resolution as compared with CT.[41,42] As a result, CT imaging continues to be one of the more commonly used techniques in imaging patients with Crohn's disease, necessitating the need to reduce the CED and consequently the associated long-term radiation risk. Cipriano and colleagues[43] evaluated the cost effectiveness of MRE as compared with CTE for routine imaging of patients with small bowel Crohn's disease to reduce patients' life-time radiation-induced cancer risk. Their results indicate that at doses of less than 6 mSv per CTE, the use of MRE had an incremental cost-effectiveness ratio of greater than $100,000 per quality-adjusted life year gained, indicating that if CTE could be provided at this low dose, then it would likely be preferred to MRE for all types of patients.[43] Several recent advances in CT scanning technique and image processing have enabled obtaining CTE examination with effective dose of less than 6 mSv.[44]

The diagnostic efficacy of CTE in the evaluation of patients with inflammatory bowel disease depends primarily on the ability to detect contrast enhancement pattern in the bowel wall and the increased mesenteric vascularity, both of which manifest as high contrast differences from background. Hence, it is possible to detect changes of active bowel inflammation on CTE despite increased image noise associated with low-dose CTE examinations. Kambadakone and colleagues[45] evaluated the impact of increased image noise of simulated low-dose CT examinations on image quality and diagnostic performance in evaluating patients with Crohn's disease. They reported that despite increased image noise, diagnostic performance was maintained on simulated low-dose CT examinations with dose reduction of 31% to 64% (volume CT dose index [$CTDI_{vol}$] of 5.76–11.04 mGy as compared with baseline $CTDI_{vol}$ of 16 mGy). Siddiki and colleagues[46] evaluated a lower dose CTE protocol in which the mean $CTDI_{vol}$ was reduced from 24 mGy to 18 mGy by reducing the tube current–time product (mAs) and found that sensitivity for detection of active inflammatory bowel disease on lower-dose CTE examinations was similar to reported sensitivity with full-dose scans.

Radiation dose from CT examination can be reduced by reducing either the tube current (mA) or the tube kilovoltage (kV).[47] Although a weight-based reduction in mAs is commonly used in pediatric patients, use of fixed mAs for scanning of the abdomen and pelvis in adults could lead to increased noise in thicker patient body regions such as the pelvis. Automated mAs modulation techniques are currently available on all CT scanners, which modulate the mAs based on the thickness of body part imaged to generate images with more homogenous noise and image quality, and should be used for all CTE examinations. Allen and colleagues[48] reported that by using weight-based quality reference mAs and automatic mAs modulation for CTE done on 64 slice MDCT, mean $CTDI_{vol}$ decreased from 15.72 mGy to 9.25 mGy without reduction in diagnostic

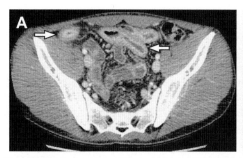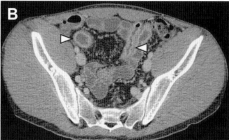

Fig. 6. Two CTE examinations obtained in a patient (weight 148 lbs., BMI of 20) within an interval of 12 months for clinically suspected acute flare of Crohn's disease done using (*A*) 80 kV with adaptive statistical iterative reconstruction and (*B*) 120 kV with filtered back projection. Mural enhancement and stratification involving 2 segments of the distal ileum and terminal ileum (*arrows in A and arrowheads in B*) are better appreciated on the 80 kV CTE examination because of higher attenuation of iodine at lower energy. The effective dose of 80 kV CTE was 2.2 mSv and that of 120 kV CTE was 4.5 mSv.

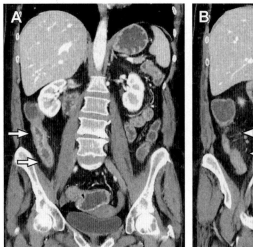
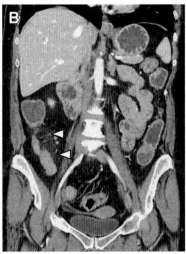

Fig. 7. (*A, B*) Coronal reformatted images of ultra-low dose CTE performed with MBIR in a patient with Crohn's disease (weight 176 lbs., BMI 27) show long segment of bowel wall thickening with mural enhancement and stratification involving the terminal ileum (*arrows*) along with adjacent mesenteric fat haziness and engorged mesenteric vascularity (*arrowheads*). Effective dose form this CTE was 3.1 mSv. Effective dose from a prior CTE done on the same patient using FBP reconstruction was 21.2 mSv.

efficiency. Reducing the tube voltage not only decreases the radiation dose but also offers the advantage of increasing the conspicuity of iodine-containing structures because of higher attenuation of iodine at lower energy.[49] Using lower kV would be beneficial for CTE in patients with inflammatory bowel disease as it would enhance the detection of bowel wall enhancement

Table 2 CTE protocol on 64-slice MDCT	
Scan Type	Helical
Detector coverage	40 mm
Slice thickness	0.625 mm
Interval	0.625 mm
Pitch	1.375:1
Speed	55 mm
Gantry rotation time	0.8 s
kVp Weight <160 lbs. Weight >160 lbs.	80 120
Auto mA (Min/Max)	100/575[a]
Noise index	30
Scan field of view	Large body
Image reconstruction algorithm	30% ASIR
Oral contrast	1350 mL total, over 1 h, 450 mL at 1 h, 450 mL at 40 min, 225 mL at 20 min and 225 mL before the scan
IV contrast	125 cc of Isovue-370 at 4 cc/s followed by 50 cc saline flush injected at a rate of 4 cc/s
Scan acquisition	65 s
Image reconstruction	Axial 2.5 mm thickness, coronal reformats at 2 mm thickness and 3D volumetric thick section in the coronal and both oblique projections.

[a] The max mA for 80 kVp scans is lowered within the following ranges based on patient weight: <100 lbs.: 200 to 300 mA, 100 to 125 lbs.: 300 to 400 mA, and 125 to 160 lbs.: 400 to 575 mA.

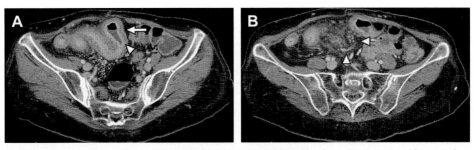

Fig. 8. (A, B) Axial images from CTE examination in a patient with ileal Crohn's disease. Mural hyperenhancement with bowel wall stratification and bowel wall edema (*arrowhead and arrow in A respectively*) and engorged adjacent mesenteric vessels (*arrowheads in B*) are consistent with active inflammatory bowel disease.

and engorged mesenteric vascularity in patients with active disease (**Fig. 6**).[44,50]

Lowering the CT radiation further and reconstructing the images using the traditional filtered back projection (FBP) techniques would lead to significantly increased image noise that would limit the diagnostic usefulness of the CT examination.

However, with recent advances in computational power, several new noise reduction image processing algorithms are currently clinically available on CT scanners through all the major manufacturers that would generate images with reduced noise on low-dose scans. Kambadakone and colleagues[45] evaluated the diagnostic performance of low-dose

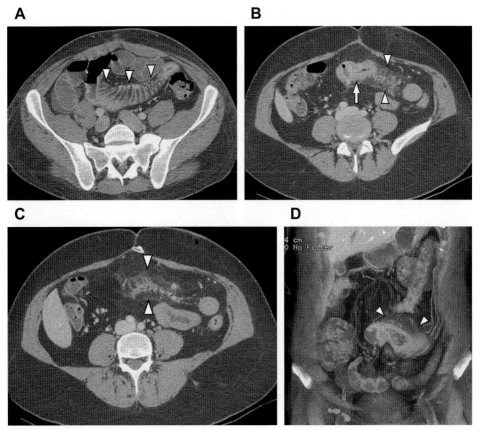

Fig. 9. Comb sign and mesenteric fat haziness. (A) Axial image from CTE examination in a patient with active ileal Crohn's disease show engorged mesenteric vessels or comb sign (*arrowheads*). (B, C) Axial and (D) coronal 3D surface-shaded CTE images in another patient with ileal active Crohn's disease (*arrow*) show increased attenuation and haziness of the mesenteric fat due to extension of the inflammation across the bowel serosal surface (*arrowheads*).

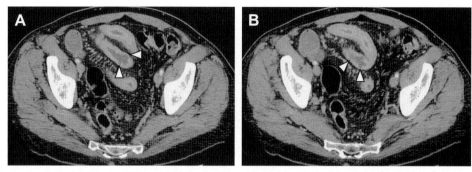

Fig. 10. Active Crohn's disease with mucosal ulcerations. (*A, B*) Axial images from CTE examination in a patient with ileal Crohn's disease showing several regions of denuded mucosal lining suggestive of mucosal ulcerations (*arrowheads*).

CTE examinations with adaptive statistical iterative reconstruction (ASIR, General Electric, Milwaukee, WI) and found the examinations to be of appropriate quality for evaluation of Crohn's disease. The use of ASIR enabled a 34% dose reduction as compared with CTE examinations done with FBP (mean $CTDI_{vol}$ of 7.7 mGy with ASIR vs 12 mGy with FBP). Lee and colleagues[51] compared standard dose CTE with FBP image reconstruction ($CTDI_{vol}$ 7.0 mGy) and 50% reduced dose CTE with iterative reconstruction in image space (IRIS, Siemens, Forchheim, Germany) ($CTDI_{vol}$ 3.5 mGy) and found that both techniques had similar performance in identifying enteric inflammation in patients with Crohn's disease. Similar dose reduction could be expected with CTE using other iterative reconstruction techniques such as iDose (Phillips, Andover, MA) and adaptive iterative dose reduction (AIDR, Toshiba, Otawara, Japan).[52] The use of noise suppression image processing would be more

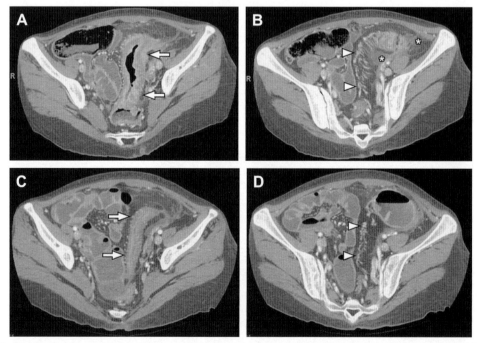

Fig. 11. (*A, B*) Axial images from CTE examination in a patient with sigmoid Crohn's disease (*arrows*) showing signs of active inflammation with significant bowel wall thickening, bowel wall stratification, bowel wall edema, and adjacent engorged mesenteric vessels (*arrowheads*) and mesenteric fat haziness and fluid (*asterisks*). (*C, D*) Follow-up examination after treatment show decrease in the bowel wall thickening (*arrows*) and reduced engorgement of the adjacent mesenteric vessels (*arrowheads*), suggesting treatment response and decrease in the degree of active inflammation.

beneficial when used with scans done at lower kV because these examinations are associated with higher image noise as compared with scans done at 120 kV. Kaza and colleagues[44] evaluated CTE done at 80 kV with ASIR image reconstruction in comparison to CTE done at 120 kV with FBP reconstruction in patients weighing less than 160 lbs. and found that both techniques had comparable diagnostic accuracy for detecting changes of inflammatory bowel disease with 71% reduction of radiation dose (mean $CTDI_{vol}$ of 6.15 mGy with 80 kV vs 20.79 mGy with 120 kV). Guimaraes and colleagues[50] evaluated image quality of 80 kV CTE after application of "projection space denoising" and concluded that image quality is close to routine dose CTE, and hence, the CTE at 80 kV with denoising can be done at 50% of routine dose levels (mean $CTDI_{vol}$ 7.9 mGy). Further advances in iterative image reconstruction such as model-based iterative reconstruction (MBIR, General Electric, Milwaukee, WI) and sinogram affirmed iterative reconstruction (SAFIRE, Siemens, Forchheim, Germany) could result in further reduction in radiation dose with CTE (Fig. 7).[52]

The CTE protocol used in the authors' department on 64 slice multidetector CT (HDCT, GE Health care) is presented in Table 2. They are in the process of further modification of CTE technique based on patient body mass index (BMI) and evaluating the use of ultra-low dose CTE using MBIR. CTE radiation dose reduction techniques must be balanced with maintaining image quality to avoid images with excessive noise, which could result in nondiagnostic examinations.[53] Application of noise reduction image processing and optimal use of lower mAs and kV tailored to patient weight and body habitus would enable obtaining diagnostic CTE examinations with the least radiation dose.

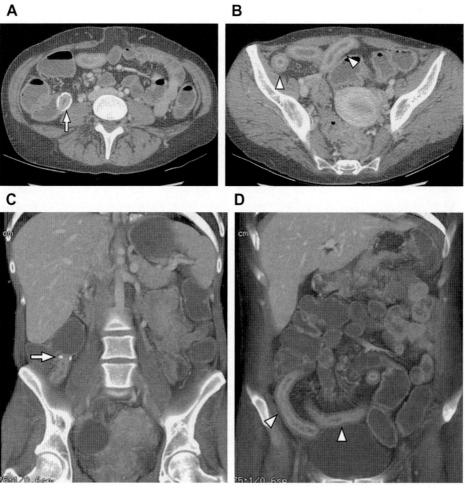

Fig. 12. (*A, B*) Axial and (*C, D*) coronal reformatted images from CTE examination in a patient with history of ileocolonic Crohn's disease after ileocecectomy presenting with disease recurrence and distal ileal active inflammation (*arrowheads*) extending proximally from the site of ileo-colic anastomosis (*arrow*).

Imaging Findings

CTE evaluation provides several advantages over traditional small bowel follow-through examinations, including more rapid acquisition requiring only few seconds to obtain the diagnostic scan (after the oral prep); assessment of longer portion of the gastrointestinal system in the same setting (stomach, duodenum, small and large bowel); assessment of the location, extent, and number of diseased segments; detection of the presence or absence of bowel obstruction; and more accurate assessment of disease activity by the presence or absence of mural inflammation, along with the added advantage of detecting extraintestinal complications.

Active inflammatory disease

The common signs of active or inflammatory Crohn's disease include bowel wall thickening, increased mural enhancement, mural stratification (reflecting increased enhancement along the mucosal and serosal surface of the bowel with intervening bowel wall edema), haziness of the surrounding mesenteric fat, and engorgement of the mesenteric vessels supplying the diseased bowel segment (**Figs. 8** and **9**). Characteristically, Crohn's disease can also demonstrate multiple skip areas of involvement with intervening unaffected segments. Bodily and colleagues[54] demonstrated that increased mural attenuation and wall thickness at CTE correlate highly with endoscopic and histologic findings of inflammatory Crohn's disease and that quantitative measures of mural attenuation are sensitive markers of small bowel inflammation. In some instances, low attenuation can be noted within the bowel wall in patients with history of long-standing Crohn's disease, which is due to fat deposition within the submucosal layer of the bowel.[55] The presence of fat does not necessarily indicate quiescent disease and may be present with signs of active inflammation. Mucosal ulceration can be seen, which indicates active inflammation (**Fig. 10**).[56] CTE can also be used to follow-up treatment response, which manifests as decreasing mural enhancement, less degree of bowel wall thickening,

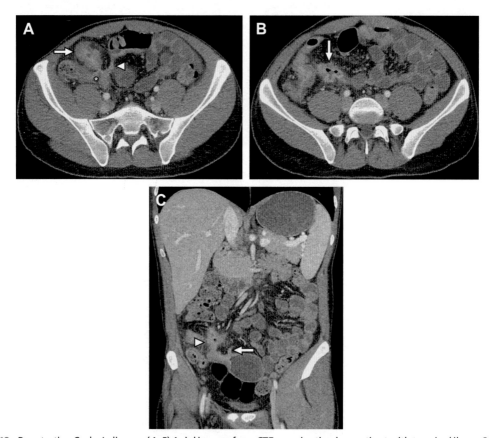

Fig. 13. Penetrating Crohn's disease. (*A, B*) Axial images from CTE examination in a patient with terminal ileum Crohn's disease (*asterisk*) and ileal active inflammatory stricture (*arrow in A*) showing ileo-colic fistula between the terminal ileum and adjacent sigmoid colon (*arrowhead in A*). There is also evidence of adjacent mesenteric abscess (*arrow in B*). (*C*) Coronal reformatted image show the mesenteric abscess (*arrowhead*) and a short adjacent sinus tract (*arrow*).

and improvement in the engorged mesenteric vascularity (**Fig. 11**).[57–59] Frequently, CTE is also used in evaluating postoperative recurrence of Crohn's disease, which is most frequently seen at or immediately proximal to the anastomotic site (**Fig. 12**). An additional potential CTE indication is its use as a baseline examination before starting new treatment, especially biologic agents that commonly causes immunosuppression to exclude abscess formation.

Fibrostenosing disease

It is imperative to differentiate active or inflammatory small bowel strictures from fibrotic small bowel strictures in patients with Crohn's disease, because the former are mostly managed medically whereas the latter may require surgical intervention (eg, balloon dilation, strictureplasty, or resection).[34] Presence of luminal narrowing without mural hyperenhancement or other signs of active inflammation such as mural stratification, mesenteric fat haziness, or engorged mesenteric vessels were considered to represent fibrostenosing Crohn's disease.[12] However, as pointed out earlier, inflammation and fibrosis often coexist in the same affected bowel segments, and as such a clear distinction between predominantly inflammatory and predominantly fibrotic strictures may not be easily distinguishable based on routine CTE findings.

Penetrating disease

The transmural inflammation in Crohn's disease coupled with increased intraluminal pressure proximal to the site of strictures can lead to extension or penetration of the inflammatory process across the serosal surface into the adjacent mesentery or structures. Blind-ending inflammatory tracts form a sinus tract that can lead to a fistula tract if it communicates with another surface or fluid cavity. CTE can assess the presence of sinus or fistula tracts that are commonly characterized by bowel tethering and visualization of linear, enhancing tracts that can

---

Box 1
CTE reporting template for Crohn's disease

- Disease distribution:
  - Stomach, duodenum, jejunum, ileum [terminal ileum], or colon
  - Skip segment(s)
- Bowel wall thickening (>3 mm)
- Length of abnormal segment(s)
- Bowel wall enhancement pattern:
  - Mural hyperenhancement
  - Mural stratification
- Stricture:
  - Luminal narrowing (luminal diameter)
  - Presence or absence of proximal bowel dilatation
- Perienteric findings:
  - Surrounding mesenteric fat stranding/haziness
  - Engorged mesenteric vessels or vasa recta (comb sign)
  - Surrounding mesenteric fibrofatty proliferation
- Penetrating disease:
  - Sinus tract (blind-ending)
  - Fistula (eg, enteroenteric, enterocolic, enterocutaneous, entero or colovesicular, colocolic, cologastric, rectovaginal and so forth)
  - Fluid collection (peritoneal, retroperitoneal, or abdominal wall)
- Extraintestinal abdominal findings (most common):
  - Gallstones, nephrolithiasis, primary sclerosing cholangitis, sacroiliitis, perianal fistula/fluid collection, or perineal disease

communicate with adjacent structures such as peritoneal or retroperitoneal spaces, skin or adjacent organs, or bowel.[60] Another sign of penetrating disease is abscess formation, which is usually contiguous to the diseased segment and is seen in the peritoneal cavity or retroperitoneal space (**Fig. 13**).

Organized reporting of imaging findings can ensure the inclusion of all pertinent pieces of information that are used to make the appropriate diagnosis and help in formulating the management plan (**Box 1**).

SUMMARY

Optimized small bowel imaging with advances in multidetector technique and use of neutral oral contrast have helped to establish the pivotal role of CTE, leading to a shift toward cross-sectional imaging rather than fluoroscopic examination in the diagnosis and management of patients with inflammatory bowel disease, namely Crohn's disease. Cross-sectional evaluation with CTE is an important noninvasive complementary diagnostic tool that is used in combination with other diagnostic modalities, such as optical or capsule endoscopy and histology for diagnosis and assessment of disease phenotype as inflammatory, fibrostenosing, or penetrating at disease presentation or follow-up. CTE has also been shown to offer high sensitivity for detection of associated complications, a significant proportion of which are clinically undetectable, and can alter patient management in significant proportion of patients. The more recent concern about the risk of cumulative radiation dose and the need of frequent imaging especially in patients with complicated disease or younger patients has led to several technologic advancements in CT dose reduction techniques, which offer the possibility of obtaining diagnostically acceptable studies at a fraction of the previously used radiation doses.

REFERENCES

1. Levine A, Griffiths A, Markowitz J, et al. Pediatric modification of the Montreal classification for inflammatory bowel disease: the Paris classification. Inflamm Bowel Dis 2011;17(6):1314–21.
2. Gasche C, Scholmerich J, Brynskov J, et al. A simple classification of Crohn's disease: report of the Working Party for the World Congresses of Gastroenterology, Vienna 1998. Inflamm Bowel Dis 2000;6(1):8–15.
3. Silverberg MS, Satsangi J, Ahmad T, et al. Toward an integrated clinical, molecular and serological classification of inflammatory bowel disease: report of a Working Party of the 2005 Montreal World Congress of Gastroenterology. Can J Gastroenterol 2005;19(Suppl A):5–36.
4. Louis E, Collard A, Oger AF, et al. Behaviour of Crohn's disease according to the Vienna classification: changing pattern over the course of the disease. Gut 2001;49(6):777–82.
5. Zisman TL, Rubin DT. Novel diagnostic and prognostic modalities in inflammatory bowel disease. Gastroenterol Clin North Am 2009;38(4):729–52.
6. Fletcher JG, Fidler JL, Bruining DH, et al. New concepts in intestinal imaging for inflammatory bowel diseases. Gastroenterology 2011;140(6): 1795–806.
7. Solem CA, Loftus EV Jr, Tremaine WJ, et al. Correlation of C-reactive protein with clinical, endoscopic, histologic, and radiographic activity in inflammatory bowel disease. Inflamm Bowel Dis 2005;11(8):707–12.
8. Adler J, Punglia DR, Dillman JR, et al. Computed tomography enterography findings correlate with tissue inflammation, not fibrosis in resected small bowel Crohn's disease. Inflamm Bowel Dis 2012; 18(5):849–56.
9. Raptopoulos V, Schwartz RK, McNicholas MM, et al. Multiplanar helical CT enterography in patients with Crohn's disease. AJR Am J Roentgenol 1997; 169(6):1545–50.
10. Wold PB, Fletcher JG, Johnson CD, et al. Assessment of small bowel Crohn disease: noninvasive peroral CT enterography compared with other imaging methods and endoscopy–feasibility study. Radiology 2003;229(1):275–81.
11. Booya F, Fletcher JG, Huprich JE, et al. Active Crohn disease: CT findings and interobserver agreement for enteric phase CT enterography. Radiology 2006;241(3):787–95.
12. Solem CA, Loftus EV Jr, Fletcher JG, et al. Small-bowel imaging in Crohn's disease: a prospective, blinded, 4-way comparison trial. Gastrointest Endosc 2008;68(2):255–66.
13. Paulsen SR, Huprich JE, Fletcher JG, et al. CT enterography as a diagnostic tool in evaluating small bowel disorders: review of clinical experience with over 700 cases. Radiographics 2006;26(3):641–57 [discussion: 657–62].
14. Hara AK, Leighton JA, Heigh RI, et al. Crohn disease of the small bowel: preliminary comparison among CT enterography, capsule endoscopy, small-bowel follow-through, and ileoscopy. Radiology 2006; 238(1):128–34.
15. Reittner P, Goritschnig T, Petritsch W, et al. Multiplanar spiral CT enterography in patients with Crohn's disease using a negative oral contrast material: initial results of a noninvasive imaging approach. Eur Radiol 2002;12(9):2253–7.
16. Vogel J, da Luz Moreira A, Baker M, et al. CT enterography for Crohn's disease: accurate preoperative

diagnostic imaging. Dis Colon Rectum 2007;50(11): 1761–9.

17. Lee SS, Kim AY, Yang SK, et al. Crohn disease of the small bowel: comparison of CT enterography, MR enterography, and small-bowel follow-through as diagnostic techniques. Radiology 2009;251(3):751–61.

18. Siddiki HA, Fidler JL, Fletcher JG, et al. Prospective comparison of state-of-the-art MR enterography and CT enterography in small-bowel Crohn's disease. AJR Am J Roentgenol 2009;193(1):113–21.

19. Jensen MD, Kjeldsen J, Rafaelsen SR, et al. Diagnostic accuracies of MR enterography and CT enterography in symptomatic Crohn's disease. Scand J Gastroenterol 2011;46(12):1449–57.

20. Higgins PD, Caoili E, Zimmermann M, et al. Computed tomographic enterography adds information to clinical management in small bowel Crohn's disease. Inflamm Bowel Dis 2007;13(3): 262–8.

21. Bruining DH, Siddiki HA, Fletcher JG, et al. Benefit of computed tomography enterography in Crohn's disease: effects on patient management and physician level of confidence. Inflamm Bowel Dis 2012; 18(2):219–25.

22. Booya F, Akram S, Fletcher JG, et al. CT enterography and fistulizing Crohn's disease: clinical benefit and radiographic findings. Abdom Imaging 2009; 34(4):467–75.

23. Elsayes KM, Al-Hawary MM, Jagdish J, et al. CT enterography: principles, trends, and interpretation of findings. Radiographics 2010;30(7):1955–70.

24. Fletcher JG. CT enterography technique: theme and variations. Abdom Imaging 2009;34(3):283–8.

25. Fletcher JG, Huprich J, Loftus EV Jr, et al. Computerized tomography enterography and its role in small-bowel imaging. Clin Gastroenterol Hepatol 2008;6(3):283–9.

26. Huprich JE, Fletcher JG. CT enterography: principles, technique and utility in Crohn's disease. Eur J Radiol 2009;69(3):393–7.

27. Tochetto S, Yaghmai V. CT enterography: concept, technique, and interpretation. Radiol Clin North Am 2009;47(1):117–32.

28. Paulsen SR, Huprich JE, Hara AK. CT enterography: noninvasive evaluation of Crohn's disease and obscure gastrointestinal bleed. Radiol Clin North Am 2007;45(2):303–15.

29. Koo CW, Shah-Patel LR, Baer JW, et al. Cost-effectiveness and patient tolerance of low-attenuation oral contrast material: milk versus VoLumen. AJR Am J Roentgenol 2008;190(5):1307–13.

30. Zhang LH, Zhang SZ, Hu HJ, et al. Multi-detector CT enterography with iso-osmotic mannitol as oral contrast for detecting small bowel disease. World J Gastroenterol 2005;11(15):2324–9.

31. Megibow AJ, Babb JS, Hecht EM, et al. Evaluation of bowel distention and bowel wall appearance by using neutral oral contrast agent for multi-detector row CT. Radiology 2006;238(1):87–95.

32. Erturk SM, Mortele KJ, Oliva MR, et al. Depiction of normal gastrointestinal anatomy with MDCT: comparison of low- and high-attenuation oral contrast media. Eur J Radiol 2008;66(1):84–7.

33. Arslan H, Etlik O, Kayan M, et al. Peroral CT enterography with lactulose solution: preliminary observations. AJR Am J Roentgenol 2005; 185(5):1173–9.

34. Maglinte DD, Sandrasegaran K, Lappas JC, et al. CT enteroclysis. Radiology 2007;245(3):661–71.

35. McCollough CH, Guimaraes L, Fletcher JG. In defense of body CT. AJR Am J Roentgenol 2009; 193(1):28–39.

36. Fuchs Y, Markowitz J, Weinstein T, et al. Pediatric inflammatory bowel disease and imaging-related radiation: are we increasing the likelihood of malignancy? J Pediatr Gastroenterol Nutr 2011;52(3): 280–5.

37. Chatu S, Subramanian V, Pollok RC. Meta-analysis: diagnostic medical radiation exposure in inflammatory bowel disease. Aliment Pharmacol Ther 2012; 35(5):529–39.

38. Peloquin JM, Pardi DS, Sandborn WJ, et al. Diagnostic ionizing radiation exposure in a population-based cohort of patients with inflammatory bowel disease. Am J Gastroenterol 2008;103(8):2015–22.

39. Desmond AN, O'Regan K, Curran C, et al. Crohn's disease: factors associated with exposure to high levels of diagnostic radiation. Gut 2008;57(11): 1524–9.

40. Gee MS, Nimkin K, Hsu M, et al. Prospective evaluation of MR enterography as the primary imaging modality for pediatric Crohn disease assessment. AJR Am J Roentgenol 2011;197(1):224–31.

41. Fidler J, Guimaraes L, Einstein D. MR imaging of the small bowel. Radiographics 2009;29(6):1811–25.

42. Dillman JR, Ladino-Torres MF, Adler J, et al. Comparison of MR enterography and histopathology in the evaluation of pediatric Crohn disease. Pediatr Radiol 2011;41(12):1552–8.

43. Cipriano LE, Levesque BG, Zaric GS, et al. Cost-effectiveness of imaging strategies to reduce radiation-induced cancer risk in Crohn's disease. Inflamm Bowel Dis 2012;18(7):1240–8.

44. Kaza RK, Platt JF, Al-Hawary MM, et al. CT enterography at 80 kVp with adaptive statistical iterative reconstruction versus at 120 kVp with standard reconstruction: image quality, diagnostic adequacy, and dose reduction. AJR Am J Roentgenol 2012; 198(5):1084–92.

45. Kambadakone AR, Prakash P, Hahn PF, et al. Low-dose CT examinations in Crohn's disease: impact on image quality, diagnostic performance, and radiation dose. AJR Am J Roentgenol 2010; 195(1):78–88.

46. Siddiki H, Fletcher JG, Hara AK, et al. Validation of a lower radiation computed tomography enterography imaging protocol to detect Crohn's disease in the small bowel. Inflamm Bowel Dis 2011;17(3): 778–86.

47. McCollough CH, Primak AN, Braun N, et al. Strategies for reducing radiation dose in CT. Radiol Clin North Am 2009;47(1):27–40.

48. Allen BC, Baker ME, Einstein DM, et al. Effect of altering automatic exposure control settings and quality reference mAs on radiation dose, image quality, and diagnostic efficacy in MDCT enterography of active inflammatory Crohn's disease. AJR Am J Roentgenol 2010;195(1):89–100.

49. Yanaga Y, Awai K, Nakaura T, et al. Hepatocellular carcinoma in patients weighing 70 kg or less: initial trial of compact-bolus dynamic CT with low-dose contrast material at 80 kVp. AJR Am J Roentgenol 2011;196(6):1324–31.

50. Guimaraes LS, Fletcher JG, Yu L, et al. Feasibility of dose reduction using novel denoising techniques for low kV (80 kV) CT enterography: optimization and validation. Acad Radiol 2010;17(10): 1203–10.

51. Lee SJ, Park SH, Kim AY, et al. A prospective comparison of standard-dose CT enterography and 50% reduced-dose CT enterography with and without noise reduction for evaluating Crohn disease. AJR Am J Roentgenol 2011;197(1):50–7.

52. Beister M, Kolditz D, Kalender WA. Iterative reconstruction methods in X-ray CT. Phys Med 2012; 28(2):94–108.

53. Leng S, Yu L, McCollough CH. Radiation dose reduction at CT enterography: how low can we go while preserving diagnostic accuracy? AJR Am J Roentgenol 2010;195(1):76–7.

54. Bodily KD, Fletcher JG, Solem CA, et al. Crohn Disease: mural attenuation and thickness at contrast-enhanced CT Enterography–correlation with endoscopic and histologic findings of inflammation. Radiology 2006;238(2):505–16.

55. Wittenberg J, Harisinghani MG, Jhaveri K, et al. Algorithmic approach to CT diagnosis of the abnormal bowel wall. Radiographics 2002;22(5): 1093–107 [discussion: 1107–9].

56. Ziech ML, Bipat S, Roelofs JJ, et al. Retrospective comparison of magnetic resonance imaging features and histopathology in Crohn's disease patients. Eur J Radiol 2011;80(3):e299–305.

57. Wu YW, Tang YH, Hao NX, et al. Crohn's disease: CT enterography manifestations before and after treatment. Eur J Radiol 2012;81(1):52–9.

58. Wu YW, Tao XF, Tang YH, et al. Quantitative measures of comb sign in Crohn's disease: correlation with disease activity and laboratory indications. Abdom Imaging 2012;37(3):350–8.

59. Hara AK, Alam S, Heigh RI, et al. Using CT enterography to monitor Crohn's disease activity: a preliminary study. AJR Am J Roentgenol 2008;190(6): 1512–6.

60. Bruining DH, Siddiki HA, Fletcher JG, et al. Prevalence of penetrating disease and extraintestinal manifestations of Crohn's disease detected with CT enterography. Inflamm Bowel Dis 2008;14(12):1701–6.

Computed Tomography of Small Bowel Obstruction

Cynthia S. Santillan, MD

KEYWORDS

- Computed tomography • Small bowel obstruction • Closed-loop obstruction • Transition zone
- Small bowel feces • Ischemia

KEY POINTS

- Careful evaluation of computed tomography in small bowel obstruction is necessary to identify patients who are likely to fail conservative management.
- Identification of the transition zone, often just distal to bowel with small bowel feces, is critical in determining the cause of the obstruction and in guiding management.
- Findings suggesting ischemia in small bowel obstruction, such as closed-loop obstruction, hypo-enhancing bowel, delayed bowel enhancement, and pneumatosis, warrant surgical management.
- Models that incorporate combinations of both clinical and imaging findings may allow identification of patients without signs of ischemia at presentation who will ultimately fail conservative management.

INTRODUCTION

Small bowel obstruction (SBO) is a significant cause of morbidity and mortality. The health care expenses are substantial, accounting for more than 300,000 hospitalizations and $3 billion in medical care per year in the United States.[1,2] Appropriate treatment of patients with SBO depends on prompt diagnosis of the obstruction and accurate identification of those patients who require surgical management. Initial assessment focuses on identifying those patients with signs and symptoms consistent with peritonitis or ischemic bowel. Surgical guidelines recommend plain radiographs as part of this initial assessment, as these can confirm the diagnosis of SBO and identify some complications such as perforation.[3,4] Those patients with an acute abdominal examination and confirmatory laboratory values and plain radiographs typically undergo emergent surgery. Plain radiographs, however, are only accurate 46% to 85% of the time, and can miss SBO in patients without air-fluid levels because of fluid-filled distended loops.[5]

Given the limitations of plain radiographs, computed tomography (CT) is frequently used for the evaluation of patients with SBO and may be the initial assessment for many patients.[6,7] CT is particularly useful in those patients who do not demonstrate clear symptoms of peritonitis or ischemia at presentation, especially if they have equivocal or negative findings on plain radiographs. Delays in surgery can result in increased morbidity and mortality, and appropriate use of abdominal CT can aid timely triage to surgical management. Mortality associated with ischemic SBO is approximately 8% if surgery is performed within 36 hours of presentation. If surgery is delayed more than 36 hours, however, mortality increases to 25%.[8] In those patients without clear indications for emergent surgery, nonoperative management with enteric tube decompression is recommended for 48 to 72 hours. However, in those patients who ultimately require surgery after failing decompression there is increased mortality and prolonged hospital stay in comparison with those undergoing more prompt surgical

Disclosure: The author is a consultant for Robarts Clinical Research.
Department of Radiology, University of California San Diego, 200 West Arbor Drive, San Diego, CA 92103, USA
E-mail address: csantillan@ucsd.edu

Radiol Clin N Am 51 (2013) 17–27
http://dx.doi.org/10.1016/j.rcl.2012.09.002

intervention, and CT may help to more appropriately risk stratify these patients.[4]

This article reviews the appropriate CT technique for assessment of SBO, common causes for obstruction, imaging findings in SBO, and the significance of those findings for determining whether a patient is likely to require surgical management for SBO.

ANATOMY AND FUNCTION

The small bowel, consisting of the duodenum, jejunum, and ileum, measures 6 to 8 m in length, and extends from the pylorus to the ileocecal valve.[9] After the duodenum, the jejunum comprises the proximal 40% of the small bowel and the ileum the remaining 60%. The normal caliber of the small bowel is less than 2.5 cm, and typically distends up to 4 cm with active distension.

The majority of the duodenum is retroperitoneal whereas the remainder of the small bowel is intraperitoneal, suspended within the mesentery. The mesenteric root extends from the left upper quadrant to the right lower quadrant, measuring 10 to 15 cm in length, with the jejunum residing predominantly in the left upper abdomen and the ileum in the right lower abdomen.[10] This mesentery allows the bowel mobility within the abdomen, and the length of the mesenteric root provides stability of the vascular supply and drainage. Shortening of the mesenteric pedicle caused by congenital malrotation or adhesions increases the risk of small bowel volvulus.[11] The vascular supply of the first and second portions of the duodenum is predominantly from the celiac artery.[12] The remainder of the small bowel is supplied by the superior mesenteric artery with drainage via the superior mesenteric vein.

The functions of the small bowel are absorption of fluid and extraction of nutrients from the lumen. The small bowel absorbs approximately 7 L of fluid each day.[9] The bulk of this fluid is salivary, biliary,

pancreatic, and intestinal secretions. Compared with disruptions of the normal function of the small bowel, which often lead to diarrhea and malabsorption disorders, an SBO will often cause nausea and vomiting, which may persist because of secretions, despite decreased oral intake. Slowed transit through the intestine can result in bacterial overgrowth, resulting in feculent vomit. Mucosal damage can appear early in the obstruction, even in the absence of ischemia, owing to alterations in perfusion.

TECHNIQUE
Scanning Parameters and Reconstructions

Imaging of SBO should be performed on a multidetector CT scanner with the ability to perform reconstructions at 3 to 5 mm. Coronal and sagittal reconstructions should be provided in all patients with a suspicion for SBO, because coronal reformats improve the ability to identify the site of obstruction (transition zone) (**Fig. 1**).[13] In addition, the overview of the bowel provided by the coronal reformat can increase confidence in diagnosing differences in bowel wall enhancement and thickness.[14]

Intravenous Contrast

Intravenous contrast is necessary for the assessment of bowel wall enhancement and vascular patency and may also aid assessment for the cause of the obstruction, such as a soft-tissue mass. Imaging should be performed in either the portal venous (approximately 80–90 seconds following contrast injection) or enteric phase (approximately 50 seconds following injection) to assess bowel wall enhancement and mesenteric vessels. In cases where there is a high concern for ischemia, delayed imaging (2–3 minutes following injection) should be considered to assess for venous occlusion or delayed bowel wall enhancement.

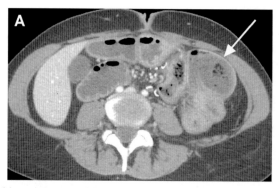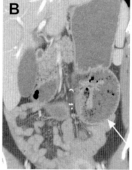

Fig. 1. Closed-loop SBO caused by an adhesion. (*A*) Axial CT demonstrates a dilated loop of small bowel with small bowel feces (*arrow*). (*B*) Coronal reformat demonstrates the C-shape of the dilated loop indicating a closed-loop obstruction (*arrow*).

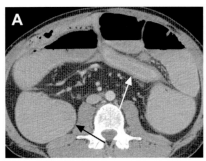
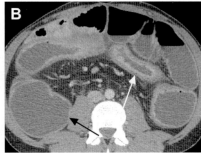

Fig. 2. Crohn's disease. A patient with a chronic SBO had a contrast-enhanced CT scan with positive oral contrast (*A*) and a follow-up examination with water as oral contrast (*B*). The examination with water demonstrates increased conspicuity of bowel wall enhancement in both normal bowel (*black arrows*) and loops with inflammation (*white arrows*).

Oral Contrast

Initial assessment of the patient with suspected SBO should be performed either without oral contrast or with a low-attenuation contrast agent such as water.[6] Patients with SBO typically have dilated or distended loops with accumulated ingested material or secretions, so administration of additional fluid may not be tolerated and is usually unnecessary. Also, positive oral contrast may limit the ability to detect abnormal bowel wall enhancement, such as hypoenhancement or mucosal hyperenhancement (**Fig. 2**).

The selection of oral contrast for follow-up of the patient with SBO is based on the indication for the examination and the patient's status. If there is concern for a complication, such as ischemia or perforation, the examination should be performed similarly to the initial assessment, with water as the oral contrast agent or without oral contrast. If the patient's condition is relatively stable and the indication is to distinguish between partial or complete obstruction, the patient may receive positive oral contrast. Rather than doing a CT, this assessment can be made by administering 100 mL of Gastrografin (Gastrografin is the trademarked name from Bracco Diagnostics), clamping the enteric tube (if present) for at least 4 hours, and performing an abdominal radiograph 12 to 24 hours later to assess for the presence of contrast in the colon.[4] If the contrast reaches the colon, there is a high likelihood that the obstruction will resolve with conservative management.[15] Alternatively, a CT scan with positive oral contrast administered at least 3 hours before the examination can be performed. Although follow-up plain radiography is recommended in surgical guidelines and results in less radiation exposure to the patient, a repeat CT scan offers the advantage of detecting signs of a complicated bowel obstruction and may be appropriate in selected patients.

ETIOLOGY OF OBSTRUCTION
Adhesions

Adhesions account for up to 80% of SBOs and typically occur in patients with a history of abdominal surgery or inflammation.[16,17] Although laparoscopic surgery has been associated with a lower risk of developing SBO than open surgery, rates of adhesiolysis in the United States have remained stable for the last 20 years, despite increasing use of laparoscopy.[2,18] Because adhesive bands are typically not visible on CT, the diagnosis of adhesions is often one of exclusion. Kinking or tethering of the bowel at the transition zone without any other identifiable cause, particularly in a patient with a history of surgery, is highly suggestive of an adhesion (**Fig. 3**).

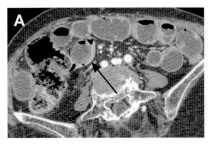
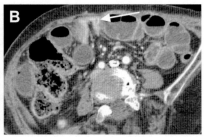

Fig. 3. Adhesion. (*A*) Axial CT demonstrates dilated loops of small bowel with a short segment of decompressed terminal ileum (*black arrow*). (*B*) Angled reconstruction demonstrates a segment of decompressed bowel closely apposed to the anterior abdominal wall (*white arrow*). After failing 1 day of conservative management because of increasing pain, surgery revealed an ileal obstruction secondary to a taut adhesive band along the anterior abdominal wall.

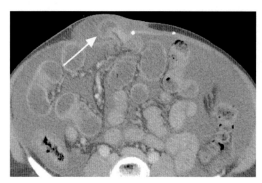

Fig. 4. External hernia. Axial CT demonstrates an incarcerated ventral hernia (*arrow*) adjacent to a previously repaired hernia. There was no evidence of bowel ischemia during the surgical repair.

Hernias

Hernias are the second most common cause of SBO.[17] External hernias, such as inguinal, umbilical, or surgical-site hernias, are easily identified by the presence of bowel extending into the subcutaneous soft tissues or abdominal wall muscles (**Fig. 4**). Internal hernias are identified by an abnormal position or orientation of bowel within the abdomen. Paraduodenal hernias account for 53% of internal hernias unrelated to prior surgery.[19] In paraduodenal hernias, the herniated bowel can appear in a sac-like configuration, and is positioned either posterior to the stomach or directly to the right of the proximal superior mesenteric artery (**Fig. 5**).

Roux-en-Y gastric bypass surgery is an important cause of internal hernia, with an estimated incidence of 5% among those undergoing laparoscopic bypass.[20] There are 3 types of hernias associated with Roux-en-Y gastric bypass surgery. Herniation of the Roux limb through the mesocolic window results in dilation of the Roux limb with inferior displacement of the transverse colon. A Petersen hernia occurs when bowel passes into the space posterior to the alimentary limb, resulting in loops of bowel positioned directly anterior to the pancreas. Hernias through the enteroenterostomy mesenteric defect (transmesenteric hernia) will displace the transverse colon superiorly (**Fig. 6**).[21]

SBO caused by hernia is often a closed-loop obstruction, and symptomatic hernias have a 28% risk of developing ischemia.[7] Therefore, all patients with symptomatic hernias should undergo surgical repair. Patients with asymptomatic or minimally symptomatic hernias may be safely observed by a surgical team or undergo elective repair.

Inflammation

Crohn's disease is increasing in frequency as a cause of SBO, and can cause obstruction through acute inflammatory narrowing or fibrostenosing disease.[16,22] In the acute phase, the affected segment of bowel will often demonstrate mural thickening, mural stratification, mucosal hyperemia, engorgement of the adjacent mesenteric vessels, and mesenteric inflammatory stranding.[23] Fibrostenosing disease can demonstrate more homogeneous enhancement of the bowel wall, and does not have associated vascular engorgement or mesenteric inflammation (**Fig. 7**).[22] Other causes of inflammation resulting in luminal narrowing include chronic ischemia, infection, and radiation enteritis.

Neoplasm

Primary malignancy of the small bowel is relatively rare, accounting for fewer than 2% of small bowel neoplasms.[17] Adenocarcinoma, carcinoid, and

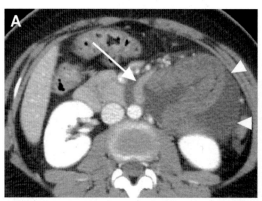
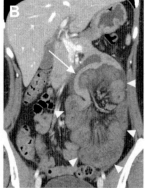

Fig. 5. Internal hernia. The patient presented with nausea, vomiting, and left upper quadrant pain. Axial CT (*A*) and coronal reformat (*B*) demonstrates that the jejunum proximal to the hernia is angulated and decompressed (*arrows*) leading into the left paraduodenal hernia sac (*arrowheads*). The bowel in the hernia is edematous and demonstrates decreased enhancement. Fluid is present in the hernia sac, and the mesentery is diffusely edematous. At surgery the bowel was edematous, but not ischemic, so no bowel was resected during the repair.

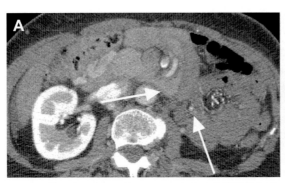
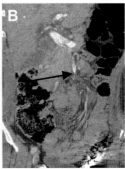

Fig. 6. Transmesenteric hernia. The patient presented with abdominal pain, nausea and vomiting, and history of gastric bypass. (A) Axial image demonstrates the mushroom sign of bowel herniating through the mesenteric defect (*white arrows*). (B) Coronal reconstruction demonstrates the herniated bowel extending into the pelvis and marked narrowing of the superior mesenteric vein (*black arrow*). The patient required resection of 30 cm of bowel because of ischemia.

gastrointestinal stromal tumors are the most common primary small bowel neoplasms. The most frequent malignancies to metastasize to the small bowel are melanoma, breast, colorectal, and ovarian. Neoplasms can cause obstruction from an intraluminal or intramural mass, extrinsic narrowing due to serosal disease, or by acting as a lead point for an intussusception. Intussusception has a very characteristic appearance, with mesenteric fat and vessels drawn into the bowel lumen (Fig. 8).[24] Although the majority of enteroenteric intussusceptions seen on CT are transient,

those that are associated with an SBO or those that have a visible lead point will likely require surgical management.[25]

DIAGNOSIS

The diagnosis of SBO can be made when there are proximal loops of small bowel measuring 2.5 cm or greater and distal loops of normal caliber or collapsed bowel (Fig. 9).[26] Note that in some cases the bowel may not be dilated proximally. This situation could occur either early in the obstruction or in very proximal obstructions where the patient has had nasogastric suctioning or has been vomiting. The presence of distal decompressed small bowel loops following a transition zone is the critical distinction between an adynamic ileus and a mechanical obstruction.

Degree of Obstruction

A complete obstruction is present when oral contrast material does not pass the site of obstruction within 3 to 24 hours after administering oral contrast.[27] Because many patients do not receive positive oral contrast because of the reasons outlined above and initial imaging of the patients often occurs before the time necessary to assess for passage of contrast beyond the site of obstruction, SBO on CT is more easily classified as either high grade (which encompasses complete) or low grade. The definitions of these grades vary in the literature. High-grade obstruction on CT has been defined as little to no gas present in the distal bowel or ascending colon (Fig. 10).[28,29] Partial obstruction is diagnosed when there is still water and fluid in the distal bowel. Other definitions regarding the discrepancy in caliber between the dilated bowel and distal bowel have been used, but the criteria vary.[17,28]

Fig. 7. Crohn's disease. Axial CT demonstrates a stricture from Crohn's disease at the patient's ileosigmoid anastomosis (*arrow*). The bowel is thickened and enhancing, and small bowel feces are present in the proximal dilated bowel.

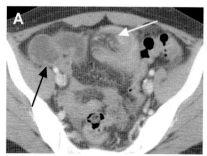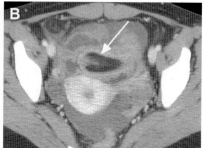

Fig. 8. Intussusception. (*A*) Axial CT image demonstrates dilated loops of small bowel (*black arrow*). Mesenteric fat and vessels are seen entering a loop of bowel consistent with an intussusception (*white arrow*). The lead point was an 8-cm lipoma (*B, white arrow*).

Although some studies have demonstrated an increased likelihood of requiring surgical management with high-grade obstruction identified on CT, studies have found overall that the presence of a high-grade obstruction has poor specificity for the need for surgical management, estimated at only 46% in one series.[7,28,30,31]

Transition Zone

Identification of the transition zone is critical in the evaluation of SBO, because the etiology of the obstruction can often be determined at the transition zone. CT can accurately localize the site of obstruction, with a 63% positive predictive value for correlation between the radiographically identified transition zone and operative findings.[32]

Although the site of transition may be clearly evident after reviewing the coronal and axial images, many cases require a more methodical approach (**Fig. 11**). In patients with a relatively small number of dilated loops suggesting a proximal obstruction, following the bowel antegrade from the stomach to the site of caliber change is recommended. If the majority of the small bowel appears dilated, a retrograde approach from the rectum should be used first.

Although the ability to identify the site of obstruction does not correlate with the likelihood of requiring surgical management, the location and number of transition zones can guide treatment and should be noted in the radiology report.[30,32] Laparoscopic surgery is more likely to succeed in patients with a single adhesive band identified on CT, compared with patients with multiple sites of adhesion.[4,33] In addition, identifying the site of obstruction may allow better placement of ports and operators at the time of laparoscopy.

Small Bowel Feces

A finding often in close proximity to the transition zone is the small bowel feces sign. This sign refers to the presence of particulate material admixed

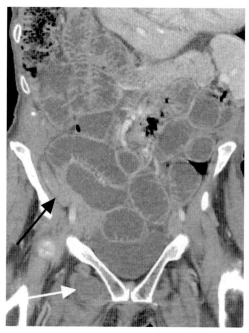

Fig. 9. Obstruction. Coronal reconstruction demonstrates dilated loops of small bowel with distal decompressed loops (*black arrow*). Obstruction was due to an obturator hernia (*white arrow*).

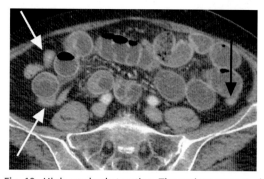

Fig. 10. High-grade obstruction. The patient presented with nausea, vomiting, and abdominal pain. Axial CT demonstrates that the small bowel (*white arrows*) and colon (*black arrow*) are completely decompressed distal to the obstruction, consistent with a high-grade SBO.

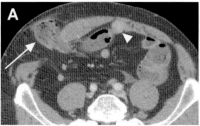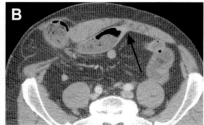

Fig. 11. Transition zone. (*A*) Axial CT image demonstrates a small bowel hernia into an ileostomy site (*white arrow*) with decompressed distal bowel (*arrowhead*). (*B*) The bowel exiting the hernia, however, is dilated and filled with feces, with a marked caliber change at the site of an adhesion to the anterior abdominal wall (*black arrow*).

with air in the small bowel (**Fig. 12**). This situation reflects the stasis of contents in the small bowel, resulting in increased resorption of fluid in bowel contents as well as possible gases released from bacterial overgrowth.[9,34,35] Although small bowel feces can be seen in patients without SBO, this finding is highly specific for obstruction when seen in combination with dilated bowel and distal decompressed loops.[36]

Small bowel feces have been found to be inversely related to ischemia and failure of conservative management.[37,38] Because this sign indicates ongoing fluid resorption, the presence of small bowel feces likely reflects preserved function and perfusion of the small bowel. This relationship is further supported by findings that patients with

longer segments of bowel with small bowel feces (>10 cm) are less likely to fail conservative management than are patients with shorter segments of small bowel feces.[29]

Closed Loop

After identification of the transition zone, it is important to determine whether the obstruction is simple or closed-loop. A closed-loop obstruction is present when the bowel is obstructed at 2 adjacent locations, which can be the case with hernias and adhesions. Typically the segment of bowel between the 2 points of obstruction is more dilated than the bowel upstream to the proximal obstruction. Because of the 2 adjacent foci of obstruction, the patient is at risk of torsion at the narrow pedicle. The loops of bowel will often be seen as U-shaped or C-shaped loops when seen in plane. If the loops are out of plane, they may be seen in an array emanating from the point of obstruction, also called "balloons on a string" (**Fig. 13**). The finding of a closed-loop obstruction, even without other evidence of ischemia, is associated with a high risk of transmural necrosis at surgery.[38]

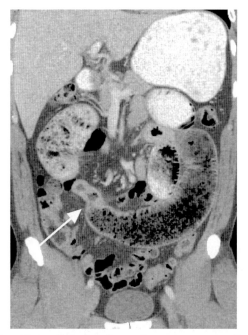

Fig. 12. Small bowel feces. Coronal reconstruction demonstrates a 16-cm segment of dilated bowel containing small bowel feces upstream to a single dense adhesion (*white arrow*). The patient required surgical exploration on a subsequent admission for SBO.

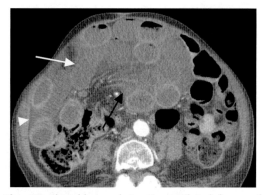

Fig. 13. Closed-loop obstruction. Dilated loops of small bowel, some of which are hypoenhancing (*white arrow*), are arranged in an array (balloons on a string) from the point of obstruction owing to a large adhesion. There is also mesenteric fluid (*arrowhead*) and edema (*black arrow*). The patient had 150 cm of ischemic bowel at surgery.

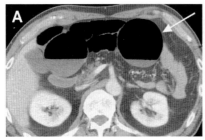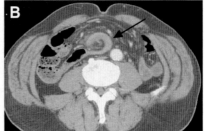

Fig. 14. Whirl sign. A patient with history of colectomy presented with a closed-loop obstruction caused by adhesions. There is a whirl sign of bowel and mesentery in the mid abdomen (*B, black arrow*). Note the nearly imperceptible wall of the dilated loops of small bowel (*A, white arrow*). The patient required resection of 20 cm of infarcted small bowel.

In a closed-loop obstruction associated with volvulus, the rotation of the bowel, vessels, and mesenteric fat at the site of obstruction is known as the whirl sign (**Fig. 14**). The whirl sign has not been shown to be sensitive or specific for SBO. In patients with clinical and radiologic findings consistent with an SBO, however, the presence of a whirl sign is associated with a markedly increased need for surgical intervention.[39] In addition, the identification of the combination of multiple transition points, the whirl sign, and a relatively posterior site of obstruction in patients with an SBO has a specificity of 100% for small bowel volvulus.[40]

Ischemia

Ischemia in SBO can arise from 2 mechanisms. The first is increasing intraluminal fluid resulting in increased pressure within the bowel wall. This pressure can result in occlusion, first of the veins and then the arteries, at a microvascular level within the wall, leading to ischemia.[7] The second cause of ischemia is direct occlusion of the mesenteric vessels resulting from torsion, hernia, or tight adhesive bands. Occlusion of the veins typically occurs first, but the arteries can also be compromised if sufficient pressure is present at the site of obstruction.[41]

Careful assessment of the bowel wall on CT is critical for patient management, as signs of ischemia warrant immediate surgical intervention.

In early ischemia, the bowel wall will often hyperenhance, an indication of vasodilation in an attempt to preserve perfusion. As the vascular supply becomes further compromised, the bowel wall will exhibit decreased or absent enhancement, which is a highly specific sign of ischemia (**Fig. 15**).[38,42,43] Delayed or prolonged enhancement of the bowel can also indicate ischemia (**Fig. 16**). Although wall thickening can indicate ischemia, this finding can be present because of edema from impaired venous outflow caused by the obstruction, and is not specific for ischemia in isolation.[12,42,44] In addition, wall thickening may not be present when ischemia has progressed to transmural infarction, as infarcted bowel loses its tone and the wall can become extremely thin (see **Fig. 14**).[12] Pneumatosis can be an important indicator of bowel ischemia and can suggest an increased risk of transmural infarction when present in combination with portal venous gas.[45] Although pneumatosis is considered specific for ischemia in the appropriate clinical setting, multiple studies have failed to identify pneumatosis as a univariate predictor of ischemia or failure of conservative management of SBO, possibly because of the relatively rare frequency of this finding in the study populations.[37,38,44,46]

Extraluminal findings can also be suggestive of ischemia in SBO. Mesenteric fluid, free fluid, and mesenteric congestion have all been assessed

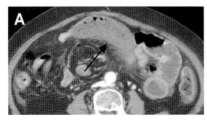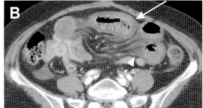

Fig. 15. Hypoenhancement. The small bowel in this closed-loop obstruction demonstrates hypoenhancement (*A, black arrow*) just distal to a segment with mucosal hyperemia (*B, white arrow*). There is mesenteric edema and fluid (*arrowhead*). The patient required resection of 20 cm of infarcted bowel.

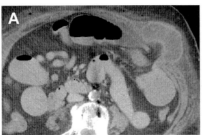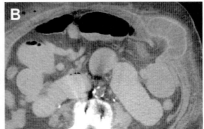

Fig. 16. Delayed enhancement. The patient presented with a SBO from a hernia into a laparoscopic trocar site. The herniated loop of bowel demonstrates persistent enhancement on the delayed phase image (*B*) compared with the portal venous phase image (*A*). The patient required resection of a small segment of bowel secondary to ischemia.

for their predictive value for ischemia in the setting of SBO. Although mesenteric fluid and free fluid are present in higher frequencies in SBOs complicated by ischemia than in uncomplicated obstructions, overall the presence of any one of these findings is not specific for the diagnosis of ischemia.[38,46,47] Because the venous obstruction that often accompanies SBO can cause mesenteric stranding, mesenteric fluid, and ascites in the absence of ischemia, these findings lack specificity for ischemia or infarction.[12] When more than 1 finding is present in a patient, however, these features may have more significance. Although one study found that the specificity of mesenteric fluid, mesenteric congestion, and free fluid for ischemia was 90%, 79%, and 76%, respectively, the specificity for ischemia increased to 94% when 2 or more of these findings were present (see **Fig. 15**).[42]

Combined Imaging and Clinical Predictive Models

The ability to identify patients who will fail conservative management despite the absence of an acute abdomen at presentation may result in better outcomes for these patients. To this end, multivariate predictive models combining imaging findings, laboratory results, and clinical findings have been developed to identify those patients requiring surgery earlier in their presentation. In a study by Schwenter and colleagues,[48] the clinical factors of pain, guarding, leukocytosis, and elevated C-reactive protein were combined with reduced wall enhancement and greater than 500 mL of free fluid on CT into a scoring system. The presence of 3 factors yielded specificity of 91% and sensitivity of 68% for surgical resection of ischemic bowel within 24 hours in comparison with successful conservative management. With 4 factors present, the specificity was 100%. Zielinski and colleagues[49] found that patients with SBO who presented with lack of flatus for at least 24 hours, mesenteric edema, and lack of small bowel feces had an 86% chance of undergoing surgical

exploration during their admission. This combination of features also had a positive predictive value of 29% for ischemic small bowel at surgery.

SUMMARY

Multidetector CT is a powerful tool for the assessment of patients with SBO. CT can provide important information about the cause and site of obstruction and the presence of a closed-loop obstruction or ischemia. Although initially recognized for its ability to accurately diagnose SBO and associated complications, there is a growing body of literature investigating the ability of CT to accurately identify those patients without clear indications for urgent surgery who will likely fail conservative management and may benefit from earlier intervention. Some of the findings under investigation include small bowel feces, mesenteric edema, mesenteric fluid, and free fluid. Models that incorporate both clinical and imaging findings may allow for further risk stratification of patients without signs of ischemia who will ultimately fail conservative management. The ability to identify these patients earlier in their course shows promise in significantly decreasing the morbidity and mortality associated with acute SBO.

REFERENCES

1. Cappell MS, Batke M. Mechanical obstruction of the small bowel and colon. Med Clin North Am 2008; 92(3):575–97, viii.
2. Scott FI, Osterman MT, Mahmoud NN, et al. Secular trends in small-bowel obstruction and adhesiolysis in the United States: 1988-2007. Am J Surg 2012; 204(3):315–20.
3. Diaz JJ Jr, Bokhari F, Mowery NT, et al. Guidelines for management of small bowel obstruction. J Trauma 2008;64(6):1651–64.
4. Catena F, Di Saverio S, Kelly MD, et al. Bologna guidelines for diagnosis and management of adhesive small bowel obstruction (ASBO): 2010 Evidence-based

guidelines of the world society of emergency surgery. World J Emerg Surg 2011;6:5.

5. Furukawa A, Yamasaki M, Furuichi K, et al. Helical CT in the diagnosis of small bowel obstruction. Radiographics 2001;21(2):341–55.

6. Taylor SA, Halligan S, Slater A, et al. Polyp detection with CT colonography: primary 3D endoluminal analysis versus primary 2D transverse analysis with computer-assisted reader software. Radiology 2006;239(3):759–67.

7. Zielinski MD, Bannon MP. Current management of small bowel obstruction. Adv Surg 2011;45:1–29.

8. Frager D. Intestinal obstruction role of CT. Gastroenterol Clin North Am 2002;31(3):777–99.

9. Feldman M, Friedman LS, Brandt LJ, editors. Sleisenger and Fordtran's gastrointestinal and liver disease. 9th edition. Philadelphia: Saunders Elsevier; 2010. No. 2.

10. Gore RM, Levine MS, editors. Textbook of gastrointestinal radiology. 3rd edition. Philadelphia: Saunders Elsevier; 2008. No. 1.

11. Pickhardt PJ, Bhalla S. Intestinal malrotation in adolescents and adults: spectrum of clinical and imaging features. Am J Roentgenol 2002;179(6):1429–35.

12. Wiesner W, Khurana B, Ji H, et al. CT of acute bowel ischemia. Radiology 2003;226(3):635–50.

13. Hodel J, Zins M, Desmottes L, et al. Location of the transition zone in CT of small-bowel obstruction: added value of multiplanar reformations. Abdom Imaging 2009;34(1):35–41.

14. Jaffe TA, Martin LC, Thomas J, et al. Small-bowel obstruction: coronal reformations from isotropic voxels at 16-section multi-detector row CT. Radiology 2006;238(1):135–42.

15. Tresallet C, Lebreton N, Royer B, et al. Improving the management of acute adhesive small bowel obstruction with CT-scan and water-soluble contrast medium: a prospective study. Dis Colon Rectum 2009;52(11):1869–76.

16. Miller G, Boman J, Shrier I, et al. Etiology of small bowel obstruction. Am J Surg 2000;180(1):33–6.

17. Silva AC, Pimenta M, Guimaraes LS. Small bowel obstruction: what to look for. Radiographics 2009; 29(2):423–39.

18. Angenete E, Jacobsson A, Gellerstedt M, et al. Effect of laparoscopy on the risk of small-bowel obstruction: a population-based register study. Arch Surg 2012;147(4):359–65.

19. Takeyama N, Gokan T, Ohgiya Y, et al. CT of internal hernias. Radiographics 2005;25(4):997–1015.

20. Nandipati KC, Lin E, Husain F, et al. Counterclockwise rotation of Roux-en-Y limb significantly reduces internal herniation in laparoscopic Roux-en-Y gastric bypass (LRYGB). J Gastrointest Surg 2012;16(4):675–81.

21. Sunnapwar A, Sandrasegaran K, Menias CO, et al. Taxonomy and imaging spectrum of small bowel obstruction after Roux-en-Y gastric bypass surgery. AJR Am J Roentgenol 2010;194(1):120–8.

22. Hara AK, Swartz PG. CT enterography of Crohn's disease. Abdom Imaging 2009;34(3):289–95.

23. Huprich JE, Fletcher JG. CT enterography: principles, technique and utility in Crohn's disease. Eur J Radiol 2009;69(3):393–7.

24. Huang BY, Warshauer DM. Adult intussusception: diagnosis and clinical relevance. Radiol Clin North Am 2003;41(6):1137–51.

25. Horton KM, Fishman EK. MDCT and 3D imaging in transient enteroenteric intussusception: clinical observations and review of the literature. AJR Am J Roentgenol 2008;191(3):736–42.

26. Fukuya T, Hawes DR, Lu CC, et al. CT diagnosis of small-bowel obstruction: efficacy in 60 patients. AJR Am J Roentgenol 1992;158(4):765–9 [discussion: 771–62].

27. Maglinte DD, Gage SN, Harmon BH, et al. Obstruction of the small intestine: accuracy and role of CT in diagnosis. Radiology 1993;188(1):61–4.

28. Hwang JY, Lee JK, Lee JE, et al. Value of multidetector CT in decision making regarding surgery in patients with small-bowel obstruction due to adhesion. Eur Radiol 2009;19(10):2425–31.

29. Deshmukh SD, Shin DS, Willmann JK, et al. Nonemergency small bowel obstruction: assessment of CT findings that predict need for surgery. Eur Radiol 2011;21(5):982–6.

30. Jones K, Mangram AJ, Lebron RA, et al. Can a computed tomography scoring system predict the need for surgery in small-bowel obstruction? Am J Surg 2007;194(6):780–3 [discussion: 783–4].

31. Tanaka S, Yamamoto T, Kubota D, et al. Predictive factors for surgical indication in adhesive small bowel obstruction. Am J Surg 2008;196(1):23–7.

32. Colon MJ, Telem DA, Wong D, et al. The relevance of transition zones on computed tomography in the management of small bowel obstruction. Surgery 2010;147(3):373–7.

33. Lee IK, Kim do H, Gorden DL, et al. Selective laparoscopic management of adhesive small bowel obstruction using CT guidance. Am Surg 2009; 75(3):227–31.

34. Mayo-Smith WW, Wittenberg J, Bennett GL, et al. The CT small bowel faeces sign: description and clinical significance. Clin Radiol 1995;50(11): 765–7.

35. Catalano O. The faeces sign. A CT finding in small-bowel obstruction. Radiologe 1997;37(5):417–9.

36. Jacobs SL, Rozenblit A, Ricci Z, et al. Small bowel faeces sign in patients without small bowel obstruction. Clin Radiol 2007;62(4):353–7.

37. Zielinski MD, Eiken PW, Bannon MP, et al. Small bowel obstruction—who needs an operation? A multivariate prediction model. World J Surg 2010; 34(5):910–9.

38. Jancelewicz T, Vu LT, Shawo AE, et al. Predicting strangulated small bowel obstruction: an old problem revisited. J Gastrointest Surg 2009;13(1):93–9.

39. Duda JB, Bhatt S, Dogra VS. Utility of CT whirl sign in guiding management of small-bowel obstruction. AJR Am J Roentgenol 2008;191(3):743–7.

40. Sandhu PS, Joe BN, Coakley FV, et al. Bowel transition points: multiplicity and posterior location at CT are associated with small-bowel volvulus. Radiology 2007;245(1):160–7.

41. Qalbani A, Paushter D, Dachman AH. Multidetector row CT of small bowel obstruction. Radiol Clin North Am 2007;45(3):499–512, viii.

42. Zalcman M, Sy M, Donckier V, et al. Helical CT signs in the diagnosis of intestinal ischemia in small-bowel obstruction. AJR Am J Roentgenol 2000;175(6):1601–7.

43. Jang KM, Min K, Kim MJ, et al. Diagnostic performance of CT in the detection of intestinal ischemia associated with small-bowel obstruction using maximal attenuation of region of interest. AJR Am J Roentgenol 2010;194(4):957–63.

44. Frager D, Baer JW, Medwid SW, et al. Detection of intestinal ischemia in patients with acute small-bowel obstruction due to adhesions or hernia: efficacy of CT. AJR Am J Roentgenol 1996;166(1):67–71.

45. Kernagis LY, Levine MS, Jacobs JE. Pneumatosis intestinalis in patients with ischemia: correlation of CT findings with viability of the bowel. AJR Am J Roentgenol 2003;180(3):733–6.

46. Sheedy SP, Earnest FT, Fletcher JG, et al. CT of small-bowel ischemia associated with obstruction in emergency department patients: diagnostic performance evaluation. Radiology 2006;241(3):729–36.

47. O'Daly BJ, Ridgway PF, Keenan N, et al. Detected peritoneal fluid in small bowel obstruction is associated with the need for surgical intervention. Can J Surg 2009;52(3):201–6.

48. Schwenter F, Poletti PA, Platon A, et al. Clinicoradiological score for predicting the risk of strangulated small bowel obstruction. Br J Surg 2010;97(7):1119–25.

49. Zielinski MD, Eiken PW, Heller SF, et al. Prospective, observational validation of a multivariate small-bowel obstruction model to predict the need for operative intervention. J Am Coll Surg 2011;212(6):1068–76.

Computed Tomography Evaluation of Gastrointestinal Bleeding and Acute Mesenteric Ischemia

Seung Soo Lee, MD, Seong Ho Park, MD*

KEYWORDS

- Small intestine • Gastrointestinal bleeding • Mesenteric ischemia • Mesenteric infarction
- Computed tomography • Enterography

KEY POINTS

- Multidetector computed tomography (MDCT) can accurately diagnose active gastrointestinal (GI) bleeding and could be the initial diagnostic tool for evaluating acute lower-GI bleeding.
- Computed tomography (CT) enterography may be incorporated into the routine diagnostic algorithm for patients with obscure GI bleeding, either as the first-line examination or as a complementary examination to capsule endoscopy.
- MDCT angiography is the preferred examination for the diagnosis of acute mesenteric ischemia.
- The CT findings of acute mesenteric ischemia are variable according to its cause, bowel perfusion status, and the severity of ischemic injury.

INTRODUCTION

Recent advances in multidetector computed tomography (MDCT) technology and powerful three-dimensional (3D) postprocessing software have expanded the role of computed tomography (CT) in the evaluation of gastrointestinal (GI) bleeding and acute mesenteric ischemia. MDCT combined with a rapid bolus injection of intravenous (IV) contrast allows for rapid dynamic contrast-enhanced scanning of the abdomen and pelvis, providing motion-free, accurately timed arterial-phase and venous-phase images with near-isometric high spatial resolution. Using 3D imaging software, CT volume data sets can be reconstructed in any anatomic plane and in various 3D displays; for example, MDCT angiography for noninvasive visualization of the mesenteric vasculature. With CT enterography, the use of neutral oral contrast agents results in better evaluation of subtle mucosal and mural abnormalities of the bowel. As a result, small bowel radiography and catheter-based mesenteric angiography, both of which were traditionally used in the diagnosis of GI bleeding and acute mesenteric ischemia, have been largely replaced by MDCT, which may also substitute for or complement diagnostic endoscopy.

GI BLEEDING

GI bleeding is a common medical problem, with an annual incidence in the United States of 40 to 150 episodes and 20 to 27 episodes per 100,000 persons for upper-GI and lower-GI bleeding, respectively.[1] Although the clinical outcome of GI bleeding is variable depending on the cause and

Disclosure: Neither of the authors has a conflict of interest.
Department of Radiology and Research Institute of Radiology, Asan Medical Center, University of Ulsan College of Medicine, 388-1 Poongnap2-Dong, Songpa-Gu, Seoul 138-040, South Korea
* Corresponding author.
E-mail address: parksh.radiology@gmail.com

the severity, it results in almost 300,000 hospitalizations per year in the United States. The reported related mortalities are 8% to 10% for upper-GI bleeding, 2% to 4% for lower-GI bleeding, and as high as 40% in hemodynamically unstable patients.[2–5] Endoscopic examinations are the mainstay in evaluating patients with GI bleeding; however, radiologic examinations, in particular state-of-the-art MDCT, have substantial complementary roles.

Clinical Presentation and Classification

The location of GI bleeding is reported with respect to the ligament of Treitz, with upper-GI bleeding occurring above the ligament and lower-GI bleeding below it. Although upper-GI bleeding is more common than lower-GI bleeding,[4] there has been a gradual trend in the opposite direction over the past 10 years, which may be related to the decrease in peptic ulcer disease and an increase in the elderly population.[6,7]

Overt GI bleeding presents as visually apparent bleeding symptoms, such as hematemesis, melena, or hematochezia.[4] Occult GI bleeding denotes a positive fecal occult blood test and/or iron-deficiency anemia without evidence of visible blood within emesis or in feces; it reflects smaller amounts of bleeding.[4,8,9] Obscure GI bleeding, although often confused with occult bleeding, specifically refers to recurrent or persistent bleeding for which no obvious cause has been identified by standard upper and lower endoscopic examinations; it can be overt or occult. Obscure bleeding accounts for approximately 5% of all cases of GI bleeding[8,10,11] and usually indicates bleeding from the small bowel. However, it can also be caused by lesions missed or overlooked in the esophagus, stomach, or colon during the initial endoscopic examination.[4,10,11]

GI bleeding is also categorized according to both the severity and the patient's hemodynamic status as massive, moderate, or minor. Massive GI bleeding is defined as the presence of resting hypotension, which can be caused by a 20% to 25% loss of total blood volume.[4] Moderate GI bleeding refers to the presence of orthostatic hypotension and tachycardia and indicates a 10% to 20% loss of total blood volume. In minor bleeding, there is no significant alteration in the patient's hemodynamic status.[4]

Causes

The causes of upper-GI and lower-GI bleeding are summarized in **Tables 1** and **2**. Peptic ulcer disease accounts for more than 50% of upper-GI bleeding,[2,4,12] whereas colonic diverticula and

Table 1
Causes of upper GI bleeding

Causes	Incidence (%)
Gastric or duodenal peptic ulcer disease	55
Esophagogastric varices	14
Arteriovenous malformations	6
Mallory-Weiss tears	5
Tumors	4
Erosions	4
Dieulafoy lesion	1
Others	11

Data from Acosta RD, Wong RK. Differential diagnosis of upper gastrointestinal bleeding proximal to the ligament of Trietz. Gastrointest Endosc Clin N Am 2011;21:555–66.

angioectasia are the 2 most common causes of lower-GI bleeding.[2–4,7] Angioectasia is overall the most common cause of small intestinal bleeding, which often presents as obscure GI bleeding. However, the causes of small intestinal bleeding vary according to patient age. For example, small bowel bleeding in patients less than 25 years of age is most commonly caused by Meckel diverticulum, whereas, in older patients, small bowel neoplasm, angioectasia, and nonsteroidal antiinflammatory drug (NSAID)–induced small bowel disease are more relevant.[10,11] Obscure GI bleeding may, rarely, have unconventional causes, such as hemobilia associated with prior liver biopsy or hepatocellular carcinoma, hemosuccus pancreaticus in patients with pancreatitis, aortoenteric fistula after abdominal aortic aneurysm repair, and ectopic small bowel varices in patients with portal hypertension.[11]

Table 2
Causes of lower GI bleeding

Causes	Incidence (%)
Diverticulosis	30–65
Angioectasia	4–15
Hemorrhoids	4–12
Ischemic colitis	4–11
Other types of colitis	3–15
Neoplasia	2–11
Postpolypectomy bleeding	2–7
Rectal ulcer	0–8

Data from Strate LL. Lower GI bleeding: epidemiology and diagnosis. Gastroenterol Clin North Am 2005;34:643–64.

General Diagnostic Approach

Endoscopy plays a major role in the evaluation of patients with GI bleeding, whereas radiological examinations are still considered supplementary, despite their proven and potential diagnostic capability (discussed later). In patients with upper-GI bleeding, the first-line diagnostic method is esophagogastroduodenoscopy (EGD), based on its high sensitivity and specificity (98% and 100%, respectively) in detecting the source of bleeding.[5] Colonoscopy is the primary method for evaluating nonurgent lower-GI bleeding and is usually performed after the cessation of a bleeding episode, with patients undergoing a full cathartic preparation of the colon. By contrast, the role of colonoscopy in urgent lower-GI bleeding is controversial given the procedural/technical challenges in this setting, including poor visibility of the colon.[4,13] When the upper and lower endoscopic examinations fail to identify the bleeding focus (ie, obscure GI bleeding), repeat EGD and colonoscopy are currently recommended as the standard next procedures to rule out any sources of bleeding in the esophagus, stomach, and colon that may have been overlooked during initial endoscopy. If the repeat examinations are negative, capsule endoscopy (CE), double-balloon enteroscopy, or nonendoscopic examinations such as CT may be used. In accordance with the diagnostic scheme, the role of radiological examinations with regard to GI bleeding has largely centered on the evaluation of acute lower-GI bleeding, especially in an emergent situation, and on obscure GI bleeding. Tagged red blood cell scintigraphy, catheter mesenteric angiography, or fluoroscopic examination are alternative nonendoscopic diagnostic examinations to diagnose GI bleeding but are not discussed in this article.

CT Techniques for the Evaluation of GI Bleeding

The CT protocol for GI bleeding should be designed to show active bleeding, if present at the time of scanning, as well as to allow for an optimized detection of the GI abnormalities that caused the bleeding, if the examination is performed after cessation of the active bleeding episodes. Biphasic scanning after a rapid bolus IV injection of contrast medium, including arterial and venous phases, is the preferred protocol.[14,15] For example, we typically inject 120 mL of nonionic iodinated contrast agent at a rate of 4 mL/s, and obtain arterial-phase imaging using a bolus-triggering method and venous-phase imaging 72 seconds after the start of the IV contrast injection. A preenhanced scan is critical because it helps in differentiating active hemorrhage or vascular lesions from high-attenuating pseudolesions in the bowel (such as orally ingested pills, residual positive oral contrast material from previous radiologic examinations, or various foreign bodies).[15,16] The administration of a neutral oral contrast agent, such as water or a sorbitol solution, is particularly useful to achieve optimal bowel distention and better lesion visibility in examinations performed after the cessation of acute bleeding episodes. However, neutral oral contrast is generally not recommended for patients with active bleeding because it can interfere with the detection of active bleeding by diluting the extravasated contrast material in the bowel lumen. Also, it should not be administered to patients with hemodynamic instability because this could result in a substantial delay of the CT examination.[16,17] In our institution, 1500 mL of a 3% sorbitol solution is orally administered continuously over 45 minutes before CT scanning, but only in those patients without active bleeding or hemodynamic instability.

Role of CT and CT Findings in the Evaluation of GI Bleeding

Patients with urgent acute GI bleeding

For patients with acute GI bleeding, CT is generally used when endoscopic examinations have failed or are difficult to perform. The primary goal of CT is to guide optimal patient treatment by determining whether there is ongoing bleeding, the location of the bleeding focus, and the cause of bleeding.[13,16,18] The diagnosis of active GI bleeding can be easily made on CT if the scan shows extravasation of contrast material into the bowel lumen; this is seen as an intraluminal focal collection or jet of contrast material that is visible in the arterial and/or venous phase but not on the preenhanced scan (**Fig. 1**). Both arterial-phase and venous-phase scans should be carefully reviewed, because slow bleeding may be visible only on the latter (**Fig. 2**). The presence of hyperattenuating intraluminal material on the preenhanced scan may indicate acute hematoma and, therefore, the site of recent bleeding (see **Fig. 1**).[18] However, this finding should be carefully interpreted with respect to the history of the recent radiologic examination, because diluted positive oral contrast or other preexisting density could have a similar appearance.

An experimental study using animal models has shown the ability of helical CT to depict active colonic bleeding at a rate as low as 0.3 mL/min.[19] Given that the detection limit of catheter mesenteric angiography is approximately 0.5 mL/min,

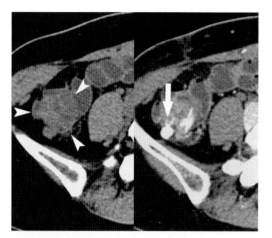

Fig. 1. Active bleeding from a cecal diverticulum in a 48-year-old woman with hematochezia. Unenhanced CT scan (*left*) shows a slightly hyperattenuating intraluminal lesion (*arrowheads*) suggesting an acute hematoma. Contrast-enhanced arterial-phase image (*right*) shows active extravasation of contrast material from the colonic diverticulum (*arrow*).

the sensitivity of CT is likely comparable with that of catheter angiography for diagnosing intestinal bleeding. Consistent with the experimental results, several clinical studies that have adopted modern CT techniques reported a fairly high accuracy for CT in the diagnosis of acute GI bleeding in clinical patients.[17,18] Yoon and colleagues[17] evaluated 26 patients with acute massive GI bleeding who underwent an arterial-phase MDCT scan. The sensitivity and specificity for the detection and localization of active bleeding were 91% and 99%, respectively, compared with catheter angiography as the reference standard. Recently, Marti and colleagues[18] reconfirmed the accuracy of MDCT in a prospective study of 47 patients with

acute lower-GI bleeding. The sensitivity and specificity of CT angiography in depicting active or recent bleeding were 100% and 96%, respectively. Furthermore, CT angiography was able to characterize the causes of bleeding accurately in 93% of the patients.[18]

Although CT is not yet regarded as the primary examination for patients with acute GI bleeding, some gastroenterologists have proposed the incorporation of CT into an early stage in the management algorithm of patients with lower-GI bleeding.[13] They suggested that, in patients with acute lower-GI bleeding, CT could be the initial diagnostic examination and therefore guide therapeutic and diagnostic decision making.[13]

Patients with obscure GI bleeding

Because most sources of obscure GI bleeding are located in the small bowel, a CT examination for obscure GI bleeding generally requires CT enterographic techniques, including the use of neutral oral contrast agent to achieve optimal small bowel distention, except, as described earlier, when contraindicated. In 2 previous studies, the sensitivity of CT enterography in identifying the causes of obscure GI bleeding was 55.2% and 88%.[15,20] CT enterography is more accurate in detecting small bowel tumors and Crohn's disease (**Figs. 3** and **4**) than in detecting Meckel diverticulum and angioectasia.[15,21,22] Angioectasia, also referred to as angiodysplasia, is the most common cause of small bowel bleeding, although it occurs more frequently in the cecum and ascending colon than in the small intestine. Angiodysplasia is characterized pathologically by dilated submucosal veins occasionally accompanied by dilated feeding arteries and draining veins in larger lesions.[4,23] On CT, angiectasia appears as a nodular or plaquelike enhancing lesion within

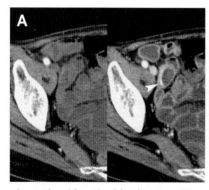
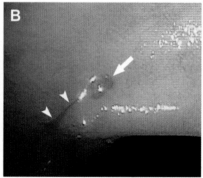

Fig. 2. Ileal angioectasia with active bleeding in a 70-year-old woman with hematochezia. (*A*) Contrast-enhanced arterial-phase image (*left*) does not show active bleeding. However, the venous-phase scan (*right*) shows a thread of extravasated contrast (*arrowhead*) in the lateral side of the distal ileal lumen, which confirms active bleeding. (*B*) Double-balloon enteroscopy shows active bleeding (*arrowheads*) from a tiny angioectasia (*arrow*) in the distal ileum.

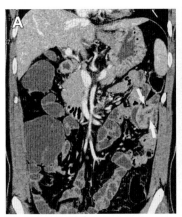
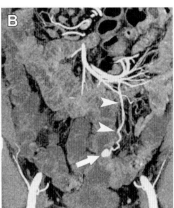
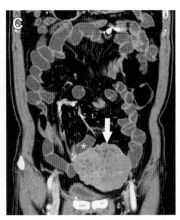

Fig. 3. Small bowel tumors diagnosed at CT. (*A*) Jejunal cancer in a 44-year-old man who presented with obscure occult GI bleeding. A coronal CT image shows an encircling mass in the proximal jejunum (*arrows*). (*B*) Capillary hemangioma in a 76-year-old man with recurrent melena. A coronal thin-slab maximal intensity projection image shows a 1-cm, well-enhancing vascular mass (*arrow*) fed by an ileal branch (*arrowheads*) of the superior mesenteric artery (SMA). (*C*) A large GI stromal tumor in the ileum that was missed by CE in a 62-year-old man with hematochezia. CE, performed as an initial diagnostic examination, only showed incidental erosions in the jejunum (not shown), whereas subsequent CT enterography shows a huge, well-enhancing mass (*arrow*) abutting the distal ileum (*asterisk*). Surgical resection of the small intestine disclosed a GI stromal tumor.

the bowel wall (**Fig. 5**).[23,24] An early draining vein is commonly seen on CT in colonic angioectasia[25] but is rarely visible on CT in small bowel angiodysplasia. Meckel diverticulum is difficult to detect at CT enterography. Because this is a true diverticulum that has all the layers of the small bowel wall, it appears as a tubular structure similar to the normal small bowel. Therefore, unless accompanied by concomitant abnormal enhancement or thickening of the diverticular wall, the only clue to

the diagnosis of Meckel diverticulum is the identification of its blind end (**Fig. 6**).

The reported diagnostic yields of CT in detecting the source of bleeding in patients with obscure GI bleeding have been variable. Although earlier studies reported high diagnostic yields of 75% to 79%,[14,26] they likely reflected the inclusion of many patients with massive bleeding. In more recent studies, in which the study population mostly comprised patients without active

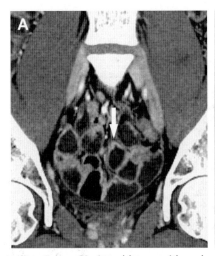
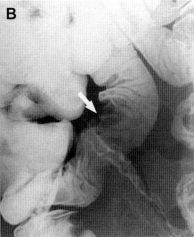

Fig. 4. Crohn's disease in a 28-year-old man with melena. (*A*) A coronal CT image shows a small ulcer (*arrow*) accompanied by subtle wall thickening, with slightly increased enhancement at the mesenteric side of the distal ileum. (*B*) A spot radiograph of a small bowel follow-through confirms a small ulceration, seen as a tiny barium collection and surrounding fold convergence (*arrow*).

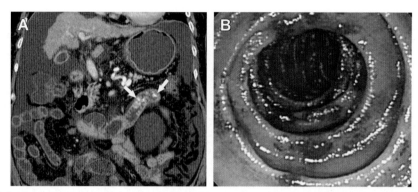

Fig. 5. Multiple duodenal angioectasias in a 66-year-old woman with hepatitis B virus liver cirrhosis and hepatocellular carcinoma. (*A*) Contrast-enhanced venous-phase coronal image shows multiple nodular enhancing lesions (*arrows*) within the bowel wall. (*B*) Endoscopic image shows multiple angioectasia, seen as slightly red vascular lesions scattered in the transverse portion of the duodenum.

bleeding, the overall diagnostic yield of CT enterography was 25% to 45%.[15,20,27,28]

The role of CT in the diagnostic algorithm for evaluating obscure GI bleeding has yet to be determined, unlike CE, which has been proposed as the primary diagnostic method in this setting.[29] However, CE has disadvantages that limit its routine use in clinical practice. For example, it is contraindicated in patients with a suspected stricture of the small bowel, swallowing disorders, or motility disorders.[21,30] In addition, CE requires lengthy examination and interpretation times and is therefore inadequate for emergent situations. It cannot definitively localize the detected abnormality, because the location of the capsule can only be roughly estimated based on its transit time.[21,30] Furthermore, although CE is highly sensitive in detecting aphthoid ulcers, whether these minute mucosal lesions are a true source of bleeding is uncertain, because such lesions can be seen in up to 7% of asymptomatic healthy subjects.[31] Earlier comparative studies obtained a higher diagnostic yield with CE than with CT in the evaluation of obscure GI bleeding,[22,32,33] but these studies may have been biased by an overestimation of the yield of CE and underestimation of that of CT. Most of the CE findings were regarded as true-positives even though further confirmation by alternative means was lacking.[22,32,33] Moreover, the CT examinations in some of these studies were not technically optimized for the evaluation of obscure GI bleeding because they were

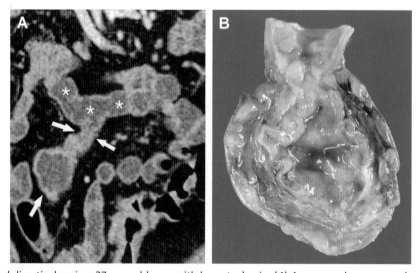

Fig. 6. Meckel diverticulum in a 37-year-old man with hematochezia. (*A*) A venous-phase, coronal, curved, multiplanar, reformatted image depicts a blind-ended tubular structure (*arrows*) connected to the ileum (*asterisks*). (*B*) Histologic examination following surgical resection of the diverticulum disclosed a true diverticulum with gastric-type mucosa.

performed without bowel distention or even after the administration of positive oral contrast agents.[21,32] To the contrary, a recent prospective comparison between state-of-the-art triple-phase CT enterography and CE found that the former has a higher sensitivity in detecting the causes of obscure GI bleeding.[20] In that study, the main advantage of CT enterography compared with CE was a higher accuracy in detecting small bowel tumors (ie, a 100% [9 of 9] sensitivity of CT enterography versus a 33% [3 of 9] sensitivity of CE).[20] Another study also showed that CT enterography has a substantial role in patients who have had nondiagnostic CE.[34] Agrawal and coworkers[34] reported that CT enterography could detect the source of bleeding in half of the patients with overt obscure GI bleeding and a nondiagnostic CE (see Fig. 3C).

Double-balloon enteroscopy (DBE) is a recently developed endoscopic technique with great potential for evaluating obscure GI bleeding. Visualization of the small bowel was possible in 42% to 86% of the patients, either as a single procedure or by the combination of per-oral and per-anal routes.[35,36] Nonetheless, although DBE is a powerful tool for evaluating the small bowel, considering its technical complexity and invasiveness, it may be more suitable for histopathologic confirmation and the treatment of detected/suspected abnormalities rather than for the initial diagnostic evaluation of patients with obscure GI bleeding.

Given the promising results obtained in recent studies in which state-of-the-art CT enterography techniques were used,[20,34] CT could now be considered to have come of age and could thus be routinely incorporated into the diagnostic algorithm for patients with obscure GI bleeding, either as the first-line examination or complementary to CE. When an urgent work-up is required, CT is likely to be the most appropriate primary diagnostic tool. It can be performed as a primary examination without the need for concern regarding unexpected small bowel stricture, and can be used to rule out bowel stricture before CE. In patients with persistent or recurrent bleeding after a negative or nondiagnostic CE, the complementary use of CT may allow the detection of a missed lesion.

ACUTE MESENTERIC ISCHEMIA

Acute mesenteric ischemia is a life-threatening abdominal emergency with an overall mortality of 60% to 80%.[37,38] Although it is uncommon, comprising only 1% of the cases of acute abdomen, the reported incidence of acute mesenteric ischemia is increasing owing to the aging population in many countries, improved diagnostic techniques, and improved awareness of this condition.[37,39,40] Because acute mesenteric ischemia may rapidly proceed to fatal intestinal infarction, its prompt diagnosis and treatment are paramount.[37–39] The survival rate is approximately 50% when the condition is diagnosed within 24 hours after the onset of symptoms, but it decreases sharply to 30% when the diagnosis is delayed.[41]

The early diagnosis of acute mesenteric ischemia requires a high index of suspicion, because the clinical presentation in most patients is nonspecific and neither the physical examination nor laboratory tests render a specific diagnosis.[37–39] Instead, radiologic examinations play a crucial diagnostic role. Mesenteric angiography was traditionally the method of choice for the diagnosis of acute mesenteric ischemia but it has now been largely replaced by CT. With the recent advances in MDCT technology, CT angiography is considered to be the first-line imaging method for the diagnosis of acute mesenteric ischemia, because it allows the assessment of the mesenteric vessels as well as ischemic changes in the bowel wall.

Causes

Acute mesenteric ischemia can be caused by arterial embolism, arterial thrombosis, mesenteric venous thrombosis, and nonocclusive mesenteric ischemia (NOMI). Among them, arterial embolism is the most common cause, accounting for approximately 50% of cases. Emboli usually originate from left atrial or ventricular thrombi, and patients frequently have heart-related risk factors, including cardiac arrhythmia, myocardial infarction, and valvular diseases. The emboli lodge at points of normal anatomic narrowing, usually immediately distal to the origin of major visceral arteries.

NOMI accounts for 20% to 30% of cases of acute mesenteric ischemia, making it the second most common cause. The pathogenesis of NOMI is poorly understood but is thought to involve mesenteric vasoconstriction in response to hypovolemia, decreased cardiac output, or hypotension.[37,39] If any of these conditions is sustained for a prolonged period, the vasoconstriction may become irreversible despite correction of the precipitating event.[37,39] Precipitating factors for NOMI may include acute myocardial infarction, congestive heart failure, arrhythmia, hypovolemic shock, dehydration, and hemodialysis.[39] Treatment options are intra-arterial papaverine infusion and surgical excision of the necrotic bowel segment.

Mesenteric arterial thrombosis is responsible for 10% to 20% of cases of acute mesenteric ischemia. It usually occurs in areas of severe atherosclerotic narrowing, typically at the origin of the superior mesenteric artery (SMA).[37,39,40,42] Up to 50% of patients with acute mesenteric ischemia caused by arterial thrombosis have previously experienced symptoms of chronic mesenteric ischemia several weeks to months before the acute event.[39]

Acute mesenteric venous thrombosis is the least common cause of mesenteric ischemia, representing up to 10% of cases.[37,39,43] Conditions that predispose to the development of acute mesenteric venous thrombosis include hypercoagulable states related to coagulation disorders, hematologic disorders, oral contraceptive usage, abdominal inflammatory diseases, postoperative state, and portal hypertension.[39,43]

CT Techniques for the Evaluation of Acute Mesenteric Ischemia

Biphasic arterial-phase and venous-phase scanning is necessary to evaluate both the arterial and the venous mesenteric systems. Positive oral contrast agent should be abandoned because it may interfere with bowel-wall enhancement and hamper visualization of the mesenteric vessels on 3D reconstructed images.[44–46] Neutral oral contrast administration may be beneficial for the assessment of bowel enhancement after intravenous contrast administration[44–49]; however, it is generally not feasible in patients with acute mesenteric ischemia because of the time delay and patient symptoms including acute abdominal pain, nausea, and vomiting, in addition to often being ineffective because of commonly occurring adynamic ileus, which delays the transit of oral contrast material.[46,50] At our institution, neutral oral contrast is not routinely administered to patients in whom acute mesenteric ischemia is suspected.

CT Findings of Acute Mesenteric Ischemia

The CT features of acute mesenteric ischemia include abnormalities in the mesenteric vessels, various morphologic changes in the bowel wall, and other miscellaneous findings such as mesenteric stranding and ascites. There is no single CT finding that is both sensitive and specific for the diagnosis of acute mesenteric ischemia. Embolic or thrombotic occlusion of the SMA and thrombosis in the superior mesenteric vein (SMV) and its tributaries are reported to be specific for diagnosing acute mesenteric ischemia, but they are not sensitive.[49,51,52] Changes in the bowel wall

are more sensitive but are less specific than the abnormalities in the mesenteric vessels.[49,51,52] Because there are differences in the CT findings according to the cause of the acute mesenteric ischemia,[46,50] in the following, the CT findings of mesenteric arterial embolism or thrombosis, mesenteric venous thrombosis, and NOMI are discussed separately.

Acute mesenteric arterial ischemia caused by embolism or thrombosis

Emboli in the SMA generally lodge a few centimeters distal to their origin from the aorta, typically near the origin of the middle colic artery (Fig. 7),[39,44] whereas SMA thrombosis usually develops within the first 2 cm after the origin of this artery.[44] Because SMA thrombosis commonly occurs in the setting of atherosclerotic disease and in patients with chronic ischemia, there is often calcified plaque adjacent to the thrombus and associated arterial collaterals.[44] A large

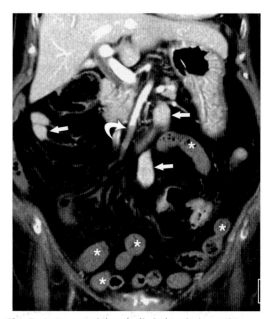

Fig. 7. Acute arterial embolic ischemia in an 85-year-old woman with atrial fibrillation who presented with acute abdominal pain and diarrhea. A coronal CT image shows embolic occlusion of the SMA from the midportion of the main trunk downwards (*curved arrow*). The ileum (*asterisks*) within the territory of the embolic occlusion is slightly dilated and shows decreased contrast enhancement compared with the normal-appearing jejunum (*arrows*) proximal to the ischemic segment. The jejunal lumen is filled with positive oral contrast material. Surgical exploration with resection of the ischemic ileum was performed the day after the CT scan. Histologic examination revealed hemorrhagic necrosis of the mucosa and submucosa of the ileum.

thrombus/embolus in the thick proximal segments of the mesenteric arteries is easily depicted by CT (see **Fig. 7**; **Fig. 8**); however, tiny emboli in the distal branches of mesenteric arteries may be difficult to detect, particularly if they are too small for the spatial resolution of CT.[45,49,51] Therefore, in some patients with embolic ischemia, CT findings may consist of nonspecific abnormalities in the bowel wall and adjacent mesenteric fat.[45] Although prior studies using single-detector CT or 4-channel MDCT reported a low detection rate (<30%) for arterial emboli or thrombus,[49] recent studies using 16-channel or greater MDCT showed the detection of arterial occlusion in 72% to 93% of patients with acute mesenteric arterial ischemia.[53] This improvement is attributed to the higher z-axis resolution of modern MDCT scanners and their faster scanning capability after bolus contrast injection.

Ischemic changes in the bowel wall as seen on CT are related to the pathophysiologic changes. The initial pathophysiologic response of the bowel to arterial occlusion is a marked increase in bowel motility and the spastic contraction of the ischemic bowel.[54] Soon thereafter, bowel motility gradually ceases,[54] leading to adynamic ileus. With prolonged arterial occlusion without subsequent reperfusion, ischemic damage in the bowel wall propagates from the mucosa to the serosa, resulting in transmural infarction.[54,55] When arterial perfusion is restored after temporary arterial occlusion and subsequent hypoxic damage to

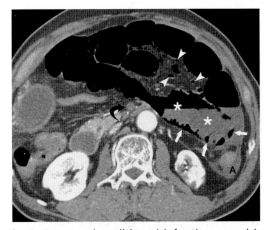

Fig. 8. Transmural small bowel infarction caused by acute thrombosis of the SMA. Axial CT images show thrombosis (*curved arrow*) of the proximal SMA. The infarcted small bowel, including the jejunum (*asterisks*), has both a paper-thin, almost imperceptible wall that lacks contrast enhancement and marked luminal dilatation. Air bubbles are noted within the bowel wall (*arrows*) and in the mesenteric veins (*arrowheads*). A small amount of ascites (A) is present.

the bowel, reperfusion injury may be superimposed on the initial hypoxic changes. An experimental study suggested that reperfusion injury is associated with increased microvascular and mucosal permeability, which ultimately leads to interstitial hemorrhage and/or edema and the leaking of fluid and biologic molecules into the bowel lumen.[54,56] Various endogenous substances, including oxygen free radicals, have been implicated in the pathogenesis of reperfusion injury.[54]

Although a time-matched correlation between the various CT findings of arterial mesenteric ischemia and the aforementioned pathophysiology of this disease is difficult to obtain in humans, empirical evidence and data from animal experiments suggest several correlations. The CT findings of the bowel wall in acute mesenteric arterial ischemia can be differentiated into 2 distinct patterns that likely represent the purely occlusive state and the reperfused state.[46,48,57,58] In acute, purely occlusive arterial ischemia, thickening of the bowel wall is rare. The ischemic bowel segment has a normal or thinner-than-normal wall thickness and a decreased or absent mural contrast enhancement on CT (see **Fig. 7**), and is frequently dilated.[46,48,59] With more prolonged arterial occlusion, the ischemic bowel wall becomes thinner and more dilated, resulting in a paper-thin appearance, which, together with a lack of mural contrast enhancement, is an ominous sign that suggests transmural bowel infarction (see **Fig. 8**).[48,51] The CT diagnosis of acute arterio-occlusive small bowel ischemia is sometimes challenging, especially when the aforementioned mural changes are mild or focal. In such cases, a nonspecific mild distention of the bowel could be misdiagnosed as simple paralytic ileus. Therefore, a high index of suspicion is necessary for the accurate diagnosis of arterio-occlusive ischemia. In particular, in elderly patients with known risk factors of arterial ischemia who present with small bowel ileus without definite obstructive causes, the possibility of acute mesenteric ischemia should be considered, requiring a meticulous evaluation of the mesenteric vessels and the bowel wall to rule out this life-threatening condition (**Fig. 9**). When there is reperfusion of blood flow after temporary arterial occlusion, the ischemic bowel wall becomes thickened, probably because of edema and hemorrhage in the mucosa and submucosa. After contrast enhancement, the bowel wall usually shows mural stratification, that is, a hyperenhancing inner layer caused by the increased microvascular permeability and inflammatory infiltration and a low-attenuating outer layer representing edema and hemorrhage (**Fig. 10**).[46,48,57,59] Previous studies suggested that this bowel-wall

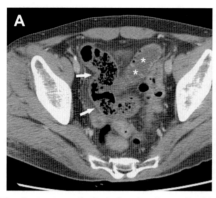
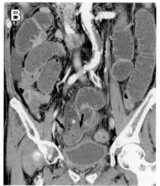
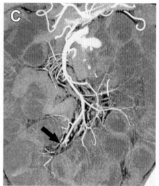

Fig. 9. Acute embolic infarction in an ileal branch of the SMA in a 62-year-old man who presented with acute abdominal pain. (*A*) An initial venous-phase CT scan at the time of the presentation shows a mildly dilated pelvic ileal segment with slightly decreased enhancement (*arrows*) compared with the normal-appearing jejunum (*asterisks*). Arterial embolus was not clearly visualized on this CT scan and a confident diagnosis of acute mesenteric ischemia could not be made based on these subtle CT findings. (*B*) A coronal image on follow-up CT obtained 2 days later shows a complete loss of enhancement in the mesenteric side of the ileal segment (*arrows*) and haziness in the adjacent mesentery (*asterisk*). (*C*) A maximal intensity projection image of the arterial-phase scan shows an abrupt cutoff of an ileal branch (*arrow*) of the SMA, representing the point of distal embolic occlusion.

pattern (slightly thickened bowel wall with hyperenhancement) indicates a good prognosis, because it shows the viability of the ischemic bowel wall.[48,51] However, the damaged bowel wall can progress to perforation and delayed stricture formation even after reperfusion.[54]

In small bowel ischemia caused by arterial occlusion, ascites and perienteric fat stranding are rare unless transmural infarction has developed (see **Figs. 8** and **9**).[46,48] The presence of pneumatosis intestinalis often indicates transmural infarction in the setting of mesenteric ischemia, particularly if associated with portomesenteric venous gas (see **Fig. 8**).[45,46,49,51] However, pneumatosis intestinalis and even portomesenteric venous gas may be seen in various nonischemic conditions, including inflammatory bowel disease, connective tissue disorder, immunosuppression, cytotoxic chemotherapy, and any condition associated with bowel distention and increased intraluminal pressure (**Fig. 11**).[60] Therefore, these findings should be interpreted carefully and with consideration for other concomitant findings of acute mesenteric ischemia, such as abnormal mural enhancement, bowel distention, and bowel-wall thickening or thinning. Isolated

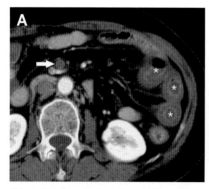
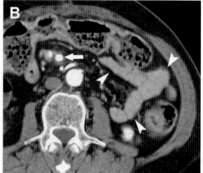

Fig. 10. Reversible arterial embolic ischemia in a 72-year-old woman with atrial fibrillation who presented with acute abdominal pain and melena. (*A*) Initial CT scan shows an embolic occlusion of the SMA (*arrow*) and an ischemic jejunum (*asterisks*) characterized by mild bowel-wall thickening, a target appearance, and mild distention. At surgical exploration, the ischemic jejunum appeared edematous but there was no definite evidence of infarction. Fogarty embolectomy was performed without bowel resection. (*B*) Follow-up CT 2 months after the operation shows the restoration of arterial flow (*arrow*) and a complete recovery from the jejunal ischemia (*arrowheads*).

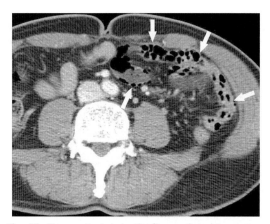

Fig. 11. Pneumatosis intestinalis unrelated to mesenteric ischemia in a 55-year-old man with gastric peptic ulcer disease. The patient was asymptomatic and had no history of a recent endoscopic examination. Pneumatosis intestinalis was incidentally found on a CT for an unrelated issue. Axial CT image shows round air densities within the ileal wall (*arrows*). Unlike acute mesenteric ischemia, the ileal segment with pneumatosis intestinalis has normal enhancement and does not show other concomitant findings of acute mesenteric ischemia, such as bowel distention, bowel-wall thickening or thinning, and ascites. Pneumatosis intestinalis disappeared on follow-up CT (not shown) without any specific treatment.

pneumatosis intestinalis with no other findings of acute mesenteric ischemia should not be regarded as acute mesenteric ischemia. One study showed that all patients with isolated pneumatosis intestinalis recovered without surgery, whereas all those with pneumatosis intestinalis accompanied by portomesenteric venous gas and other findings of mesenteric ischemia had transmural bowel infarction.[61]

Acute mesenteric venous ischemia caused by mesenteric venous thrombosis

In patients with acute mesenteric venous ischemia caused by thrombosis, contrast-enhanced CT usually identifies the mesenteric venous thrombus, which appears as a hypoattenuating tubular filling defect within the affected vein (**Figs. 12 and 13**).[43,50,62] Acute thrombus may show a high attenuation on nonenhanced CT.

CT findings of acute mesenteric venous ischemia reflect the pathophysiologic processes of acute mesenteric venous thrombosis. At an early period after mesenteric venous occlusion, arterial blood flow to the affected bowel segment may continue because of the higher arterial pressure. This blood flow causes an increase in the intravascular hydrostatic pressure of the mesentery and bowel segment. In turn, the increased hydrostatic pressure results in the extravasation of plasma and blood into the bowel wall, and serosanguineous fluid sequestration into the adjacent mesentery or peritoneal cavity.[55] With prolonged venous occlusion, arterial inflow may cease because of increased intravascular/interstitial pressure in the bowel wall and vasoconstriction, which may lead to bowel-wall hypoxia and necrosis.[50,54,55] Bacterial translocation into the bowel wall through the damaged mucosa, and mural inflammation, with neutrophil infiltration, fibropurulent exudates, and resultant peritonitis, may follow in advanced disease.[55]

Bowel-wall thickening is the most common CT finding in acute mesenteric venous ischemia. Unlike acute arterial ischemia, acute mesenteric venous ischemia typically leads to prominent (>1 cm) bowel-wall thickening.[50,63] At an earlier stage of bowel ischemia, when arterial inflow is

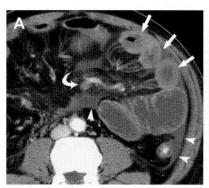
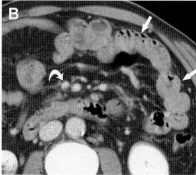

Fig. 12. Reversible acute mesenteric venous ischemia secondary to mesenteric venous thrombosis in a 50-year-old man. (*A*) Initial CT scan shows a thrombus in the SMV (*curved arrow*) and marked bowel-wall thickening of the jejunum with mural stratification (*arrows*). There is a small amount of ascites (*arrowheads*) in the paracolic gutter and small bowel mesentery. Intravenous anticoagulation was initiated immediately after the CT scan. (*B*) Follow-up CT 3 months after the initial CT scan shows a resolution of the thrombus in the SMV (*curved arrow*) and complete recovery from the ischemic changes in the jejunum (*arrows*).

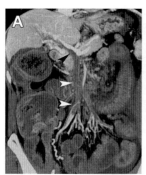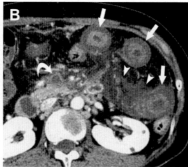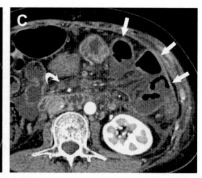

Fig. 13. Transmural infarction of the jejunum secondary to acute mesenteric venous thrombosis in a 54-year-old woman with systemic lupus erythematosus. (*A*) Coronal maximal intensity projection image of the initial CT scan shows extensive thrombosis of the portomesenteric vein and its tributaries (*arrowheads*). (*B*) Axial CT image from the initial CT scan shows thrombosis in the SMV (*curved arrow*), severe bowel-wall thickening of the jejunum with mural stratification (*arrows*), and marked mesenteric edema (*arrowheads*). Intravenous anticoagulation was performed as initial treatment. (*C*) However, a follow-up CT scan 2 weeks after the initial CT scan shows persistent thrombosis of the SMV (*curved arrow*), despite anticoagulation. The ischemic jejunum (*arrows*) has become thinner and dilated, with poor enhancement and an indistinct margin of the bowel wall. Surgical exploration performed after the second CT disclosed transmural infarction of the jejunum.

preserved and the bowel wall is still viable, the affected bowel usually shows thickening with mural stratification (ie, an enhancing inner layer, a hypoattenuating middle layer, and an enhancing outer layer; see **Figs. 12** and **13**). As ischemic injury progresses to transmural infarction, the enhancement decreases and becomes more uniform, whereas the lumen may show marked distention.[50] At a later stage, when transmural infarction has developed, the bowel wall becomes thinner (see **Fig. 13**). According to a study of patients with acute mesenteric venous thrombosis, uniformly decreased mural enhancement and a luminal diameter greater than 2 cm on CT suggests the development of transmural infarction.[50] The degree of bowel-wall thickening does not correlate well with the severity of bowel ischemia.[48,50] Unlike arterial ischemia, mesenteric haziness and ascites are present in almost all patients with acute mesenteric venous ischemia and therefore do not necessarily suggest severe disease.

NOMI

As discussed earlier, mesenteric ischemia or infarction in the presence of patent mesenteric vessels is referred to as NOMI.[39,56] SMA angiography is the method of choice in the diagnosis of this condition and provides the route for intra-arterial papaverine infusion for therapy.[64] Typical angiographic findings include narrowing and irregularities of the origins of the major branches of the SMA, spasm of the mesenteric arcades, and impaired filling of the intramural vessels.[64,65]

The CT findings in patients with NOMI are still poorly understood. Some review articles have

loosely categorized shock bowel as a subtype of NOMI[40,44,46,66] and thereby described similar CT findings, including fluid-filled dilatation, diffuse mural thickening, and intense mural enhancement of the small bowel[67,68]; however, this categorization may not be appropriate. To our knowledge, there have only been 2 published papers, with a total of 6 cases, that specifically addressed the CT findings of surgically and pathologically proven NOMI.[69,70] The reported CT findings of NOMI consisted of diffuse narrowing of the SMA, poor visualization of its secondary branches, bowel distension, a thin and poorly enhancing bowel wall, and pneumatosis intestinalis,[69,70] which are similar to the findings of acute arterio-occlusive ischemia, except for the absence of thrombus/embolus in NOMI.

SUMMARY

Recent technical advances in MDCT, including better spatial resolution, dynamic contrast enhancement, enterography techniques, and robust 3D imaging, have contributed greatly to the improved diagnostic CT evaluation of patients with GI bleeding or suspected acute mesenteric ischemia. Thus, with the state-of-the-art imaging techniques and a sound knowledge of the pathophysiology of GI bleeding and acute mesenteric ischemia, MDCT is better able to contribute to the management of these patients.

REFERENCES

1. Manning-Dimmitt LL, Dimmitt SG, Wilson GR. Diagnosis of gastrointestinal bleeding in adults. Am Fam Physician 2005;71:1339–46.

2. Peura DA, Lanza FL, Gostout CJ, et al. The American College of gastroenterology bleeding registry: preliminary findings. Am J Gastroenterol 1997;92:924–8.

3. Longstreth GF. Epidemiology and outcome of patients hospitalized with acute lower gastrointestinal hemorrhage: a population-based study. Am J Gastroenterol 1997;92:419–24.

4. Rockey DC. Gastrointestinal bleeding. In: Feldman M, Friedman LS, Brandt LJ, editors. Sleigenger and Fordtran's gastrointestinal and liver disease. 8th edition. Philadelphia: Saunders; 2006. p. 255–99.

5. Liu R, Kalva SP. Multidetector CT for GI bleeding: first-line diagnostic study? J Clin Gastroenterol 2012;46:6–7.

6. Lanas A, Garcia-Rodriguez LA, Polo-Tomas M, et al. The changing face of hospitalisation due to gastrointestinal bleeding and perforation. Aliment Pharmacol Ther 2011;33:585–91.

7. Strate LL. Lower GI bleeding: epidemiology and diagnosis. Gastroenterol Clin North Am 2005;34:643–64.

8. Zuckerman GR, Prakash C, Askin MP, et al. AGA technical review on the evaluation and management of occult and obscure gastrointestinal bleeding. Gastroenterology 2000;118:201–21.

9. Rockey DC. Gastrointestinal bleeding. Gastroenterol Clin North Am 2005;34:581–8.

10. Lin S, Rockey DC. Obscure gastrointestinal bleeding. Gastroenterol Clin North Am 2005;34:679–98.

11. Raju GS, Gerson L, Das A, et al. American Gastroenterological Association (AGA) Institute technical review on obscure gastrointestinal bleeding. Gastroenterology 2007;133:1697–717.

12. Acosta RD, Wong RK. Differential diagnosis of upper gastrointestinal bleeding proximal to the ligament of Trietz. Gastrointest Endosc Clin N Am 2011;21:555–66.

13. Copland A, Munroe CA, Friedland S, et al. Integrating urgent multidetector CT scanning in the diagnostic algorithm of active lower GI bleeding. Gastrointest Endosc 2010;72:402–5.

14. Scheffel H, Pfammatter T, Wildi S, et al. Acute gastrointestinal bleeding: detection of source and etiology with multi-detector-row CT. Eur Radiol 2006;17:1555–65.

15. Lee SS, Oh TS, Kim HJ, et al. Obscure gastrointestinal bleeding: diagnostic performance of multidetector CT enterography. Radiology 2011;259:739–48.

16. Yoon W, Jeong YY, Kim JK. Acute gastrointestinal bleeding: contrast-enhanced MDCT. Abdom Imaging 2006;31:1–8.

17. Yoon W, Jeong YY, Shin SS, et al. Acute massive gastrointestinal bleeding: detection and localization with arterial phase multi-detector row helical CT. Radiology 2006;239:160–7.

18. Marti M, Artigas JM, Garzon G, et al. Acute lower intestinal bleeding: feasibility and diagnostic performance of CT angiography. Radiology 2012;262:109–16.

19. Kuhle WG, Sheiman RG. Detection of active colonic hemorrhage with use of helical CT: findings in a swine model. Radiology 2003;228:743–52.

20. Huprich JE, Fletcher JG, Fidler JL, et al. Prospective blinded comparison of wireless capsule endoscopy and multiphase CT enterography in obscure gastrointestinal bleeding. Radiology 2011;260:744–51.

21. Hara AK, Leighton JA, Sharma VK, et al. Imaging of small bowel disease: comparison of capsule endoscopy, standard endoscopy, barium examination, and CT. Radiographics 2005;25:697–711 [discussion: 711–8].

22. Hara AK, Walker FB, Silva AC, et al. Preliminary estimate of triphasic CT enterography performance in hemodynamically stable patients with suspected gastrointestinal bleeding. Am J Roentgenol 2009;193:1252–60.

23. Huprich JE. Multi-phase CT enterography in obscure GI bleeding. Abdom Imaging 2008;34:303–9.

24. Grassi R, di Mizio R, Romano S, et al. Multiple jejunal angiodysplasia detected by enema-helical CT. Clin Imaging 2000;24:61–3.

25. Junquera F, Quiroga S, Saperas E, et al. Accuracy of helical computed tomographic angiography for the diagnosis of colonic angiodysplasia. Gastroenterology 2000;119:293–9.

26. Miller F. An initial experience: using helical CT imaging to detect obscure gastrointestinal bleeding. Clin Imaging 2004;28:245–51.

27. Huprich JE, Fletcher JG, Alexander JA, et al. Obscure gastrointestinal bleeding: evaluation with 64-section multiphase CT enterography–initial experience. Radiology 2008;246:562–71.

28. Shin JK, Cheon JH, Lim JS, et al. Long-term outcomes of obscure gastrointestinal bleeding after CT enterography: does negative CT enterography predict lower long-term rebleeding rate? J Gastroenterol Hepatol 2011;26:901–7.

29. Pasha SF, Hara AK, Leighton JA. Diagnostic evaluation and management of obscure gastrointestinal bleeding: a changing paradigm. Gastroenterol Hepatol (N Y) 2009;5:839–50.

30. Maglinte DD, Sandrasegaran K, Chiorean M, et al. Radiologic investigations complement and add diagnostic information to capsule endoscopy of small-bowel diseases. AJR Am J Roentgenol 2007;189:306–12.

31. Goldstein JL, Eisen GM, Lewis B, et al. Video capsule endoscopy to prospectively assess small bowel injury with celecoxib, naproxen plus omeprazole, and placebo. Clin Gastroenterol Hepatol 2005;3:133–41.

32. Saperas E, Dot J, Videla S, et al. Capsule endoscopy versus computed tomographic or standard

angiography for the diagnosis of obscure gastrointestinal bleeding. Am J Gastroenterol 2007;102:731–7.

33. Voderholzer WA, Ortner M, Rogalla P, et al. Diagnostic yield of wireless capsule enteroscopy in comparison with computed tomography enteroclysis. Endoscopy 2003;35:1009–14.

34. Agrawal JR, Travis AC, Mortele KJ, et al. Diagnostic yield of dual-phase CT enterography in patients with obscure gastrointestinal bleeding and a nondiagnostic capsule endoscopy. J Gastroenterol Hepatol 2012;27:751–9.

35. Heine GD, Hadithi M, Groenen MJ, et al. Double-balloon enteroscopy: indications, diagnostic yield, and complications in a series of 275 patients with suspected small-bowel disease. Endoscopy 2006;38:42–8.

36. Yamamoto H, Kita H, Sunada K, et al. Clinical outcomes of double-balloon endoscopy for the diagnosis and treatment of small-intestinal diseases. Clin Gastroenterol Hepatol 2004;2:1010–6.

37. Oldenburg WA, Lau LL, Rodenberg TJ, et al. Acute mesenteric ischemia: a clinical review. Arch Intern Med 2004;164:1054–62.

38. Yasuhara H. Acute mesenteric ischemia: the challenge of gastroenterology. Surg Today 2005;35:185–95.

39. Brandt LJ. Intestinal ischemia. In: Feldman M, Friedman LS, Brandt LJ, editors. Sleigenger and Fordtran's gastrointestinal and liver disease. 8th edition. Philadelphia: Saunders; 2006. p. 2563–85.

40. Gore RM, Yaghmai V, Thakrar KH, et al. Imaging in intestinal ischemic disorders. Radiol Clin North Am 2008;46:845–75, v.

41. Boley SJ, Feinstein FR, Sammartano R, et al. New concepts in the management of emboli of the superior mesenteric artery. Surg Gynecol Obstet 1981;153:561–9.

42. Wyers MC. Acute mesenteric ischemia: diagnostic approach and surgical treatment. Semin Vasc Surg 2010;23:9–20.

43. Kumar S, Sarr MG, Kamath PS. Mesenteric venous thrombosis. N Engl J Med 2001;345:1683–8.

44. Horton KM, Fishman EK. CT angiography of the mesenteric circulation. Radiol Clin North Am 2010;48:331–45, viii.

45. Levy AD. Mesenteric ischemia. Radiol Clin North Am 2007;45:593–9, x.

46. Furukawa A, Kanasaki S, Kono N, et al. CT diagnosis of acute mesenteric ischemia from various causes. Am J Roentgenol 2009;192:408–16.

47. Wasnik A, Kaza RK, Al-Hawary MM, et al. Multidetector CT imaging in mesenteric ischemia–pearls and pitfalls. Emerg Radiol 2011;18:145–56.

48. Wiesner W, Khurana B, Ji H, et al. CT of acute bowel ischemia. Radiology 2003;226:635–50.

49. Kirkpatrick ID, Kroeker MA, Greenberg HM. Biphasic CT with mesenteric CT angiography in the evaluation of acute mesenteric ischemia: initial experience. Radiology 2003;229:91–8.

50. Lee SS, Ha HK, Park SH, et al. Usefulness of computed tomography in differentiating transmural infarction from nontransmural ischemia of the small intestine in patients with acute mesenteric venous thrombosis. J Comput Assist Tomogr 2008;32:730–7.

51. Taourel PG, Deneuville M, Pradel JA, et al. Acute mesenteric ischemia: diagnosis with contrast-enhanced CT. Radiology 1996;199:632–6.

52. Aschoff AJ, Stuber G, Becker BW, et al. Evaluation of acute mesenteric ischemia: accuracy of biphasic mesenteric multi-detector CT angiography. Abdom Imaging 2009;34:345–57.

53. Ofer A, Abadi S, Nitecki S, et al. Multidetector CT angiography in the evaluation of acute mesenteric ischemia. Eur Radiol 2009;19:24–30.

54. Patel A, Kaleya RN, Sammartano RJ. Pathophysiology of mesenteric ischemia. Surg Clin North Am 1992;72:31–41.

55. Mitsudo S, Brandt LJ. Pathology of intestinal ischemia. Surg Clin North Am 1992;72:43–63.

56. Paterno F, Longo WE. The etiology and pathogenesis of vascular disorders of the intestine. Radiol Clin North Am 2008;46:877–85.

57. Chou CK. CT manifestations of bowel ischemia. AJR Am J Roentgenol 2002;178:87–91.

58. Grassi R. MRI of bowel ischemia on rat models [abstract SF 10 AB-04]. In: The 67th Korean Congress of Radiology and Annual Delegate Meeting of the Korean Society of Radiology. Seoul (Korea), October 29, 2011.

59. Romano S, Lassandro F, Scaglione M, et al. Ischemia and infarction of the small bowel and colon: spectrum of imaging findings. Abdom Imaging 2005;31:277–92.

60. St Peter SD, Abbas MA, Kelly KA. The spectrum of pneumatosis intestinalis. Arch Surg 2003;138:68–75.

61. Kernagis LY, Levine MS, Jacobs JE. Pneumatosis intestinalis in patients with ischemia: correlation of CT findings with viability of the bowel. AJR Am J Roentgenol 2003;180:733–6.

62. Bradbury MS, Kavanagh PV, Bechtold RE, et al. Mesenteric venous thrombosis: diagnosis and noninvasive imaging. Radiographics 2002;22:527–41.

63. Kim JY, Ha HK, Byun JY, et al. Intestinal infarction secondary to mesenteric venous thrombosis: CT-pathologic correlation. J Comput Assist Tomogr 1993;17:382–5.

64. Boley SJ, Sprayregan S, Siegelman SS, et al. Initial results from an aggressive roentgenological and surgical approach to acute mesenteric ischemia. Surgery 1977;82:848–55.

65. Siegelman SS, Sprayregen S, Boley SJ. Angiographic diagnosis of mesenteric arterial vasoconstriction. Radiology 1974;112:533–42.

66. Rha SE, Ha HK, Lee SH, et al. CT and MR imaging findings of bowel ischemia from various primary causes. Radiographics 2000;20:29–42.

67. Sivit CJ, Taylor GA, Bulas DI, et al. Posttraumatic shock in children: CT findings associated with hemodynamic instability. Radiology 1992;182:723–6.

68. Mirvis SE, Shanmuganathan K, Erb R. Diffuse small-bowel ischemia in hypotensive adults after blunt trauma (shock bowel): CT findings and clinical significance. AJR Am J Roentgenol 1994;163:1375–9.

69. Woodhams R, Nishimaki H, Fujii K, et al. Usefulness of multidetector-row CT (MDCT) for the diagnosis of non-occlusive mesenteric ischemia (NOMI): assessment of morphology and diameter of the superior mesenteric artery (SMA) on multi-planar reconstructed (MPR) images. Eur J Radiol 2010;76:96–102.

70. Kazui T, Yamasaki M, Abe K, et al. Non-obstructive mesenteric ischemia: a potentially lethal complication after cardiovascular surgery: report of two cases. Ann Thorac Cardiovasc Surg 2012;18(1):56–60.

Computed Tomography of Miscellaneous Regional and Diffuse Small Bowel Disorders

Douglas S. Katz, MD[a,b,*], Christopher D. Scheirey, MD[c,d],
Ritu Bordia, MBBS[a], John J. Hines, MD[e,f],
Bruce R. Javors, MD[a], Francis J. Scholz, MD[c]

KEYWORDS

- Small bowel • Small bowel disorders • Computed tomography • Gastrointestinal infection
- Gastrointestinal inflammation

KEY POINTS

- The differential diagnosis of regional and diffuse small bowel disorders is broad, and the computed tomography (CT) findings are often nonspecific.
- CT findings of regional and diffuse small bowel disease commonly include varying degrees of small bowel wall thickening, the halo or target sign, and ancillary findings, including ascites, peritoneal thickening, mesenteric edema, and lymphadenopathy.
- Correlation with the history, clinical, and laboratory findings in each specific case of regional or diffuse small bowel disease as identified on CT is critical for accurate diagnosis.

INTRODUCTION

This article reviews the computed tomography (CT) findings of miscellaneous regional and diffuse small bowel disorders. CT technique and potential pitfalls are briefly discussed. An overview of several categories of regional and diffuse small bowel conditions is presented, with representative CT images shown. Conditions to be discussed and shown on CT include peritonitis, chemotherapy-related and radiation therapy–related enteritis, sclerosing peritonitis (SP), a variety of infectious processes involving the small bowel, celiac disease (CD), angioedema related to angiotensin-converting enzyme (ACE) inhibitors and other causes, spontaneous intramural hematoma, lupus and other vasculitides, and amyloidosis. Some of these conditions are common, whereas others are uncommon or rare. These disorders often have nonspecific CT appearances, and correlation with the history, clinical, and laboratory findings in each specific case is critical. However, in selected conditions, the CT findings are highly specific (eg, in SP, in which calcium deposits along the peritoneum and small bowel serosa in a patient on peritoneal dialysis), and in intramural hematoma, if noncontrast CT is performed in a patient on an anticoagulant or with an underlying coagulopathy who presents with abdominal pain. Small bowel ischemia and Crohn's disease are covered elsewhere in this issue by Mahmoud and colleagues, and are not specifically discussed, nor are focal disorders such as small bowel diverticulitis, trauma, or malignancy. It is not possible to cover every previously described cause of regional or diffuse small intestinal disease which

[a] Department of Radiology, Winthrop-University Hospital, 259 First Street, Mineola, NY 11501, USA; [b] State University of New York, Stony Brook School of Medicine, Stony Brook, 101 Nicholls Road, NY 11794, USA; [c] Tufts University School of Medicine, 136 Harrison Avenue, Boston, MA 02111, USA; [d] Department of Radiology, Lahey Clinic, 41 Mall Road, Burlington, MA 01805, USA; [e] Department of Radiology, Long Island Jewish Medical Center, 270-05 7th Avenue, New Hyde Park, NY 11040, USA; [f] Department of Radiology, Hofstra University School of Medicine, 1000 Fulton Avenue, Hempstead, NY 11549, USA
* Corresponding author.
E-mail address: dkatz@winthrop.org

Radiol Clin N Am 51 (2013) 45–68
http://dx.doi.org/10.1016/j.rcl.2012.09.004
0033-8389/13/$ – see front matter © 2013 Elsevier Inc. All rights reserved.

may present either acutely or subacutely/chronically on abdominal and pelvic CT, and some of these entities are rarely encountered in clinical practice (eg, Waldenström macroglobulinemia, graft-versus-host disease). However, the imaging literature of a representative number of the common as well as some of the less common entities is reviewed, and clues to narrowing the differential diagnosis are also provided.

CT TECHNIQUE, NORMAL FINDINGS, GENERAL APPROACH, AND POTENTIAL PITFALLS AND VARIANTS
CT Technique

Because patients with regional or diffuse small bowel disease present with nonspecific acute, or subacute to chronic, abdominal and pelvic signs and symptoms, unless the clinical suspicion is particularly high for a specific disorder (eg, intramural small bowel hematoma/hemorrhage [ISBH], when noncontrast CT should be performed), or when follow-up is being performed for a known or suspected small bowel disease, such patients typically undergo the routine abdominal/acute abdominal CT protocol of an institution or practice.[1–3] At our institutions, for example, such patients typically undergo 16 to more than 64 multidetector CT during the portal venous phase of intravenous (IV) contrast (assuming IV contrast can be administered), either with or without positive oral contrast administration. Slice reconstruction is usually 3 mm in the axial plane, and coronal reformations are usually routinely performed and reviewed. Occasionally, water is given as a neutral oral contrast agent. However, CT angiography is not performed (unless mesenteric ischemia is

suspected), nor is CT enterography usually performed in such patients. To our knowledge, the usefulness of CT enterography in the disorders discussed later has not been well studied and is not known, although it may clarify and help to characterize equivocal cases of bowel wall thickening on routine CT, for example in patients with known or suspected CD. Excluding inflammatory bowel disease, there is little published in the literature to our knowledge on CT enterography of regional or diffuse small bowel disorders.

Normal CT Findings/Potential Pitfalls and Variants

The appearance of the small bowel on CT varies with the degree of luminal distention, which can make evaluation difficult. When the lumen is well distended, the normal small bowel wall should be imperceptible or thin (1–2 mm).[4] When the lumen is nondistended or underdistended, the wall may appear mildly symmetrically thickened, measuring between 2 and 3 mm, and is comparable with other similarly distended segments.[5] Enhancement after IV contrast administration normally occurs to some degree, and depends on the amount of contrast administered, the rate of contrast administration, and the timing of the acquisition. Enhancement is normally more prominent along the mucosa, and is more readily seen in loops filled with low attenuation fluid.[4,5]

A variety of pitfalls may lead the radiologist to misdiagnose small bowel disease when normal findings are present. The classic example of this misdiagnosis is the otherwise normal mildly prominent folds of the proximal and mid jejunum (Fig. 1).[5,6] Distinguishing this finding from true

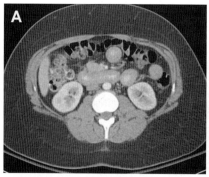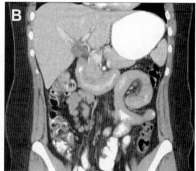

Fig. 1. Prominent but presumably normal duodenal and jejunal folds. 26-year-old woman with left lower quadrant abdominal pain, with prominent proximal small bowel folds on representative axial (A) and coronal (B) images from an abdominal and pelvic CT performed with oral and IV contrast. Prominence of the valvulae conniventes of the proximal to midjejunum to varying degrees on CT is a common, normal finding, which may be confused with disease. This particular case, although the proximal small bowel folds are prominent, was still believed to be within the range of normal, because the patient presented with acute pain related to epiploic appendagitis of the sigmoid colon on the CT (images not shown), and had no other medical history.

disease may be difficult in some cases (even for experienced radiologists), particularly when the bowel is collapsed, but a target appearance of the bowel wall, with submucosal edema, and associated inflammation of the adjacent fat, are signs of true abnormality, as opposed to just mildly prominent but otherwise normal jejunal folds. Prominent submucosal fat (the fat halo sign), which is identifiable on CT, may be a sign of true disease, such as chronic radiation enteritis or inflammatory bowel disease, but alternatively submucosal fat is a normal and common finding in many patients undergoing CT for unrelated reasons, especially in the distal small bowel (and particularly in the colon) when collapsed, and is more common in obese individuals. Submucosal fat may also be confused with a true target sign (**Fig. 2**).[5–10] Other potential pitfalls include confusing admixture of positive oral contrast and fluid/small bowel contents with wall thickening, particularly at the leading or trailing edge of the contrast column.[6,11]

General Approach to Regional and Diffuse Small Bowel Diseases on CT

The principles espoused by Balthazar in 1991[4] on the analysis of bowel disease using CT remain true. The presence of homogeneous, circumferential thickening, particularly when associated with a halo or target appearance of the small (or large) bowel, indicates submucosal edema and a nonneoplastic process, although the differential is broad and includes infection, ischemia, and a variety of immunologic and inflammatory processes. The length of involvement (ie, segmental/regional if <40 cm, and diffuse if >40 cm), the severity of wall thickening, and the location(s) of thickening should be noted by the radiologist, as well as the attenuation pattern of the bowel wall thickening, which layer(s) of the wall appear thickened (mucosal,

submucosal, or serosal), and the presence or absence of symmetric/circumferential thickening, as well as ancillary findings with respect to the adjacent fat, lymph nodes, and vasculature.[2,4,11] Then, as emphasized throughout this article, because this particular category of CT findings can be nonspecific, close correlation with a particular patient's detailed history and medications (ie, a history of radiation therapy, a known connective tissue disorder, a history of immunosuppression, or use of an ACE inhibitor), with relevant previous imaging examinations if available, and with the patient's laboratory evaluation (ie, evidence of infection, hemorrhage/anemia, or an inflammatory/immunologic process), is critical, because these CT findings cannot be interpreted in a vacuum.[2,3]

ACUTE PERITONITIS AND NONSPECIFIC PROCESSES

A variety of processes may cause acute peritonitis (eg, bowel perforation related to inflammation, trauma, a fistula, or an anastomatic leak; bacterial peritonitis related to peritoneal dialysis; other types of infection) and associated dilatation and thickening of the small bowel on CT to varying extents. On CT, in addition to the small bowel findings, there is some combination of free intraperitoneal gas or fluid, mesenteric edema, and peritoneal thickening. With focal perforation of the gastrointestinal tract (eg, related to a gastric or duodenal ulcer [**Fig. 3**]), the specific site of perforation is identifiable on CT in upwards of 85% to 90% of cases.[12,13] In addition to visualizing the site of perforation directly on CT, associated findings to look for include a concentration of extraluminal gas bubbles in the vicinity of the perforation as well as abscess formation (**Fig. 4**).[12,13] In a recent study of peritonitis related to gastrointestinal perforation, the attenuation of

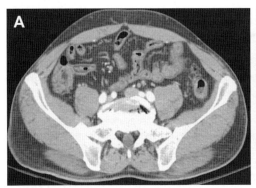
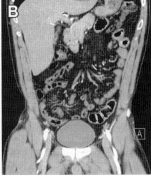

Fig. 2. Submucosal fat in otherwise normal small bowel loops. 46-year-old man with suspected aortic dissection. Axial (*A*) and coronal (*B*) images from the abdominal and pelvic portion of CT angiography through chest, abdomen, and pelvis shows diffuse submucosal fat in the walls of otherwise normal, collapsed mid to distal small bowel loops, as well as in the cecal wall.

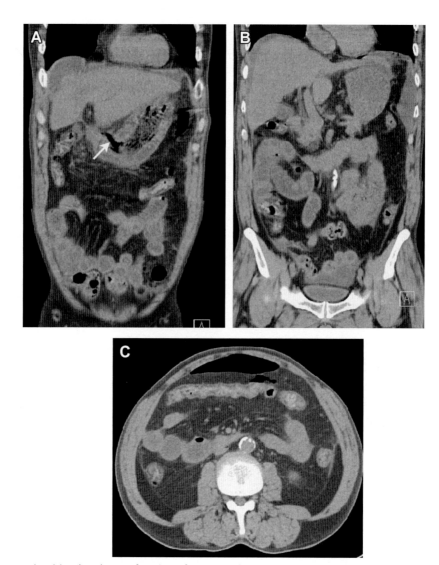

Fig. 3. Acute peritonitis related to perforation of a gastric ulcer. 53-year-old man with acute abdominal pain and free intraperitoneal air on chest radiography (not shown). (*A, B*) Coronal CT images without oral or IV contrast show a defect in the superior wall of the distal stomach (*arrow, A*), with extension of air into the adjacent soft tissues. There is ascites adjacent to the liver, and mild dilatation and thickening of the small bowel, reflecting a secondary ileus and relatively mild peritonitis related to the perforated gastric ulcer. (*C*) Axial CT image through the midabdomen also shows anterior free intraperitoneal gas, as well as the dilated small bowel.

the peritoneum on noncontrast CT was significantly lower (presumably reflecting a greater degree of edema) in patients with severe disease and a poorer outcome.[14]

In other patients, despite the best efforts of the clinicians and the radiologists, and correlation with the specific history and with appropriate laboratory or other workup, segmental or diffuse thickening of the small bowel is identified on CT for which a specific cause is never discovered. These processes may be infectious or immunologic/inflammatory. These patients should be followed clinically, as well as radiologically as needed. In

our experience, this is a frequent occurrence (**Fig. 5**). Other patients may have diffuse, mild circumferential small bowel thickening on CT related to ascites or anasarca, which is a common scenario in a variety of underlying conditions, including hypoproteinemia, heart failure, and portal hypertension (**Fig. 6**).[6,15]

CHEMOTHERAPY-RELATED AND RADIATION THERAPY–RELATED ENTERITIS

Chemotherapy-related enteritis, without a clear infectious or other cause to explain small bowel

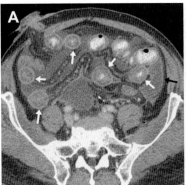
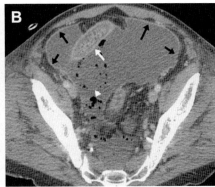

Fig. 4. Peritonitis. 66-year-old man 11 days after a low anterior resection with a colorectal anastomosis, loop ileostomy, and possible anastomotic leak on previous abdominal CT (not shown). (*A, B*) Axial images from a CT examination of the abdomen and pelvis with oral and IV contrast show marked submucosal edema with a target appearance of multiple pelvic small bowel loops (*white arrows*). Note pockets of extraluminal gas (*arrowhead, B*) secondary to anastomotic leak, and smooth thickening and enhancement of the peritoneal lining (*black arrows, A* and *B*), manifestations of the patient's peritonitis.

abnormalities on CT, is common, and has been shown on CT to be otherwise nonspecific, with regional or diffuse small bowel wall thickening causing the target sign, as well as small bowel dilatation, which may be associated with mesenteric vascular engorgement and edema (**Fig. 7**).[16] A variety of chemotherapy agents, including cytotoxic agents in long-standing use (such as 5-fluorouracil plus leucovorin), as well as epidermal growth factor-targeted therapies, have been reported to cause diarrhea commonly and to cause enteritis, which is evident on CT examinations less frequently. Additional clinical findings include abdominal pain, bloating, and diarrhea. The enteritis may be diffuse or predominantly involve the distal ileum.[16] Rarely, small bowel perforation may occur. The differential diagnosis includes a wide variety of infectious processes as well as radiation enteritis.

Radiation enteritis (acute and then chronic) can develop at radiation doses of 4500 to 5000 cGy or more. This finding has been attributed to an endarteritis obliterans, with diffuse collagen deposition and a progressive, occlusive vasculitis. In addition to the radiation dose, the amount of small bowel in the radiation field, and the fractionation of the dose, are also related to the potential development of radiation enteritis.[17] Over time, narrowing of the small intestinal lumen occurs, with dilatation of the more proximal bowel, and thickening of the small bowel wall. Symptoms are often nonspecific and include abdominal pain and vomiting.

Malabsorption, ulceration, necrosis, stricture, fistula formation, and frank small bowel perforation may further complicate radiation enteritis.[17–19] The pelvic small bowel is most often affected. Chronic radiation enteritis has been reported in up to 20% or more of patients who have received pelvic radiation. Predisposing factors include a low body mass index (calculated as weight in kilograms divided by the square of height in meters), previous abdominal surgery, concomitant chemotherapy, and a smoking history. Significant morbidity and mortality are reported in chronic

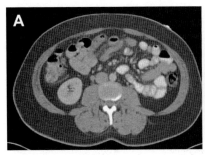
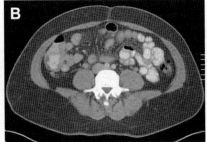
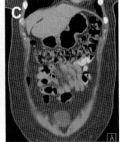

Fig. 5. Nonspecific small bowel thickening, for which no cause was identified. 42-year-old previously healthy woman with abdominal pain and vomiting. Axial (*A, B*) and coronal (*C*) CT images show mild small bowel wall thickening with mild edema of the adjacent mesentery.

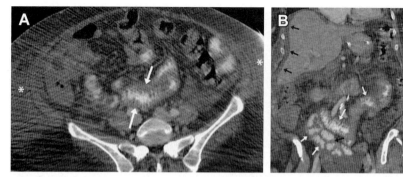

Fig. 6. Small bowel thickening because of hypoproteinemia. 57-year-old woman with autoimmune hepatitis. CT of the abdomen and pelvis with oral and IV contrast (*A*, axial image; *B*, coronal image) shows diffuse smooth fold thickening throughout the small intestine (*white arrows*). Note the anasarca (*asterisks, A*), and the ascites (*black arrows, B*).

radiation enteritis, although many patients are asymptomatic and the enteritis is discovered during routine imaging performed as surveillance for their underlying malignancy (**Fig. 8**).[13,17–20]

CT findings of radiation enteritis depend on the chronicity of the process, and include small bowel wall edema and fold thickening, submucosal fat deposition, effacement of the mucosal fold pattern, small mucosal ulcerations, stenoses, and fistulas, as well as mesenteric edema.[3,19–21] As with other regional or generalized small bowel disorders, the CT findings may be nonspecific unless the patient is known to have received radiation therapy.[3,20] In symptomatic patients, treatment is supportive and is generally ineffective.[17,18]

SP

SP, also known as encapsulating SP or sclerosing encapsulating peritonitis, is a serious complication of chronic ambulatory peritoneal dialysis (CAPD), characterized by diffuse thickening of the peritoneum and adjacent serosa, particularly of the small bowel, with deposition of fibrinous tissue and inflammatory infiltrates, and in many cases, associated calcium deposition. The involved bowel loops are adherent and may become completely encapsulated.[22–26]

The initial clinical presentation of SP may be nonspecific, findings may include decreased ultrafiltration and bloody dialysis effluent, and eventually abdominal pain and bowel motility abnormalities develop, with recurrent intestinal obstruction and associated complications. The exact cause is unknown, although it has been ascribed to chronic irritation of the peritoneum related to the CAPD. The incidence of SP is low at the start of CAPD, but increases progressively with 6 years or more of CAPD.[22,25,26]

CT findings of SP include smooth and diffuse thickening and increased enhancement of the serosa of the bowel wall and the peritoneum, often in association with curvilinear calcium deposition as well as more confluent focal areas of

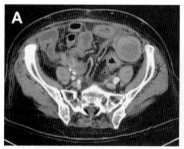
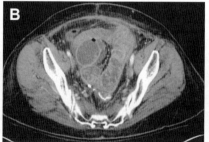
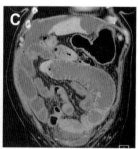

Fig. 7. Chemotherapy-related enteritis. 58-year-old woman with metastatic adenocarcinoma of the sigmoid colon, after resection, now on chemotherapy. Images from the most recent CT examination show diffuse small bowel wall thickening without a clear explanation clinically or radiographically other than chemotherapy-related enteritis. Axial (*A, B*) and coronal (*C*) images from the most recent CT examination performed with IV contrast show a long segment of significant, continuous small bowel thickening/edema, small bowel dilatation more proximally, and some ascites. There are also postsurgical changes in the posterior pelvis. The findings were similar to those on previous CT examinations performed over the course of several months (not shown).

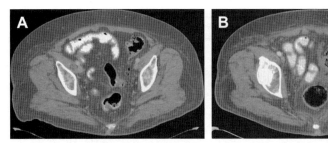

Fig. 8. Radiation therapy-related enteritis. 60-year-old woman with no abdominal symptoms underwent serial CT for routine follow-up of endometrial carcinoma. The patient had received radiation therapy to the pelvis in the past. (*A, B*) Axial CT images of the pelvis with oral and IV contrast show mild thickening of the walls and of the folds of the visualized small bowel loops.

calcification. There are usually loculated fluid collections, there is bowel dilatation, and there may be envelopment of a portion or all of the small bowel by a cocoon (**Figs. 9** and **10**).[22,23,26] Complications of SP include bowel perforation. Progression of CT findings seem to correlate worsening of clinical symptoms.[23] Although the prognosis of SP is generally poor, CT can reveal the diagnosis earlier, which traditionally was established only at surgery.[22,26]

SP may be alternatively be idiopathic, presenting with an abdominal cocoon formed by congregated loops of small bowel with a thickened membrane and thickening of the walls of these small bowel loops, as is identifiable on CT. Such patients have classically been reported in young women from tropical and subtropical zones, although cases have also been reported in temperate zones. There is also a long list of rare causes and associations of SP.[25] Treatment

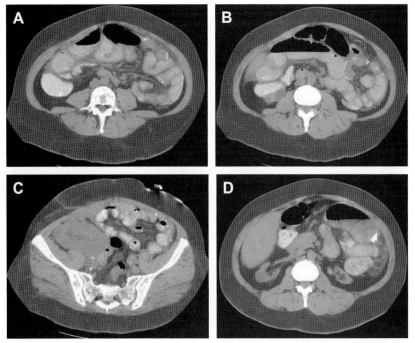

Fig. 9. SP. 41-year-old woman with a failed renal transplant, on peritoneal dialysis, with acute abdominal pain. (*A–C*) CT of the abdomen and pelvis with oral contrast only shows diffuse calcification along the serosa of the small bowel, which was not present on previous CT examinations (not shown), as well as dilatation and thickening of small bowel loops in the right abdomen. Also note the atrophic native kidneys (*D*) and the renal transplant (*C*), as well as the dense bones. Although SP is often an end-stage process with a poor prognosis, this patient was still alive 7 years later.

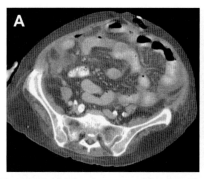
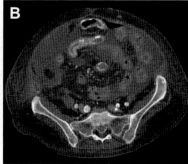
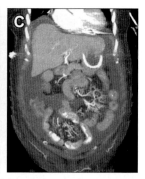

Fig. 10. Rapid development of fatal SP. 73-year-old woman on peritoneal dialysis. (*A*) Axial image from an initial CT with oral and IV contrast shows thickened small bowel, but without identifiable wall calcification. CT performed a week later with IV contrast only, for worsening abdominal pain (*B*, axial image; *C*, coronal slab image) shows the marked interval development of diffuse calcification within and along the wall of several loops of small bowel, as well as a substantial amount of ascites. The patient developed cecal perforation and died rapidly thereafter.

options are generally limited but include nutritional support, surgery, and, if the disorder is caught in time, changing to hemodialysis.[26]

SMALL BOWEL INFECTION
Clostridium difficile

Clostridium difficile is increasingly being recognized as an infection that can involve the small bowel, although colonic involvement is more common. Risk factors are similar to those for *C difficile* colitis, including recent antibiotic treatment, recent hospitalization, gastrointestinal surgery, and old age.[27] The pathogenesis is not entirely understood. Presenting symptoms are also similar to the colitic form, including fever, increased white blood cell count, and high-volume diarrhea, as well as watery ileostomy output.[28] The treatment is similar to that for colonic infection, including IV hydration and antibiotics. The CT findings of *C difficile* enteritis include ascites, mesenteric fat stranding, and fluid-filled, distended small bowel loops. Mural thickening is present in most cases, with predominant involvement of the terminal ileum (**Fig. 11**).[29] Radiologists must correlate the CT findings with the clinical presentation and make the association with previous colectomy, inflammatory bowel disease, or antibiotic therapy to establish the correct diagnosis.

Other Ileal Infectious Enteritides

Acute infectious bacterial enteritides involving the ileum, other than *C difficile* also present with diarrhea, fever, and right lower quadrant abdominal pain. The most frequently encountered organisms include *Campylobacter*, *Yersinia*, and *Salmonella* species. If initial stool cultures are not sent, the underlying cause may not be determined, but the most common infections are caused by *Campylobacter* species (**Fig. 12**). CT findings are nonspecific and include circumferential small bowel thickening, with fat stranding and adjacent adenopathy.[30] Although the diagnosis can be established by stool cultures or serologies, radiologists should recognize that the CT appearance of these infectious processes may overlap with early Crohn's disease, although marked luminal narrowing, fissures, and fistulas are usually absent in infection.[31] Alternatively, when the small bowel thickening is more proximal, in the clinical setting of suspected infection, giardiasis should be

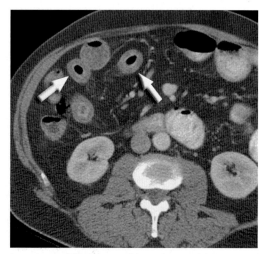

Fig. 11. *C difficile* enteritis. 58-year-old man with nausea, vomiting, and diarrhea, after a visit to a nursing home. Abdominal CT image with oral and IV contrast reveals circumferential small bowel wall thickening in the distal ileum (*arrows*), with sparing of the colon. Stool cultures were positive for *C difficile*.

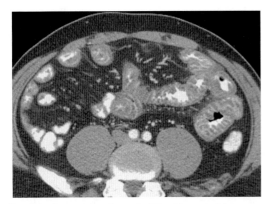

Fig. 12. *Campylobacter* enteritis. 49-year-old woman with abdominal pain and diarrhea. CT with oral and IV contrast shows extensive, diffuse small bowel fold thickening, which is most pronounced in the jejunum.

considered in the differential diagnosis (**Fig. 13**), amongst other possibilities.

Tuberculosis

The risk of reactivation of latent abdominal *Mycobacterium tuberculosis* is most often seen in patients with altered immune status. Patients typically present with abdominal pain, weight loss, anemia, and fever with night sweats. Patients may also present with obstruction, right lower quadrant pain, or a mass in the right iliac fossa.[32] The abdominal findings are often disseminated, with associated peritoneal involvement, ascites, and lymphadenopathy, as well as bowel involvement.[33] There is a predominance for involvement of the distal ileum and the cecum.[34] In early-stage disease, there is mild bowel wall thickening, with haziness of the pericecal fat and

prominent adjacent nodes.[35] There is then progressive involvement of the regional nodes, with more marked thickening of the cecum and distal ileum.[36] The lymph nodes are characteristically described as having central low density on CT, as a result of caseating necrosis.[37] Chest radiographs are normal in half or more of patients.[38] Many of the features of ileocecal tuberculosis overlap with Crohn's disease as well as with primary and metastatic tumor. Patients require definitive diagnosis, and should undergo endoscopy with deep biopsy to reach the submucosa.

Mycobacterium avium-intracellulare

Mycobacterium avium and *Mycobacterium intracellulare* are acid-fast mycobacteria which form the *Mycobacterium avium-intracellulare* complex. Patients with AIDS with low CD4 counts may develop disseminated disease after inhalation or ingestion. Typically, the organism spreads through the mucosal surfaces and infects the macrophages in the submucosa, with subsequent spread to the lymph nodes, leading to disseminated involvement, which can affect the liver, spleen, and bone marrow. Abdominal involvement typically presents with night sweats, diarrhea, abdominal pain, and weight loss.[39] On CT, there is small bowel fold thickening, which can be focal or diffuse, but which has a tendency to affect the jejunum.[40] In addition, patients frequently have mesenteric and retroperitoneal adenopathy, which is more likely to be solid than necrotic (as opposed to in *M tuberculosis* or Whipple disease). There can also be hepatomegaly and splenomegaly, with focal lesions in solid abdominal organs occurring less frequently.[39,40]

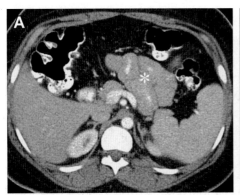
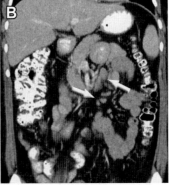

Fig. 13. Giardiasis of the jejunum. 24-year-old woman with abdominal pain. Axial (*A*) and coronal (*B*) CT images of the abdomen and pelvis show mild, nonspecific jejunal wall thickening (*asterisk*), with associated prominent mesenteric lymph nodes (*arrows*). Stool cultures were positive for *Giardia lamblia*. The patient was subsequently diagnosed with common variable immune deficiency.

Whipple Disease

Whipple disease is a rare systemic infectious process caused by the gram-positive bacillus *Tropheryma whippelli* and is generally believed to be related to an altered immune response to the micro-organism, with a propensity toward male involvement.[41,42] Affected individuals often present with nonspecific malabsorptive symptoms, including weight loss and diarrhea, but frequently also have systemic symptoms, including joint and central nervous system involvement, as well as cardiac disease. Classically Whipple disease involves the proximal small bowel, manifested by diffuse jejunal fold thickening.[43] In addition, there are usually numerous low-density mesenteric lymph nodes, as a result of obstructed lymphatics and lipid-laden macrophages within the nodes.[44] Because of its propensity to involve the small bowel and produce low-density nodes, there is overlap with the CT appearance of mycobacterial infections, as noted earlier (**Fig. 14**). The diagnosis is usually made on biopsy of the involved small bowel segments.

Cryptosporidiosis

Cryptosporidiosis is a parasitic protozoan infection that causes a self-limiting diarrheal state in immunocompetent individuals who have had exposure to the feces of infected animals, and in immunocompromised individuals, particularly patients with AIDS with a low CD4 count. *Cryptosporidium parvum* can cause an intractable diarrhea lasting for months.[45] The CT features are nonspecific, with fluid-filled, diffusely thickened small bowel loops, with a relative absence of adenopathy. The stomach and proximal small bowel tend to be involved, with relative sparing of the ileum.[46]

Cytomegalovirus

Cytomegalovirus (CMV) is a DNA virus belonging to the herpes viral group. Although more frequently identified in immunocompromised patients, diarrheal infection can be seen in immunocompetent individuals, with scattered case reports of severe infections and even fatalities related to the disease. In immunocompromised patients, disease may be related to reactivation of latent infection or to primary acute infection. Symptoms are often nonspecific, and are similar to those for other small intestinal infection, including fever and abdominal pain, as well as weight loss and diarrhea, but occasionally, there are more severe presentations, with small bowel hemorrhage and perforation. The pathophysiology in these severe cases is related to vascular endothelial injury, with resultant ischemia and ulceration.[47] CMV may affect any segment of the gastrointestinal tract, but there is a predilection for the distal small bowel and the right colon. CT shows circumferential small bowel thickening and adjacent edema, and in more severe cases, ulcerations.[48] Pseudopolyps and pseudomembranes may also occur in severe disease.[47]

Celiac Disease

The most common lifetime disorder of the small bowel is celiac disease (CD), occurring in about 1% of the adult population, with a recent increasing prevalence,[49,50] yet radiologists rarely establish or even suggest the diagnosis. Fewer than 10% of individuals with CD are currently diagnosed,[51] with a diagnostic delay of more than 10 years from onset of symptoms. CD produces significant but subtle and insidious morbidity, and has variable severity depending on multiple factors. It is now well known that CD accelerates many human disease processes, with earlier onset of heart disease, cataracts, and osteoporosis,

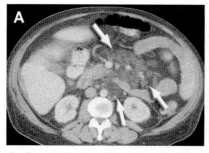
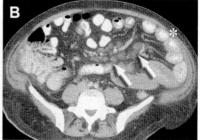

Fig. 14. Whipple disease. 42-year-old man presenting with lower extremity swelling and malabsorptive symptoms, including a 23-kg (70-pound) weight loss. (*A*) Upper abdominal CT image shows confluent low-density mesenteric and retroperitoneal adenopathy (*arrows*), characteristic of Whipple disease. (*B*) A lower CT image shows mild jejunal wall thickening (*asterisk*), in addition to mesenteric adenopathy (*arrows*). Lymph node biopsy confirmed the diagnosis of Whipple disease.

amongst other sequelae. Delayed menarche, early menopause, secondary amenorrhea, infertility, and intrauterine growth retardation are now recognized complications of untreated CD.[52]

In past decades, radiologists suggested malabsorption diseases using barium examinations.[53,54] At present, abdominal CT is often performed for unexplained abdominal pain and for other patient signs and symptoms, as well as for iron-deficiency anemia, which may be caused by underlying CD. Recognizing the individual findings of CD and the patterns that they produce on CT may prompt further evaluation and earlier correct diagnosis. An inexpensive blood test for increased antibodies to tissue transglutaminase is usually all that is required to diagnose CD.

CD is an autoimmune process that attacks the small bowel mucosal cells in genetically susceptible individuals who are exposed to dietary gluten. There is resultant progressive villus inflammation and destruction, which begins in the duodenum and progresses to the ileum.[55] Loss of cells shortens and eventually destroys the villi, and stimulates hypertrophy of the cell-generating crypts at the base of the mucosal layer. There are 5 pathologic stages of severity, from 0 to 4, with 0 being a normal appearance in treated patients with CD. Stage 4 represents advanced disease, with complete loss of crypts and total mucosal atrophy. Stages 1 to 4 can be conceptualized as 2 phases: the attack and the destroyed phases. The attack phase is an early inflammatory period, with lymphocytes flooding the duodenum and jejunum, inflaming and thickening the mucosa. The walls and mucosa appear thick and fluffy in the jejunum on CT. This phase has not been previously recognized by radiologists. In the destroyed phase, there is a thin jejunal wall with widely spaced folds and reversal of the jejunoileal fold pattern, as inflammation progresses to the ileum. The ileal folds now become prominent and fluffy. This latter stage of CD is what has most often been previously encountered on barium examinations.[56]

Small intestinal crypts secrete fluid, and their hypertrophy in CD leads to larger volumes of fluid secretion. Continuous increased fluid production and lack of fluid absorption result in large volumes of small bowel fluid, which chronically strains and stretches the musculature, resulting in dilatation and impairing peristalsis and therefore digestion and absorption of nutrients. The colon can compensate by absorbing excess fluid, and only in the most advanced cases is diarrhea a major presenting complaint. Chronic fluid overload is therefore the basis of the main small bowel imaging findings in CD. CT findings include excess fluid within the small bowel, with dilatation, oral contrast dilution, flocculation, and laminar flow.[57] Individual features of CD, such as intramural fat, increased splanchnic circulation, mesenteric adenopathy, jejunoileal fold reversal, and intussusception, have been described on CT (**Figs. 15–18**).[57–63] However, a comprehensive description of the CT patterns of undiagnosed and untreated patients has rarely been attempted.[56,64] To establish the diagnosis of CD, radiologists must seek not isolated findings but patterns of clustered findings in a disease that has a spectrum from early inflammation to end-stage advanced malabsorption. One or 2 findings alone do not constitute a pattern; many findings creating a pattern are seen in symptomatic patients, in our experience.

Additional CT findings in CD beyond those in the small bowel may be useful (see **Fig. 16**; **Fig. 19**). Mesenteric nodes are always prominent in number, and they may be moderately enlarged in untreated cases. These nodes can be best appreciated on coronal reformations. Undigested and unabsorbed food affects the appearance of the colon, producing dilatation with gas, liquid, or solid fat-density stool, wall encrustation from adherent unemulsified fatty debris, and geodes of fat-density stool, which may have calcified walls from saponification of fat. Advanced CD can present with a colon filled only with pure fluid, as the absorptive capacity of the colon becomes overwhelmed.[56] Additional clues occasionally seen to the diagnosis of CD include a small spleen, fat-density lymph nodes, fatty infiltration of the liver, prominent mesenteric vascularity, fold prominence in the distal small bowel loops, and absent body fat.[58,65,66] Other disorders producing a malabsorption pattern share clinical and imaging features seen in CD, including diseases of pancreatic, hepatic, and biliary insufficiency, diseases diminishing effective bowel length through resection, bypass, or other intrinsic small bowel disease (eg, Crohn's disease), and a variety of other conditions.[67,68]

SMALL BOWEL ANGIOEDEMA

Angioedema is a process characterized by episodes of increased vascular permeability and weeping of serum into the interstitial spaces of the skin and mucus membranes.[69] There are a variety of causes of angioedema, ranging from hereditary to acquired forms, including idiopathic and drug-induced. The pathologic basis depends on the underlying cause, and is not completely understood. Patients with hereditary angioedema have inhibition of the first component of the complement system, C1-esterase inhibitor.[70]

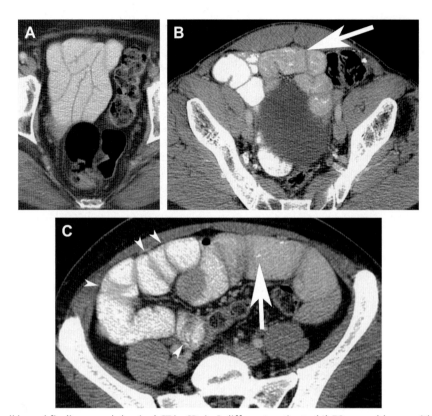

Fig. 15. Small bowel findings on abdominal CT in CD, in 3 different patients. (*A*) 56-year-old man with abdominal pain and weight loss; CD was diagnosed 2 years after initial presentation. There is conformation of flaccid pelvic loops of small bowel, with all space between them obliterated. The mucosal folds are normal, not yet visibly affected with inflammation. There is slight prominence of stool and gas in the colon. (*B*) 70-year-old man with abdominal pain. The diagnosis of CD was established based on CT at initial presentation. There is laminar flow of oral contrast and fluid (*arrow*). This finding is caused by flaccid loops with occasional peristaltic contractions pushing pooled fluid or oral contrast distally, creating longitudinal streaks of contrast and fluid. This condition can be mistaken for intussusception. After this peristaltic wave passes, the contrast settles out as flocculated barium. (*C*) 45-year-old woman with bloating and abdominal pain; further testing after CT led to the diagnosis of CD. There are flocculated dots of barium (*arrow*) in dilated small bowel loops with telescoping of folds (*arrowheads*).

There is also an acquired form, most commonly seen in association with lymphoproliferative disorders, but which can also be associated with a variety of autoimmune, neoplastic, and infectious diseases.[70] These patients have hyperactivation of the complement system.[71] Laboratory analysis, as well as personal and family history, may help distinguish amongst these forms. Drug-induced reactions, including ACE inhibitor–induced angioedema (ACE-IA), may be related to altered levels of circulating bradykinin.[72]

Regardless of the underlying cause, these patients present with recurrent bouts of angioedema, which can elude proper diagnosis.[69,73–75] In particular, patients may have episodes of intestinal angioedema, which can lead to recurrent presentations to clinicians or emergency departments. Their clinical and radiographic findings are often mistaken for other conditions, including ischemia, Crohn's disease, and vasculitis. This situation often necessitates an extensive diagnostic workup, and occasionally unnecessary surgery.

Patients with small intestinal angioedema present with abdominal pain, nausea, vomiting, and diarrhea. The pain can be severe and mimic life-threatening intestinal ischemia.[73] These patients usually have abrupt symptom onset as well as abrupt symptom cessation, in contradistinction to other conditions in the differential diagnosis. Reports of patients on ACE-IA therapy indicate that the initial episode may be seen years after initiation of therapy, and not necessarily in close temporal relationship to the start of therapy, and the episode then often resolves spontaneously while the patient remains on the medication.[73,76,77]

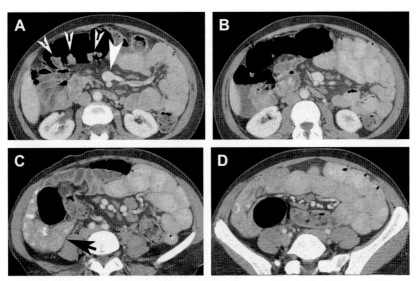

Fig. 16. 42-year-old woman with abdominal pain and diarrhea, prospectively diagnosed with CD based on CT findings. (*A–D*) The small bowel is dilated, with dilution that grays the oral contrast material. The small bowel walls conform to each other, obliterating all space between them. Distal small bowel loops are fluid-filled with flocculated oral contrast (*arrow, C*). Numerous mesenteric lymph nodes surround the proximal mesenteric vessels. The mesenteric vessels are enlarged (*arrowhead, A*), with the superior mesenteric vein larger than the aorta. A large-diameter colon has voluminous gas. The right colon is fluid-filled, and a high loop of sigmoid has discrete round geodes of stool (*notched arrowheads, A*).

Patients usually have a mild increase of the white blood cell count, but the lack of fever and the presence of severe abdominal pain are clues to the correct diagnosis.[73]

Radiographic descriptions of intestinal angioedema are similar, regardless of their underlying cause. The CT appearance is that of contiguous long-segment small bowel wall thickening, with marked submucosal edema and a target sign (**Fig. 20**).[73,78–81] Patients given positive oral contrast should have no evidence of small bowel obstruction, and often have rapid contrast transit

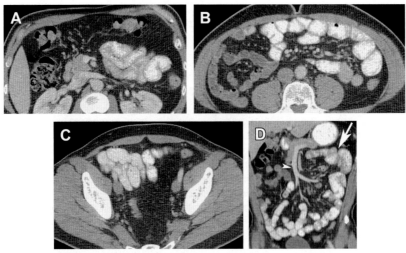

Fig. 17. Multiple features of the malabsorption pattern on abdominal CT, in a 49-year-old man with left lower quadrant pain, who was prospectively diagnosed with CD based on CT findings (*A–D*). The small bowel is dilated with fluid-filled distal loops. Proximal jejunal loops show conformation. Proximal mesenteric lymph nodes and large caliber of the superior mesenteric vessels (*arrowhead, D*) are noted. The folds in the proximal small bowel are increased (*arrow, D*), a sign that the inflammation is still ongoing in the jejunum. Sometimes individual findings may be less evident on axial views, and better summated on coronal views (*D*).

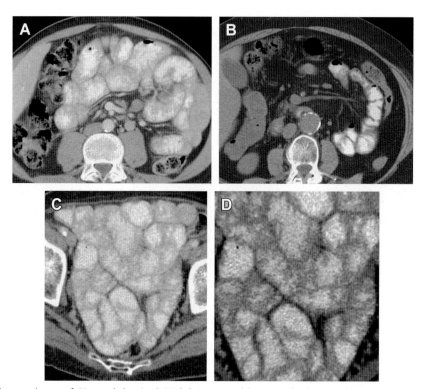

Fig. 18. Different phases of CD on abdominal CT. (*A*) 57-year-old man with abnormal liver function tests, and adenopathy on CT, which initiated a workup that led to the diagnosis of CD. There is active inflammation, likely Marsh stage 1 or 2. The early or attack phase of CT exaggerates folds in the jejunum, creating a fluffy appearance of luminal contrast. Note the prominent size and number of proximal mesenteric lymph nodes. (*B*) 70-year-old woman with known CD, recently noncompliant with a gluten-free diet. CT was performed for severe right upper quadrant pain. Late or destroyed mucosal phase, likely Marsh stage 3 or 4, associated with the reversal of fold pattern in the jejunum. Note fewer than 3 folds per inch in the jejunum, indicated complete villous atrophy. The folds may represent ring strictures from jejunal ulcerations, a well-known barium appearance in CD. (*C, D*; *D*, close-up detail) 76-year-old woman with iron-deficiency anemia, diagnosed by antibody test with CD just before CT. There are inflammatory changes that have progressed into the ileum, producing thick folds, identical to the changes that are usually noted initially in the jejunum. The reversal of the jejunal-ileal fold pattern in CD is caused by progression of the immune attack distally after the jejunum has been destroyed.

to the colon, related to the underlying diarrheal state. Our recent study of 20 patients with a diagnosis of ACE-IA also described straightening of the affected small bowel segment(s) (**Fig. 21**).[73] Virtually all descriptions of small bowel angioedema also report ascites. Because ACE-IA may be confused with small bowel ischemia, radiologists should document the patency of the mesenteric arteries and veins on CT, as well as the absence of pneumatosis and pneumoperitoneum, which should not be present in patients with ACE-IA. Should follow-up CT be deemed necessary, these patients typically have rapid resolution of the initial findings.[73]

EOSINOPHILIC ENTERITIS

Eosinophilic enteritis (or gastroenteritis) is an unusual (but likely underrecognized) disease of

unknown cause characterized by the nonneoplastic infiltration of the wall of the gastrointestinal tract by eosinophils. It is not associated with parasitic or extraintestinal diseases.[67] Some but not all patients have peripheral eosinophilia, and atopy is common.[43] This chronic relapsing disorder usually affects adults in the third decade of life, but may also occur in older patients. The stomach and proximal small bowel are most often affected, as is the esophagus. The clinical findings depend on which layer(s) of the small bowel wall are involved. As would be expected, when mucosal disease predominates, protein-losing enteropathy and malabsorption may occur. When mural involvement is the main finding, then intestinal obstruction may be identified. If the serosa is involved, then ascites may be present. Overlapping clinical manifestations may be seen because often more than 1 layer of bowel is involved.[67]

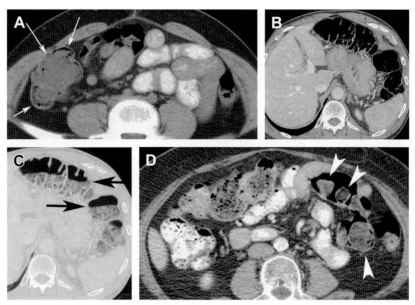

Fig. 19. The colon in CD on CT. (A) 45-year-old woman with left lower quadrant pain, who was not compliant with a gluten-free diet. Undigested carbohydrates and fat passing from the small bowel into the colon undergo rapid bacterial degradation, producing prominent gas. Fluid entering the colon is visible as a cecal fluid plume, surrounded by a thin rim of gas (arrows), rapidly produced by bacteria. (B, C) 64-year-old man with abdominal pain. The prospective diagnosis of CD was made using CT findings. A large-volume colon, which seems to be filled with gas on the abdominal window (B), is seen to have an air-fluid level with liquid fat (arrows), when using a lung window (C). Unemulsified fat is more slowly processed by bacteria than are carbohydrates. (D) 61-year-old woman with alternating constipation and diarrhea, diagnosed with CD shortly after CT was performed. A colon chronically distended by air cannot form normal stool. Liquefied fatty stool is dehydrated passing through the colon, but stool is not compacted and rather rolls, leading to geodes, or round areas of stool seen here in the left colon (arrowheads).

Patients with small bowel involvement have wall thickening on CT, ranging from 6 to 12 mm in 1 series (Fig. 22). Mucosal thickening with positive oral contrast caught between thickened folds was described in half of the affected patients, luminal narrowing was present in 75%, and the halo sign was commonly identified. One patient had enlarged mesenteric lymph nodes with peripheral rim enhancement and central necrosis.[82] Differentiation from other causes of malabsorption

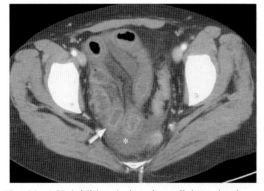

Fig. 20. ACE inhibitor-induced small bowel edema. 61-year-old woman on lisinopril therapy and acute abdominal pain. Axial CT image of the pelvis with IV contrast shows a large amount of ascites (asterisk), mild distention of the small bowel, and long-segment small bowel wall thickening with submucosal edema producing a target sign (arrow).

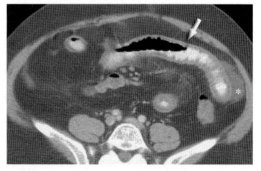

Fig. 21. ACE inhibitor-induced small bowel edema. 56-year-old woman on lisinopril therapy with acute abdominal pain. Axial CT image of the pelvis shows long-segment small bowel thickening, mild distention, and straightening of the affected segment (arrow). Ascites (asterisk) is also noted.

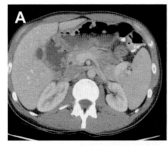
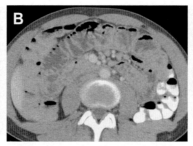
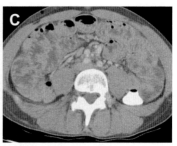

Fig. 22. Eosinophilic gastroenteritis. Young man with endoscopically proven eosinophilic gastroenteritis, and subacute abdominal pain. CT of the abdomen with oral and IV contrast shows generalized thickening of the gastric wall (*A*), and generalized mild thickening and distension of the proximal and mid small bowel (*B, C*).

and bowel wall thickening must be based on clinical presentation, abnormal laboratory values, and if necessary, bowel wall biopsy.

SPONTANEOUS ISBH

The CT appearance of spontaneous ISBH (ie, intramural bleeding without specific external trauma, and not related to a procedure such as endoscopy or to surgery) was first described in 1982 as hyperdense bowel wall with Hounsfield units ranging from +50 to +80.[83] There is usually a known underlying risk factor, particularly anticoagulation with warfarin (but not heparin), leukemia, or a bleeding disorder such as hemophilia. Patients usually present with nonspecific abdominal pain, and may have nausea and vomiting, as well as anemia. Hemorrhage into the lumen of the small bowel, which then presents clinically as gastrointestinal hemorrhage, is seen in only a few cases.[84] The diagnosis may not be specifically suspected clinically, but if there is prospective suspicion for ISBH, then CT without oral contrast,

and particularly without IV contrast, should be performed, to maximize detection of the intramural hematoma, because IV contrast may obscure the diagnosis and the findings may then simulate other types of disorders (**Fig. 23**).[84,85]

Although any portion of the small bowel may be affected, the proximal jejunum and the duodenum are most often involved. This finding has been ascribed to the high vascularity of the more proximal small bowel, as well as the relatively fixed nature of the duodenum, which seems to predispose patients with relevant risk factors, after seemingly minor events such as cough and Valsalva maneuvers, to ISBH.[84,85] Most frequently, a single contiguous segment of small bowel is affected, which in 1 series of 13 patients averaged an estimated 23 cm in length.[85]

CT findings of ISBH, in addition to hyperattenuation in the bowel wall, include circumferential wall thickening with a halo or target appearance (especially if IV contrast was administered), luminal narrowing, mesenteric edema, and obstruction proximal to the level of the hematoma, the last of

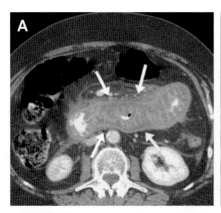
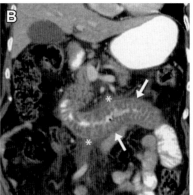

Fig. 23. Spontaneous ISBH in a patient with a supratherapeutic warfarin level. 72-year-old woman with epigastric pain. CT of the abdomen with oral and IV contrast (*A*, axial image; *B*, coronal image) shows marked mural thickening of the distal duodenum and proximal jejunum with a target sign appearance (*arrows*) caused by intramural hematoma, although the nature of the wall thickening is not so clear given the presence of the IV contrast. Note a small amount of hemorrhagic fluid surrounding the involved small bowel (*asterisks, B*).

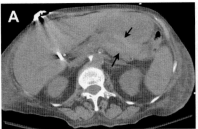
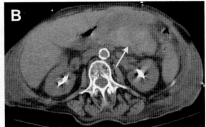

Fig. 24. Spontaneous ISBH in a patient on warfarin. 76-year-old woman with acute abdominal pain and upper gastrointestinal bleeding. (*A, B*) Axial noncontrast CT images shows proximal intramural hematoma of the jejunum. There is hyperdense thickening of the anterior and posterior jejunal wall (*arrows*), which improved on follow-up CT (not shown) after conservative management. There are bilateral ureteral stents in the kidneys.

which is common (see **Fig. 23**; **Figs. 24** and **25**). The individual small bowel folds can be substantially thickened, producing a CT appearance analogous to the classic plain film/fluoroscopic findings of the stack-of-coins or picket-fence appearance.[86,87] In a few cases, there is associated hemorrhagic peritoneal fluid, intramesenteric hemorrhage, or retroperitoneal hemorrhage.[4,84–87] Over the following 10 days to 2 weeks, the hematoma evolves and becomes less dense on repeat CT, and the associated obstruction usually resolves. Conservative management is generally indicated, including nasogastric tube placement, correction of the coagulopathy, and fluid and blood replacement as needed. The prognosis is usually good, unless a very long segment of small bowel is affected. In a few cases, there can be extension to the right colon, involvement of more than 1 contiguous segment of small bowel, or the need for surgical intervention.[84,85]

ISBH is relatively rare, although it may be underdiagnosed because of the presence of contrast material in some patients, as noted earlier. The differential diagnosis of ISBH includes secondary hemorrhage related to complicated small bowel obstruction or ischemia, as well as vasculitis. In 1 series of 19 patients with small bowel ischemia compared with 16 patients with ISBH, there was some overlap of the CT features, including of the CT target sign, although wall thickness of greater than 1 cm was more typical of ISBH, whereas ischemia usually produced less wall thickening but involved a longer segment of abnormal small bowel.[86]

LUPUS AND OTHER VASCULITIS/CONNECTIVE TISSUE DISORDERS INVOLVING THE SMALL BOWEL
Lupus

Lupus (also known as systemic lupus erythematosus [SLE]) is an autoimmune disorder of unknown cause in which tissue damage occurs because of deposition of autoantibodies and immune complexes. Most cases occur in women of childbearing age. The disease is characterized by exacerbations and remissions.[88] Abdominal pain is the most common gastrointestinal symptom, and lupus enteritis is the most common cause of acute abdominal pain in lupus, although the clinical differential diagnosis for abdominal pain in patients with known SLE is relatively long.[89] Small bowel disease can be multifactorial, but is usually related to an underlying vasculitis component, and there is often a resultant element of

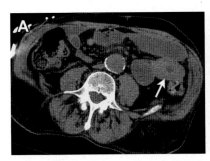
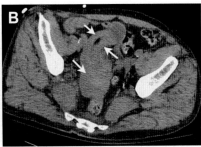

Fig. 25. Spontaneous ISBH in a patient on warfarin. 79-year-old man with hypotension, gastrointestinal bleeding, and an abdominal aortic aneurysm. Axial noncontrast CT images show intramural hematoma in both the proximal (*A*) and distal (*B*) small bowel wall (*arrows*), in association with proximal small bowel obstruction (note the dilated loops of anterior left abdominal small bowel, *A*).

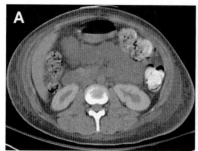
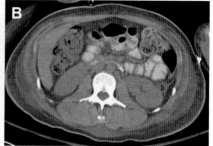

Fig. 26. Lupus enteritis. 21-year-old woman with lupus, acute abdominal pain, and renal failure, with marked jejunal edema on abdominal CT. Axial noncontrast abdominal CT image shows marked thickening of the proximal small bowel (A). There is substantial anasarca, and there is retained IV contrast in the kidneys from a CT examination performed 3 days earlier for suspected pulmonary embolism (as well as contrast in the colon, which was excreted via the biliary tract). Pleural and pericardial effusions were also present (not shown), and the patient had a recent pericardial window. Representative axial image from a CT obtained several weeks earlier with oral contrast only (B), shows just mild thickening of the proximal small bowel folds.

ischemia, although frank infarction is unusual.[90] Patients can also be affected by associated antiphospholipid antibodies, with subsequent vascular thrombosis.[89,91,92]

Typical CT findings of lupus enteritis include circumferential and symmetric bowel wall thickening, particularly of the jejunum and the ileum, with a target appearance, and variable lengths of bowel involvement, which do not necessarily correspond to a single vascular territory. Ascites is usually present, with associated mesenteric edema, and prominence of the adjacent mesenteric vessels (comb sign) (Figs. 26–28).[89,90] There may also be peritoneal enhancement, as well as involvement of the colon. Patients respond well to high-dose steroid therapy, and follow-up CT usually shows marked resolution of findings.[89,90] Unusual complications of lupus enteritis potentially identifiable on CT include intramural hemorrhage as well as bowel infarction and perforation. Associated abnormalities, including thickening of other segments of bowel, lymphadenopathy, pancreatitis, and nephritis, may also be identified.[88,91]

Henoch-Schönlein Purpura

Henoch-Schönlein purpura (HSP) is a small-vessel systemic vasculitis related to IgA (with immune complex deposition and a leukocytoclastic vasculitis). HSP is the most common systemic vasculitis in childhood. Affected individuals are typically between 3 and 10 years, but a few are adults. There are associations with infection, particularly *Streptococcus* (which may explain the reported winter predominance of the disorder) as well as associations with medications, although the cause is not well established.[93,94] The typical skin findings are a rash on the buttocks and lower extremities, which evolves into palpable purpura. There may be involvement of the joints, kidneys, and bowel. In approximately 10% to 15% of patients, the gastrointestinal and other findings may precede the onset of skin lesions, making correct diagnosis more difficult.[93,94]

Gastrointestinal bleeding in HSP is usually occult. Patients with HSP with gastrointestinal tract involvement present with abdominal pain, which is usually colicky. They also present with

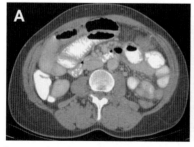
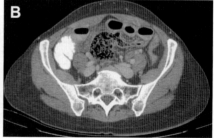

Fig. 27. Mixed connective tissue disorder with a lupus component, and enteritis related to underlying vasculitis. 67-year-old woman with severe abdominal pain and thickening of multiple loops of small bowel on CT (A, B), associated with dilatation, and mild mesenteric edema as well as mild dilatation of the mesenteric vessels. Subsequent catheter angiography (not shown) confirmed mesenteric vasculitis.

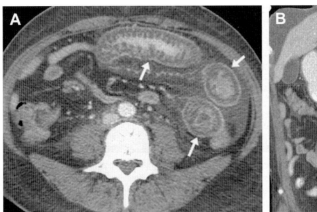
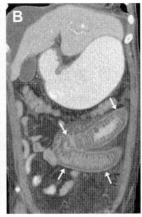

Fig. 28. Lupus enteritis. 31-year-old woman with lupus and abdominal pain. Axial (A) and coronal (B) images from a CT examination of the abdomen and pelvis with oral and IV contrast shows marked submucosal edema with a target appearance of multiple pelvic small bowel loops (arrows). There is involvement of a long segment of jejunum, with associated mesenteric edema and fluid.

vomiting, and occasionally with hematemesis or lower gastrointestinal bleeding. The duodenum, jejunum, and ileum can be involved to varying extents, and multicentric regions of small bowel thickening with skip lesions are common.[94] There are characteristic ringlike petechiae as well as diffuse hemorrhagic erosions at endoscopy. A small percentage of patients with HSP with gastrointestinal involvement have complications requiring surgery, including intussusception (which may be ileoileal or ileocolic), bowel perforation, bowel infarction, or some combination of these.[93] However, most patients respond to conservative therapy, which includes steroid administration.

There is surprisingly little in the imaging literature on the CT findings in HSP, consisting primarily of case reports and small series.[94,95] CT reveals edema/hemorrhage of the small bowel wall/folds, as well as small bowel dilatation, with hemorrhage more evident if IV and oral contrast are not administered (**Figs. 29** and **30**). There may be associated mesenteric edema, ascites, pleural effusions, mild adenopathy, and as noted earlier, complications including intussusception or perforation, as well as infarctions in the spleen and kidneys. In a series of 7 patients with HSP, the length of small bowel involvement was variable, but all patients had circumferential and symmetric thickening.[94]

Other Vasculitis and Connective Tissue Disorders

A variety of other vasculitis and connective tissue disorders can affect the small intestine. Polyarteritis nodosa, in addition to producing the characteristic multiple aneurysms of small and medium-sized vessels, can directly involve the small intestine. Similarly, Wegener granulomatosis,

microscopic polyangiitis, and Behçet syndrome can also involve the small bowel.[91] Scleroderma can cause widespread bowel motility disturbance, with resultant small bowel dilatation, proximal small bowel fold crowding, and pseudodiverticulae.[96]

SMALL INTESTINAL AMYLOIDOSIS

Amyloid may be primary, from a malignant clone (myeloma), or from a nonproliferative population of plasma cells (plasmacellular dyscrasia). It may alternatively be secondary, after or coexisting with a wide variety of chronic disorders, including tuberculosis, rheumatoid arthritis, chronic infection, and other malignancies (eg, renal cell carcinoma). The small bowel is the most frequently affected site of involvement within the abdomen.[97]

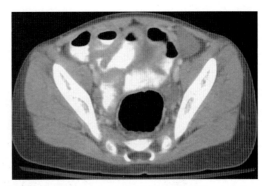

Fig. 29. HSP. 5-year-old girl with intermittent abdominal pain, bloody diarrhea, and rash. Axial CT image of the pelvis with oral and IV contrast shows ileal thickening and mild dilatation, and some ascites in the left anterior pelvis, without associated intussusception.

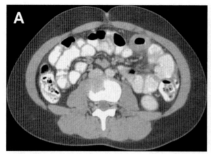

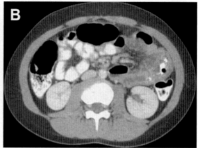

Fig. 30. HSP. 10-year-old girl with periumbilical pain and lower gastrointestinal hemorrhage. (A, B) Axial CT images with oral and IV contrast show substantial focal/regional thickening of the jejunum, without associated bowel obstruction. It is difficult to determine whether there is ISBH, given the presence of IV contrast. Free intraperitoneal fluid was also present in the pelvis (not shown).

In amyloidosis of the small bowel (as well as in other abdominal organs, when they are involved), there is deposition of abnormal fibrillar protein between connective tissue cells, in parenchymal cells, and within and around blood vessels, which compresses and replaces normal tissue, causing organ dysfunction. Resultant motor dysfunction and bowel ischemia, when it occurs, is multifactorial, but is usually caused by muscle deposition and vascular occlusion. Malabsorption, diarrhea, impaired motility, ulceration, obstruction, infarction, perforation, and hemorrhage can occur in small bowel amyloidosis.[97–99] The manifestations of amyloidosis clinically and radiologically in the abdomen are numerous and variable, which makes accurate diagnosis difficult.[98]

CT findings of small bowel involvement in amyloidosis include symmetric diffuse wall thickening. Focal masslike thickening is rare (the so-called amyloidoma). Nodular fold thickening, which can be identified on fluoroscopic examinations, is difficult to appreciate on CT (Figs. 31 and 32). There may be bowel dilatation, and delay of oral contrast transit, depending on the degree of motility disorder. Less frequently, there can be adenopathy, as well as mesenteric or omental masses, which may calcify. The CT findings with respect to the small bowel may otherwise be nonspecific, if an underlying predisposing condition is not known to be present. Other portions of bowel can be affected, and there may be varying degrees of hepatosplenomegaly.[3,97–100]

MASTOCYTOSIS

Mastocytosis is a rare disorder that results in the growth of an excessive number of mast cells within the bone marrow, skin, and other viscera. Mastocytosis is usually idiopathic, but may be associated with underlying hematologic malignancy. Subtyping of mastocytosis is based on how aggressive this proliferation is, what organs are involved, and how symptomatic the patient is. The aggressive lymphadenopathic form is the most severe form of the disorder. Because mast cells produce histamine, symptoms may include flushing, urticarial pigmentosa, abdominal pain, vomiting, and diarrhea. Episodes of histamine release vary from mild to life-threatening.[101,102] Abdominal CT may show hepatosplenomegaly and mesenteric, periportal, and retroperitoneal adenopathy. Omental thickening is also observed.[101,102] The small bowel may show mural thickening, with prominent and occasionally

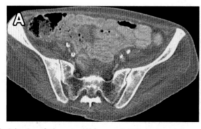

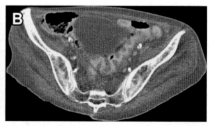

Fig. 31. Amyloidosis of the small bowel. 56-year-old woman with diarrhea related to known small bowel amyloid associated with underlying myeloma. Small bowel series 2 months earlier (not shown) revealed nodular fold thickening of the jejunum. Pelvic CT performed with oral and IV contrast shows mild generalized small bowel wall thickening (A), marked anasarca, and rectosigmoid thickening (B).

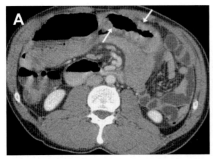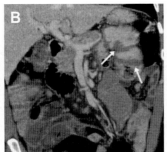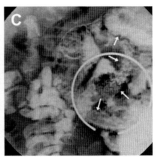

Fig. 32. Amyloidosis of the small bowel. 58-year-old man with a history of prostate cancer presented with vomiting. CT of the abdomen with oral and IV contrast (*A*, axial image; *B*, coronal image) shows mural and fold thickening of the jejunum (*arrows*). (*C*) Spot image of the left upper quadrant from a small bowel series shows diffuse nodular fold thickening of the jejunum (*arrows*).

nodular folds.[101] To our knowledge, there are few reports on the CT findings of small bowel involvement in mastocytosis.

LYMPHANGIECTASIA

Lymphangiectasia is a rare disease most often identified in children and young adults, but which can be secondary to other processes in adults. Dilation of lymphatics within the small bowel mesentery and within the small bowel itself results in lymphatic edema. Clinical findings include protein-losing enteropathy, ascites, and pleural effusions.[103,104] CT findings include dilated small bowel, with mesenteric edema, which may be prominent. Diffusely thickened bowel wall with a prominent halo sign has been reported.[103–105] Because the clinical presentation and findings differentiate lymphangiectasia from other causes of malabsorption and small bowel thickening, the major role of CT may be in excluding other underlying causes for lymphatic blockage.[103]

SUMMARY

Patients presenting with regional or diffuse acute as well as more chronic small bowel disorders other than Crohn's disease, or ischemia related to typical causes, have a wide variety of potential causes. The CT findings may be specific in selected cases, as in ISBH related to anticoagulation or an underlying coagulopathy, with high attenuation in the bowel wall, which is most evident on noncontrast CT, or in SP, in which the presence of calcification and associated findings in a patient with peritoneal dialysis are identified. Other disorders, such as radiation therapy–related enteritis or ACE-inhibitor-related small bowel angioedema, present with CT findings, which are suggestive if the patient's clinical history is known. Other disorders may be problematic and

nonspecific on CT, and close correlation with the history and appropriate laboratory evaluation are otherwise necessary. Some of these conditions are common and are well known to radiologists, whereas others, including ACE-inhibitor-related small bowel angioedema, are uncommon but only recently have begun to be recognized with greater frequency. Others, such as small bowel amyloidosis, are rare. Additional disorders, particularly celiac disease, are common, but are presently underrecognized on CT examinations. The radiologist therefore needs to be aware of this broad spectrum of regional and diffuse small bowel conditions, and to place the CT findings in the correct clinical context.

REFERENCES

1. Patak MA, Mortele KJ, Ros PR. Multidetector row CT of the small bowel. Radiol Clin North Am 2005; 43:1063–77.
2. Macari M, Megibow AJ, Balthazar EJ. A pattern approach to the abnormal small bowel: observations at MDCT and CT enterography. AJR Am J Roentgenol 2007;188:1344–55.
3. Horton KM, Corl FM, Fishman EK. CT of nonneoplastic diseases of the small bowel: spectrum of disease. J Comput Assist Tomogr 1999;23:417–28.
4. Balthazar EJ. CT of the gastrointestinal tract: principles and interpretation. AJR Am J Roentgenol 1991;156:23–32.
5. James S, Balfe DM, Lee JK, et al. Small-bowel disease: categorization by CT examination. AJR Am J Roentgenol 1987;148:863–8.
6. Anderson SW, Soto JA. Sources of error when imaging acute abdominal pain. Syllabus, categorical course, pitfalls in clinical imaging. Reston (VA): American Roentgen Ray Society; 2012. p. 209–14.
7. Muldowney SM, Balfe DM, Hammerman A, et al. "Acute" fat deposition in bowel wall submucosa: CT

appearance. J Comput Assist Tomogr 1995;19: 390–3.

8. Harisinghani MG, Wittenberg J, Lee W, et al. Bowel wall fat halo sign in patients without intestinal disease. AJR Am J Roentgenol 2003;181:781–4.

9. Jones B, Fishman EK, Hamilton SR, et al. Submucosal accumulation of fat in inflammatory bowel disease: CT/pathologic correlation. J Comput Assist Tomogr 1986;10:759–63.

10. Wittenburg J, Harisinghani MG, Jhaveri K, et al. Algorithmic approach to CT diagnosis of the abdominal bowel wall. Radiographics 2002;22: 1093–109.

11. Macari M, Balthazar EJ. CT of bowel wall thickening: significance and pitfalls of interpretation. AJR Am J Roentgenol 2001;176:1105–16.

12. Hainaux B, Agneessens E, Bertinotti R, et al. Accuracy of MDCT in predicting site of gastrointestinal tract perforation. AJR Am J Roentgenol 2006;187: 1179–83.

13. Ghekiere O, Lesnik A, Hoa D, et al. Value of computed tomography in the diagnosis of the cause of nontraumatic gastrointestinal tract perforation. J Comput Assist Tomogr 2007;31:169–76.

14. Tsujimoto H, Yaguchi Y, Hiraki S, et al. Peritoneal computed tomography attenuation values reflect the severity of peritonitis caused by gastrointestinal perforations. Am J Surg 2011;202:455–60.

15. Karahan OK, Dodd GD 3rd, Chintapalli KN, et al. Gastrointestinal wall thickening in patients with cirrhosis: frequency and patterns at contrast-enhanced CT. Radiology 2000;215:103–7.

16. Torrisi JM, Schwartz LH, Gollub MJ, et al. CT findings of chemotherapy-induced toxicity: what radiologists need to know about the clinical and radiologic manifestations of chemotherapy toxicity. Radiology 2011;258:41–56.

17. Theis VS, Sripadam R, Ramani V, et al. Chronic radiation enteritis. Clin Oncol (R Coll Radiol) 2010;22:70–83.

18. Nguyen NP, Antoine JE, Dutta S, et al. Current concepts in radiation enteritis and implications for future clinical trials. Cancer 2002;95:1151–63.

19. Mendelson RM, Nolan DJ. The radiological features of radiation enteritis. Clin Radiol 1985;36:141–8.

20. Bluemke DA, Fishman EK, Kuhlman JE, et al. Complications of radiation therapy: CT evaluation. Radiographics 1991;11:581–600.

21. Chen S, Harisinghani MG, Wittenberg J. Small bowel CT fat density target sign in chronic radiation enteritis. Australas Radiol 2003;47:450–2.

22. Krestin GP, Kaci G, Hauser M, et al. Imaging diagnosis of sclerosing peritonitis and relation of radiologic signs to the extent of the disease. Abdom Imaging 1995;20:414–20.

23. Stafford-Johnson DB, Wilson TE, Francis IR, et al. CT appearance of sclerosing peritonitis in patients on chronic ambulatory peritoneal dialysis. J Comput Assist Tomogr 1998;22:295–9.

24. Kim MY, Koo JH, Yeon JW, et al. Ileal obstruction caused by idiopathic sclerosing encapsulated peritonitis. Abdom Imaging 1999;24:82–4.

25. Tannoury JN, Abboud BN. Idiopathic sclerosing encapsulating peritonitis: abdominal cocoon. World J Gastroenterol 2012;18:1999–2004.

26. George C, Al-Zwae K, Nair S, et al. Computed tomography appearances of sclerosing encapsulating peritonitis. Clin Radiol 2007;62:732–7.

27. Freiler JF, Durning SJ, Ender PT. Clostridium difficile small bowel enteritis occurring after total colectomy. Clin Infect Dis 2001;33:1429–31.

28. Lundeen SJ, Otterson MF, Binion DG, et al. Clostridium difficile enteritis: an early postoperative complication in inflammatory bowel disease patients after colectomy. J Gastrointest Surg 2007;11:138–42.

29. Wee B, Poels JA, McCafferty IJ, et al. A description of CT features of Clostridium difficile infection of the small bowel in four patients and a review of the literature. Br J Radiol 2009;82:890–5.

30. Hoeffel C, Crema MD, Belkacem A, et al. Multi-detector row CT: spectrum of diseases involving the ileocecal area. Radiographics 2006; 26:1373–90.

31. Rubesin SE. Inflammatory disorders of the small bowel other than Crohn's. In: Gore RM, Levine MS, editors. Textbook of gastrointestinal radiology. 3rd edition. Philadelphia: Saunders; 2008. p. 807–24.

32. Kapoor VK. Abdominal tuberculosis. Postgrad Med J 1998;74:459–67.

33. Sinan T, Sheikh M, Ramadan S, et al. CT features in abdominal tuberculosis: 20 years experience. BMC Med Imaging 2002;2:3.

34. Carrera GF, Young S, Lewicki AM. Intestinal tuberculosis. Gastrointest Radiol 1976;1:147–55.

35. De Backer AI, Mortelé KJ, De Keulenaer BL, et al. CT and MR imaging of gastrointestinal tuberculosis. JBR-BTR 2006;89:190–4.

36. Balthazar EJ, Gordon R, Hulnick D. Ileocecal tuberculosis: CT and radiologic evaluation. AJR Am J Roentgenol 1990;154:499–503.

37. Epstein BM, Mann JH. CT of abdominal tuberculosis. AJR Am J Roentgenol 1982;139:861–6.

38. Marshall JB. Tuberculosis of the gastrointestinal tract and peritoneum. Am J Gastroenterol 1993; 88:989–99.

39. Nyberg DA, Federle MP, Jeffrey RB, et al. Abdominal CT findings of disseminated Mycobacterium avium-intracellulare in AIDS. AJR Am J Roentgenol 1985;145:297–9.

40. Radin DR. Intra-abdominal Mycobacterium tuberculosis vs. Mycobacterium avium-intracellulare infections in patients with AIDS: distinction based on CT findings. AJR Am J Roentgenol 1991;156:487–91.

41. Relman DA, Schmidt TM, MacDermott RP, et al. Identification of the uncultured bacillus of Whipple's disease. N Engl J Med 1992;327:293–301.

42. Durand DV, Lecomte C, Cathébras P, et al. Whipple disease. Clinical review of 52 cases. The SNFMI Research Group on Whipple Disease. Société Nationale Française de Médecine Interne. Medicine (Baltimore) 1997;76:170–84.

43. Levine MS, Rubesin SE, Laufer I. Pattern approach for diseases of mesenteric small bowel on barium studies. Radiology 2008;249:445–60.

44. Rubesin SE. Malabsorption. In: Gore RM, Levine MS, editors. Textbook of gastrointestinal radiology. 3rd edition. Philadelphia: Saunders; 2008. p. 825–44.

45. Phillips AD, Thomas AG, Walker-Smith JA. Cryptosporidium, chronic diarrhea, and the proximal small intestinal mucosa. Gut 1992;33:1057–61.

46. Berk RN, Wall SD, McArdle CB, et al. Cryptosporidiosis of the stomach and small intestine in patients with AIDS. AJR Am J Roentgenol 1984;143:549–54.

47. Goodgame RW. Gastrointestinal cytomegalovirus disease. Ann Intern Med 2003;119:924–35.

48. Balthazar EJ, Martino JM. Giant ulcers in the ileum and colon caused by cytomegalovirus in patients with AIDS. AJR Am J Roentgenol 1996;166:1275–6.

49. Rubio-Tapia A, Kyle RA, Kaplan EL, et al. Increased prevalence and mortality in undiagnosed celiac disease. Gastroenterology 2009;137:88–93.

50. Rubio-Tapia A, Murray JA. Celiac disease. Curr Opin Gastroenterol 2010;26:116–22.

51. Catassi C, Krysak D, Louis-Jacques O, et al. Detection of celiac disease in primary care: a multicenter case-finding study in North America. Am J Gastroenterol 2007;102:1454–60.

52. Soni S, Badawy SZ. Celiac disease and its effect on human reproduction: a review. J Reprod Med 2010;55:3–8.

53. Anderson CM, Astley R, French JM, et al. The small bowel pattern in celiac disease. Br J Radiol 1952; 25:526–30.

54. Herlinger H. Radiology in malabsorption. Clin Radiol 1992;45:73–8.

55. Marsh MN. Gluten, major histocompatibility complex, and the small intestine. A molecular and immunobiologic approach to the spectrum of gluten sensitivity. Gastroenterology 1992;102:330–54.

56. Scholz FJ, Afnan J, Behr S. CT findings of adult celiac disease. Radiographics 2011;31:977–92.

57. Moser PP, Smith JK. CT findings of increase splanchnic circulation in a case of celiac sprue. Abdom Imaging 2004;29:15–7.

58. Reddy D, Salomon C, Demos TC, et al. Mesenteric lymph node cavitation in celiac disease. AJR Am J Roentgenol 2002;178:247.

59. Jones B, Bayless TM, Fishman EK, et al. Lymphadenopathy in celiac disease: computed tomographic observations. AJR Am J Roentgenol 1984;142:1127–32.

60. Tomei E, Marini M, Messineo D. CT of small bowel in adult celiac disease: the jejunoileal fold pattern reversal. Eur Radiol 2000;10:119–22.

61. Scholz FJ, Behr S, Scheirey CD. Intramural fat in the duodenum and proximal small intestine in patients with celiac disease. AJR Am J Roentgenol 2007;189:786–90.

62. Strobl PW, Warshauer DM. CT diagnosis of celiac disease. J Comput Assist Tomogr 1995;19:319–20.

63. Soyer P, Boudiaf M, Dray X, et al. CT enteroclysis features of uncomplicated celiac disease: retrospective analysis of 44 patients. Radiology 2009; 253:416–24.

64. Tomei E, Diacinti D, Marini M. Abdominal CT findings may suggest coeliac disease. Dig Liver Dis 2005;37:402–6.

65. Robinson PJ, Bullen AW, Hall R, et al. Splenic size and function in adult coeliac disease. Br J Radiol 1980;53:532–7.

66. Burrell HC, Trescoli C, Chow K, et al. Mesenteric lymph node cavitation, an unusual complication of coeliac disease. Br J Radiol 1994;67:1139–40.

67. Herlinger H, Metz DS. Malabsorption states. In: Herlinger H, Maglinte DD, Birnbaum DA, editors. Clinical imaging of the small intestine. 2nd edition. New York: Springer-Verlag; 1999. p. 331–76.

68. Rubesin SE, Rubin SA, Herlinger H. Small bowel malabsorption: clinical and radiologic perspectives. Radiology 1992;184:297–305.

69. Agostoni A, Aygoren-Pursun E, Binkley KE, et al. Hereditary and acquired angioedema: problems and progress: proceedings of the third C1 esterase inhibitor deficiency workshop and beyond. J Allergy Clin Immunol 2004;114:S51–131.

70. Agostoni A, Cicardi M. Hereditary and acquired C1-inhibitor deficiency: biological and clinical characteristics in 235 patients. Medicine 1992;71: 206–15.

71. Melamed J, Alper CA, Cicardi M, et al. The metabolism of C1 inhibitor and C1q in patients with acquired C1-inhibitor deficiency. J Allergy Clin Immunol 1986;77:322–6.

72. Gainer JV, Morrow JD, Loveland A, et al. Effect of bradykinin-receptor blockade on the response to angiotensin-converting enzyme inhibitor in normotensive and hypertensive subjects. N Engl J Med 1998;339:1285–92.

73. Scheirey CD, Scholz FJ, Shortsleeve MJ, et al. Angiotensin-converting enzyme inhibitor-induced small-bowel angioedema: clinical and imaging findings in 20 patients. AJR Am J Roentgenol 2011;197:393–8.

74. Brown NJ, Snowden M, Griffin MR. Recurrent angiotensin-converting enzyme inhibitor-associated angioedema. JAMA 1997;278:232–3.

75. Pavletic A. Late angioedema caused by ACE inhibitors underestimated. Am Fam Physician 2002;66: 956–8.

76. Pavletic AJ. Angioedema after long-term use of an angiotensin-converting enzyme inhibitor. J Am Board Fam Pract 1997;10:370–3.

77. Orr KK, Myers JR. Intermittent visceral edema induced by long-term enalapril administration. Ann Pharmacother 2004;38:825–7.

78. De Backer AI, De Schepper AM, Vandevenne JE, et al. CT of angioedema of the small bowel. AJR Am J Roentgenol 2001;176:649–52.

79. Fisher AJ, Fleishman MJ, Hancock D. Angioedema of the small bowel: CT appearance. AJR Am J Roentgenol 2000;175:554.

80. Byrne TJ, Douglas DD, Landis ME, et al. Isolated visceral angioedema: an underdiagnosed complication of ACE inhibitors? Mayo Clin Proc 2000;75: 1201–4.

81. Abdelmalek MF, Douglas DD. Lisinopril-induced isolated visceral angioedema: review of ACE-inhibitor-induced small bowel angioedema. Dig Dis Sci 1997;42:847–50.

82. Zhen X, Cheng J, Pan K, et al. Eosinophilic enteritis: CT features. Abdom Imaging 2008;33:191–5.

83. Plojoux O, Hauser H, Wettstein P. Computed tomography of intramural hematoma of the small intestine. Radiology 1982;144:559–61.

84. Lane MJ, Katz DS, Mindelzun RE, et al. Spontaneous intramural small bowel haemorrhage: importance of non-contrast CT. Clin Radiol 1997;52: 378–80.

85. Abbas MA, Collins JM, Olden KW. Spontaneous intramural small-bowel hematoma: imaging findings and outcome. AJR Am J Roentgenol 2002; 179:1389–94.

86. Macari M, Chandarana H, Balthazar EJ, et al. Intestinal ischemia versus intramural hemorrhage: CT evaluation. AJR Am J Roentgenol 2003;180: 177–84.

87. Balthazar EJ, Hulnick D, Megibow AJ, et al. Computed tomography of intramural intestinal hemorrhage and bowel ischemia. J Comput Assist Tomogr 1987;11:67–72.

88. Byun JY, Ha HK, Yu SY, et al. CT features of systemic lupus erythematosus in patients with acute abdominal pain: emphasis on ischemic bowel disease. Radiology 1999;211:203–9.

89. Lee CK, Ahn MS, Lee EY, et al. Acute abdominal pain in systemic lupus erythematosus: focus on lupus enteritis (gastrointestinal vasculitis). Ann Rheum Dis 2002;61:547–50.

90. Ko SF, Lee TY, Cheng TT, et al. CT findings at lupus mesenteric vasculitis. Acta Radiol 1997;38:115–20.

91. Ha HK, Lee SH, Rha SE, et al. Radiologic features of vasculitis involving the gastrointestinal tract. Radiographics 2000;20:779–94.

92. Kim JK, Ha HK, Byun JY, et al. CT differentiation of mesenteric ischemia due to vasculitis and thromboembolic disease. J Comput Assist Tomogr 2001;25:604–11.

93. Ebert EC. Gastrointestinal manifestations of Henoch-Schonlein purpura. Dig Dis Sci 2008;53: 2011–9.

94. Jeong YK, Ha HK, Yoon CH, et al. Gastrointestinal involvement in Henoch-Schönlein syndrome: CT findings. AJR Am J Roentgenol 1997;168:965–8.

95. Demirci A, Cengiz K, Baris S, et al. CT and ultrasound of abdominal hemorrhage in Henoch-Schönlein purpura. J Comput Assist Tomogr 1991;15:143–5.

96. Weston S, Thumshirn M, Wiste J, et al. Clinical and upper gastrointestinal motility features in systemic sclerosis and related disorders. Am J Gastroenterol 1998;93:1085–9.

97. Araoz PA, Batts KP, MacCarty RL. Amyloidosis of the alimentary canal: radiologic-pathology correlation of CT findings. Abdom Imaging 2000;25: 38–44.

98. Urban BA, Fishman EK, Goldman SM, et al. CT evaluation of amyloidosis: spectrum of disease. Radiographics 1993;13:1295–308.

99. Mainenti PP, Segreto S, Mancini M, et al. Intestinal amyloidosis: two cases with different patterns of clinical and imaging presentation. World J Gastroenterol 2010;16:2566–70.

100. Kala Z, Valek V, Kysela P. Amyloidosis of the small intestine. Eur J Radiol 2007;63:105–9.

101. Nguyen BD. CT and scintigraphy of aggressive lymphadenopathic mastocytosis. AJR Am J Roentgenol 2002;178:769–70.

102. Avila NA, Ling A, Worobec AS, et al. Systemic mastocytosis: CT and US features of abdominal manifestations. Radiology 1997;202:367–72.

103. Holzknecht N, Helmberger T, Beurers U, et al. Cross-sectional imaging findings in congenital intestinal lymphangiectasia. J Comput Assist Tomogr 2002;26:526–8.

104. Mazzie JP, Maslin PI, Moy L, et al. Congenital intestinal lymphangiectasia: CT demonstration in a young child. Clin Imaging 2003;27:330–2.

105. Stevens RL, Jones B, Fishman EK. The CT halo sign: a new finding in intestinal lymphangiectasia. J Comput Assist Tomogr 1997;21:1005–7.

CT Colonography
Pitfalls in Interpretation

Perry J. Pickhardt, MD*, David H. Kim, MD

KEYWORDS

- CT colonography • Virtual colonoscopy • Pitfalls • Technique • Polyps

KEY POINTS

- A wide array of potential pitfalls exists for interpretation of CTC.
- Interpretive pitfalls at CTC can be divided in those related to technique and those related to anatomic considerations, although considerable overlap exists.
- Recognition and understanding of the major interpretive pitfalls are the most important steps in avoiding many of them.
- Robust preparation, distention, scanning, and interpretation techniques greatly minimize or avoid many pitfalls at CTC.

INTRODUCTION

CT colonography (CTC) has rapidly evolved into a highly effective minimally invasive test for detecting colorectal polyps and cancers.[1,2] With attention to detail and proper technique in terms of colonic preparation, distention, scanning, and interpretation,[3,4] excellent results can be expected. However, even when proved state-of-the-art techniques are consistently applied, there are several potential pitfalls that may be encountered at interpretation. When suboptimal techniques are applied, the number and severity of interpretive pitfalls can rapidly multiply, underscoring the need for high-quality practice standards. At first glance, the laundry list of potential pitfalls at CTC may seem daunting (**Box 1**). However, some of these pitfalls pose little challenge after they are fully appreciated. These can largely be divided into two main categories: pitfalls related to technical factors, and pitfalls related to specific anatomic features. With proper awareness, these potential pitfalls can be effectively managed so as to minimize any negative impact on diagnostic performance. Common interpretive pitfalls are reviewed, with illustrations to demonstrate the typical appearances. A more extensive review with hundreds of illustrations can be found in our dedicated referenced textbook.[5]

POTENTIAL PITFALLS RELATED TO TECHNIQUE
Retained Solid Fecal Material

Residual stool represents a fundamental diagnostic challenge for CTC interpretation, even when cathartic agents are used. Although laxatives and lavages generally remove the major bulk of fecal volume, residual adherent debris can closely mimic the appearance of soft tissue polyps, especially if not tagged by oral contrast. Unlike formed stool, which typically contains foci of near-air density, smaller particulate fecal matter can more closely approximate uniform soft tissue attenuation. This underscores the critical need for oral contrast tagging, which is highly effective for internally labeling otherwise nonspecific residual adherent stool (**Figs. 1 and 2**), thus allowing for clear distinction from true soft tissue polyps.[6,7]

We discovered early on that, although diatrizoate (Gastrograffin) is extremely valuable for its cathartic-like effect and ability to uniformly opacify luminal fluid, barium sulfate (2% wt/vol) is much more effective for internal tagging of solid residue.

Department of Radiology, University of Wisconsin School of Medicine and Public Health, E3/311 Clinical Science Center, 600 Highland Avenue, Madison, WI 53792–3252, USA
* Corresponding author.
E-mail address: ppickhardt2@uwhealth.org

Radiol Clin N Am 51 (2013) 69–88
http://dx.doi.org/10.1016/j.rcl.2012.09.005
0033-8389/13/$ – see front matter © 2013 Elsevier Inc. All rights reserved.

As such, we continue to use both of these contrast agents in their CTC bowel preparation. At primary three-dimensional evaluation, translucency rendering can rapidly demonstrate internal tagging of fecal material (see **Figs. 1** and **2**),[8] which can reduce the number of time-consuming two-dimensional correlations. Nonetheless, it is the two-dimensional display that provides the most definitive assessment for equivocal findings seen on three-dimension.

A false-positive interpretation caused by residual stool is extremely rare when using our dedicated cathartic preparation with the dual-contrast tagging regimen. Untagged stool, however, continues to be a major issue at same-day completion CTC after incomplete optical colonoscopy (OC). Although diatrizoate is typically administered in this setting, it lacks the ability of 2% barium given the evening before in terms of solid stool tagging. Incomplete tagging of solid stool also will likely be an important issue facing noncathartic approaches.[9]

Retained Luminal Fluid

Untagged residual luminal fluid can obscure even large polyps and masses when they are submerged. Early on, some advocated for the routine use of intravenous contrast to help identify submerged lesions,[10] but we have found it much simpler, safer, and probably more effective to "enhance" the surrounding fluid with oral contrast instead.[3] Iodinated contrast agents undoubtedly tag luminal fluid more effectively and homogeneously than barium preparations.[7,11] Therefore, we continue to believe that barium and iodinated contrasts agents are extremely useful in tandem for adequate tagging of solid and liquid residuals, respectively.[3] In cases where a relevant colorectal lesion is submerged under opacified fluid, soft tissue windowing may completely obscure the finding, necessitating the wider "polyp window" (W: 2000 HU, L: 0 HU) for detection (**Fig. 3**).

Although we initially performed electronic cleansing on the tagged fluid before interpretation very early on in our CTC experience, we discontinued this practice in 2003 because of the

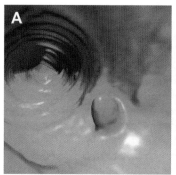
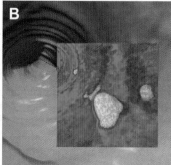
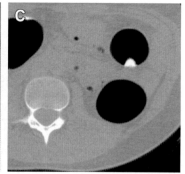

Fig. 1. Tagged adherent stool simulating a sessile polyp on three-dimensional imaging. (*A*) Three-dimensional endoluminal CTC image shows a polypoid lesion and smaller adjacent diminutive foci. Three-dimensional translucency rendering (*B*) and two-dimensional correlation (*C*) show dense internal contrast tagging, easily excluding a polyp. Note that the adherent stool is nondependent on this prone two-dimensional view, which could simulate a true lesion if untagged. (*From* Pickhardt PJ, Kim DH. Potential pitfalls at CTC Interpretation. In: Pickhardt PJ, Kim DH, editors. CT colonography: principles and practice of virtual colonoscopy. Philadelphia: Saunders; 2010; with permission.)

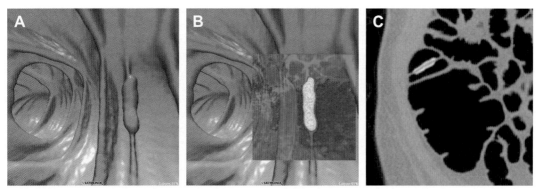

Fig. 2. Tagged stool mimicking a flat polyp on three-dimensional imaging. (*A*) Three-dimensional endoluminal CTC image shows an elongated flat lesion on a colonic fold. However, three-dimensional with translucency rendering (*B*) and coronal two-dimensional correlation (*C*) show dense internal contrast tagging, excluding a flat polyp. Care must be taken in such cases to ensure a true flat soft tissue polyp does not lie deep to the contrast.

troublesome artifacts that were introduced (discussed later).[7] Instead, we prefer to concentrate on the submerged regions on the two-dimensional evaluation. Because of the complementary shifting of luminal fluid between supine and prone positions, it is extremely rare to have a significant polyp completely submerged on both views with our standard CTC preparation.[12] The most common scenario where we may still encounter larger volumes of residual luminal fluid is in the setting of

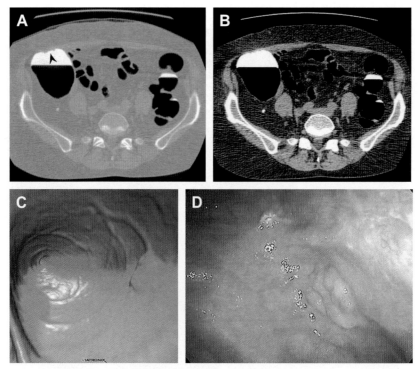

Fig. 3. Flat lesion obscured by densely opacified fluid on soft tissue windows. (*A*) Prone transverse two-dimensional CTC image with polyp windowing shows a flat cecal polyp (*arrowhead*), which is submerged under opacified fluid but is nonetheless detectable. (*B*) On the soft tissue window setting, however, the lesion is obscured by the dense surrounding fluid. This windowing phenomenon is also the reason why two-dimensional lesion measurement must take place on the wider polyp window setting. (*C*) Three-dimensional endoluminal CTC image in the supine position shows the flat lesion outlined by air. (*D*) The lesion was confirmed at subsequent OC and proved to be a tubulovillous adenoma.

same-day tagging after failed OC. In this setting, we administer 30 mL of diatrizoate after the patient has adequately recovered from sedation, and wait up to 2 to 3 hours before scanning. In the future, a better approach might be to give diatrizoate as part of the original OC preparation, which would allow for a reduction in the amount of cathartic needed and also provide fluid tagging for CTC in the event of an incomplete OC examination.[13]

Inadequate Luminal Distention

Inadequate luminal distention impacts both two- and three-dimensional evaluation at CTC. The minimum requirement for a diagnostic CTC evaluation is to have all segments at least partially distended on at least one view. Because of the complementary nature of supine and prone positioning in terms of preventing luminal collapse, nondiagnostic examinations are fortunately uncommon (<1% of cases in the authors' experience). Cases with focal or segmental partial but incomplete collapse may be suboptimal but are often diagnostic. Compared with excellent luminal distention, such cases generally require more scrutiny, because the luminal narrowing is compounded by

dynamic thickening of the colonic folds, which makes interpretation more challenging. However, because relevant colorectal lesions require detection on just one view, confirmation on the lesser quality view is generally achievable even in cases of inadequate distention (**Fig. 4**).

For cases in which complete focal collapse persists at the same point on supine and prone displays, a decubitus view usually allows for diagnostic assessment.[14] The region of nondiagnostic evaluation from focal collapse typically accounts for just a tiny fraction of the total colonic length. Because the sigmoid and descending colon account for most such cases, typically related to underlying diverticular disease (discussed later), a right lateral decubitus view is typically performed (**Fig. 5**). Online assessment of the two-dimensional images for adequate left-sided distention during CTC examination should be made by the technologist at the CT console because the scout view alone can be unreliable or misleading.[15] Depending on the specific patient population, a decubitus rate of approximately 10% can be expected, although the frequency generally is increased in the setting of an incomplete OC, among other factors.[14]

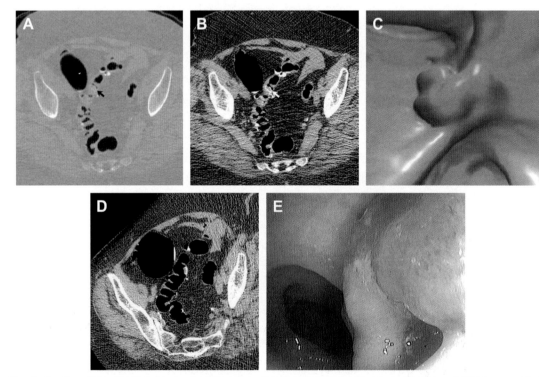

Fig. 4. Confirmation of polyp on poorly distended colonic segment. Supine two-dimensional CTC images (*A, B*) show long-segment collapse of the sigmoid colon, largely obscuring a 15-mm polyp (*arrows*), which is easily identified on the alternate position (*C, D*). This proved to be a tubular adenoma after resection at OC (*E*). (*From* Pickhardt PJ, Kim DH. Potential pitfalls at CTC Interpretation. In: Pickhardt PJ, Kim DH, editors. CT colonography: principles and practice of virtual colonoscopy. Philadelphia: Saunders; 2010; with permission.)

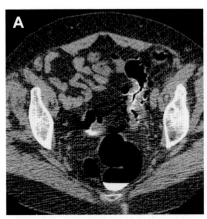 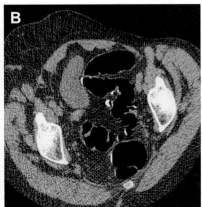

Fig. 5. Right lateral decubitus position for salvaging adequate luminal distention. (*A*) Supine two-dimensional CTC image shows long-segment collapse of the sigmoid colon, related to diverticular disease. The prone view had a similar appearance (not shown). (*B*) Luminal distention on the decubitus view, however, was excellent and allowed for a diagnostic examination.

We have not found spasmolytics to be necessary in our CTC practice, because less than 1% of cases have a persistent area of luminal collapse. Additional reasons include that glucagon is generally not effective, Buscopan is not available in the United States, and several of these difficult cases actually represent fixed pathologic strictures. For cases of truly nondiagnostic evaluation in the sigmoid or descending colon, unsedated same-day flexible sigmoidoscopy may be performed to complete the screening evaluation.

Automated low-pressure CO_2 delivery provides for adequate distention on a more consistent basis than manual room air insufflation, and should be considered the standard of care.[16] However, the lower pressures and increased resorption with CO_2 can also result in partial collapse, particularly in the transverse colon in the prone position and rectosigmoid junction in the supine position. This issue is exacerbated in morbidly obese patients, where the low-pressure CO_2 cannot overcome extracolonic pressures. In such cases, decubitus positioning or even conversion to manual room air may be necessary (**Fig. 6**).

Imaging Artifacts and Distortion

There are many potential artifacts related to CT scanning, image reconstruction, and postprocessing that can result in interpretive challenges. Most radiologists with ample experience in body CT interpretation, including advanced visualization techniques, are adept at handling these imaging artifacts. The larger concern stems from potential interpretation by nonradiologists with minimal CTC training and little or no familiarity with either general CT interpretation or the basic physics of medical imaging. Although computer-aided detection (CAD) has been advanced as a way to compensate for inadequate training, this notion ignores the fact that poor specificity would lead to an unacceptable false-positive rate.

Artifacts related to respiratory and other patient motion are much less common with multidetector CT scanners having 16 or more channels, because of shorter acquisition times. However, we have noticed a common artifact at CTC relating to the active intrascan flow of opacified luminal fluid, which we refer to as the "dense waterfall" sign.[17] This artifact is characterized by alternating bright and dark curvilinear bands, which can cause substantial distortion on two- and three-dimensional images (**Fig. 7**). Dynamic spilling of the opacified fluid between differential air-fluid levels is almost always apparent. Beam-hardening artifacts related to metallic objects, such as spinal hardware or hip prostheses, are accentuated by the low-dose CTC technique (**Fig. 8**). Polyp windowing reduces the impact of the beam-hardening artifact, and may allow for lesion detection. Novel reconstruction algorithms should reduce the effect of beam hardening in the near future.

Several important artifacts result from postprocessing of the multidetector CT source data. Chief among these are the geometric distortions that are introduced in creating nonstandard three-dimensional displays, such as the 360-degree virtual dissection view.[18] The primary motivation for developing these alternate views is to reduce the time needed to visualize the entire luminal surface. However, geometric distortion is the unavoidable trade-off, which can greatly compromise polyp recognition. Polyp size is also difficult to judge on the 360-degree virtual dissection

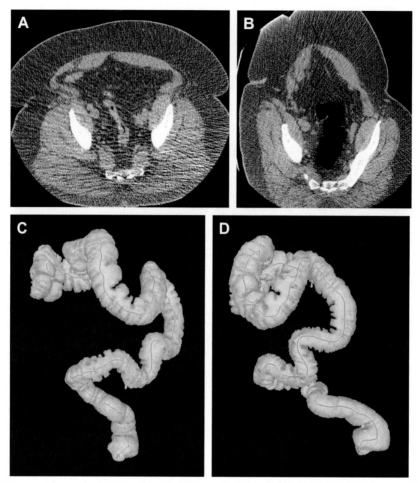

Fig. 6. Decubitus position in morbidly obese individual. Supine two-dimensional CTC image (A) in a 350-lb patient shows complete collapse of the sigmoid colon. An equilibrium pressure of 20 mm Hg was used for the automated CO_2. Decubitus positioning (B) and increase to 25 mm Hg resulted in good luminal distention of this segment, as shown by frontal (C) and lateral (D) three-dimensional colon maps.

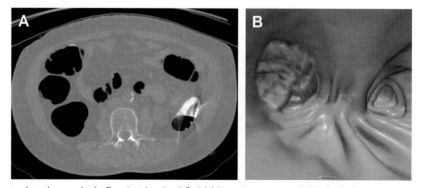

Fig. 7. Artifact related to actively flowing luminal fluid (the "dense waterfall" sign). (A) Prone two-dimensional CTC image shows multiple arciform streaks off the air-fluid level in the descending colon, which is caused by the intrascan flow of fluid. Note the lack of motion or artifacts elsewhere on the image. (B) The artifacts are also evident on the three-dimensional endoluminal view.

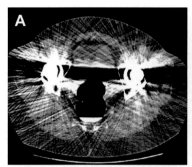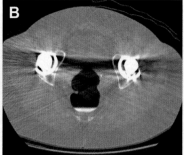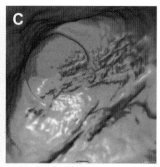

Fig. 8. Beam-hardening artifact from bilateral total hip arthroplasties. (*A, B*) Two-dimensional CTC images through the pelvis show marked beam-hardening artifact, which appears more severe on the soft tissue windows. (*C*) Streak artifact across the rectum is also apparent on the three-dimensional endoluminal view.

view, because areas are either stretched or compressed to fit a standard width. We prefer a milder form of distortion that simply consists of widening the field-of-view angle to 120 degrees on the more stable three-dimensional endoluminal view. By decreasing the number of fly-throughs from four down to two on well-distended cases, one can decrease interpretation time without introducing troublesome spatial distortion.[19,20]

Another important potential source of postprocessing artifacts come from digital fluid subtraction or "electronic cleansing" of tagged luminal fluid.[7] Because of volume averaging effects at the interfaces between luminal gas, tagged fluid, and the colonic wall, pseudopolyps are a common result of the digital subtraction process. Submerged semisolid stool that approaches soft tissue density can appear polypoid. Interrogating these pseudopolyps not only increases interpretation time, it also has the potential to decrease specificity if such lesions are mistaken for true pathology. With our current bowel preparation, the fluid level almost never overlaps between supine and prone positioning.[12] Therefore, primary three-dimensional evaluation without digital fluid extraction generally covers the entire luminal surface, and navigation is much faster without the troublesome artifacts. Furthermore, true lesions are detectable on two-dimensional imaging within tagged fluid pools without subtraction. As digital fluid subtraction techniques continue to improve, the various artifacts will perhaps be minimized or eliminated.

Low-Dose CT Technique

Concerns regarding potential harms from radiation dose exposure related to CT have increased recently in the United States. Although any health risks related to CT-level doses in adults are too small to measure,[21] it nonetheless behooves

radiology as a specialty to minimize dose to the lowest levels possibly that maintain diagnostic accuracy. Fortunately for CTC, there are several factors that further reduce the concern for radiation. The study is generally performed on older adults and excludes most of the chest. Furthermore, the inherent characteristics of the colon wall-air interface allow for substantial dose reduction at CTC compared with standard abdominal CT imaging. However, at extremely low dose levels, image noise can become an issue even for CTC, especially with the use of traditional filtered back projection for image reconstruction. Noise is especially problematic when reading thin images in obese patients, particularly when viewing soft tissue windows. It is critical not to mistake the image noise within a true lesion on two-dimensional soft tissue windowing (or three-dimensional translucency rendering) as low-attenuation heterogeneity from stool or fat. Image noise is much better tolerated on the wider two-dimensional polyp windows. On the three-dimensional endoluminal view, image noise from low-dose technique manifests as surface mottling when mild to luminal streaks when severe (**Fig. 9**).

With a fixed milliampere low-dose technique, image noise can be accentuated inferiorly because of the bony pelvis but may be unnecessarily low for the upper abdomen. Tube current modulation can avoid this discordance by boosting the milliampere only as needed to maintain a static noise level. Some CTC protocols target more aggressive dose reduction on the prone view because much of the information is redundant to the supine view. Perhaps the most significant dose reduction will come from the implementation of the newer iterative reconstructions techniques, some of which allow for routine submillisievert scanning for CTC (see **Fig. 9**).[22,23] Some of these newer techniques need to be validated before widespread clinical implementation.

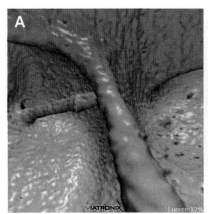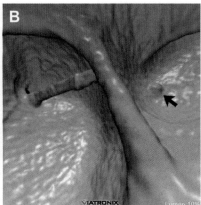

Fig. 9. Ultra-low-dose CTC using newer iterative reconstruction algorithms. (*A*) Three-dimensional endoluminal CTC image from ultra-low-dose scan (0.3 mSv) reconstructed with traditional filtered back projection technique shows significant image noise. The rectal catheter is visible but the rectal polyp is largely obscured. (*B*) When the same CT image data are reconstructed with a newer iterative reconstruction algorithm, the polyp (*arrow*) becomes much more conspicuous.

Contrast Coating of Polyps

One potential pitfall that has actually become a useful interpretive asset is the tendency for true soft tissue polyps, particularly flat and villous lesions, to demonstrate a thin surface coating of adherent positive oral contrast (**Fig. 10**).[24] This contrast etching is generally not seen with the surrounding normal colonic mucosa or adherent stool. On two-dimensional imaging, contrast coating of polyps is easy to distinguish from internal tagging of stool, which is a critical distinction. In effect, this thin surface coating of contrast serves as a beacon for polyp detection. One notable pitfall is that small coated polyps may mimic tagged stool on the three-dimensional translucency view, because the underlying soft tissue signature may be obscured by the overlying shell of contrast.

Two-Dimensional–only Polyp Detection

Early CTC studies relied on polyp detection by using only two-dimensional images, with three-dimensional endoluminal imaging reserved for "problem solving,"[25–27] which may largely explain the often disappointing performance. The search pattern for detecting polyps on two-dimensional imaging, especially small 6- to 9-mm lesions, is simply too onerous to maintain acceptable performance. In contrast, lesion conspicuity at three-dimensional imaging is greatly enhanced but requires adequate CTC software for execution. Subsequent CTC trials adding primary three-dimensional detection alongside two-dimensional review showed markedly improved sensitivity for polyps.[1,28] In fact, when a large subset of cases from the Department of Defense CTC trial were retrospectively interpreted using only two-dimensional review for initial detection (and three-dimensional for problem solving) by radiologists with more CTC experience and training than those involved in the original trial, there was a significant drop-off in sensitivity that paralleled the earlier two-dimensional trials.[29] In practice, the ease of polyp detection at three-dimensional compared with two-dimensional imaging is obvious to anyone who has interpreted more than a few CTC examinations.

Polyp Measurement

Although CTC is the most accurate method available for polyp measurement,[30] inaccurate size assessment remains an important potential pitfall because it could lead to inappropriate patient management. In our experience, a CTC measurement that combines two- and three-dimensional assessment can closely match a very careful OC measurement.[31] Two-dimensional measurement of polyps should be carried out on the wider "polyp" window setting (W: 2000 HU, L: 0 HU), because the lesion is undersized on the soft tissue window setting (**Fig. 11**). Two-dimensional polyp size is also artifactually decreased for lesions submerged under densely opacified fluid (see **Fig. 11**). It is important to recognize that two-dimensional polyp measurement on the standard orthogonal views (ie, transverse, coronal, and sagittal) undersizes lesions whenever the long axis of the polyp does not align perfectly with an orthogonal plane (**Fig. 12**).[32] This is a more relevant issue for lesions with an irregular or elongated morphology. Polyp measurement on the three-dimensional endoluminal view can also be problematic if care is not taken

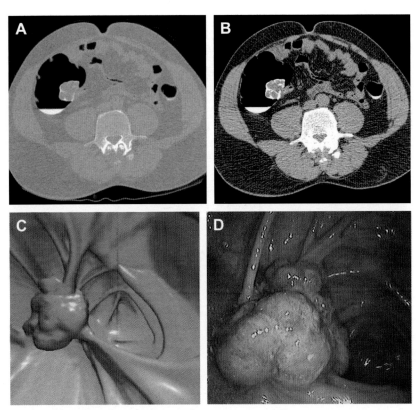

Fig. 10. Large contrast-coated tubulovillous adenoma involving the ileocecal valve. Transverse two-dimensional CTC images with polyp (*A*) and soft tissue (*B*) window settings show a multilobulated mass occupying the expected location of the ileocecal valve. Note the distinct contrast etching that outlines the surfaces of the lesion. Three-dimensional endoluminal (*C*) and OC (*D*) images show the mass, which involved the ileocecal valve. (*From* Pickhardt PJ, Kim DH. Potential pitfalls at CTC Interpretation. In: Pickhardt PJ, Kim DH, editors. CT colonography: principles and practice of virtual colonoscopy. Philadelphia: Saunders; 2010; with permission.)

to optimize the vantage point. Incorrect caliper placement, partially submerged polyps, and thick contrast coating of polyps can also lead to erroneous three-dimensional measurement. Oversizing diminutive lesions on three-dimensional imaging is a common pitfall that can lead to overaggressive management if not carefully correlated with the two-dimensional polyp size. Over time, one can generally learn to appreciate lesions that are clearly diminutive in size without the need to formally measure each one.

For suspected polyps approaching 5 to 6 mm or greater detected at CTC, we recommend performing a careful combined two- and three-dimensional size assessment. For most polyps, the two- and three-dimensional measurements are within 1 mm of each other. Unless the lesion is at or near a critical size threshold (ie, 6 and 10 mm), the final reported size is not a major issue. However, if the lesion is bordering one of these two important thresholds, or there is a large discrepancy between the two- and three-dimensional assessments, then a judgment call is necessary to determine the most

appropriate size to report. Polyp size need only be reported to the nearest millimeter. Beyond CTC, OC with use of a calibrated probe is probably the next best method, whereas visual estimation at OC is less accurate, and pathologic ex vivo measurement is least accurate of all.[30,31,33] Given its ability to better assess interval change in polyp size, volume assessment will likely play an increasingly important role in the future.[34–36]

POTENTIAL PITFALLS RELATED TO ANATOMY
Thickened Colonic Folds

Fold thickening at CTC is largely caused by inadequate luminal distention, underlying diverticular disease, or a combination of the two. At two-dimensional evaluation, it can be challenging to distinguish an unimportant thickened fold from relevant pathology. However, as long as the lumen is at least partially distended, primary three-dimensional evaluation can generally make this distinction, because the smooth, uniform, and often circumferential nature of incidental fold thickening is readily

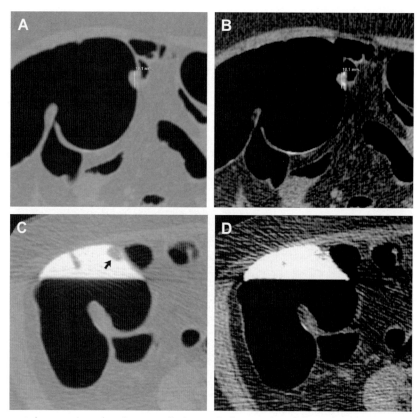

Fig. 11. Apparent decrease in polyp size on soft tissue window setting. (*A*) Supine transverse two-dimensional CTC image with polyp window setting (2000/0) shows a 10-mm sessile polyp in the cecum (*calipers*). (*B*) On a soft tissue window setting (350/40), the polyp appears to decrease in size to less than 10-mm. Polyp measurement on soft tissue windows could lead to inappropriate management. (*C, D*) On the prone two-dimensional CTC images, the polyp (*arrow*) is submerged under densely opacified fluid, which further decreases the apparent polyp size. (*D*) Note how the lesion is barely perceptible on the soft tissue window setting. (*From* Pickhardt PJ, Kim DH. Potential pitfalls at CTC Interpretation. In: Pickhardt PJ, Kim DH, editors. CT colonography: principles and practice of virtual colonoscopy. Philadelphia: Saunders; 2010; with permission.)

apparent (**Fig. 13**). Atypical thickened folds occasionally need confirmation at OC; biopsy is sometimes necessary, but often yields only normal mucosa. Without the associated features of contrast coating or a lobulated contour, the diagnostic yield of sending isolated "thick folds" to OC is too low to justify. Other causes of apparent focal soft tissue thickening at two-dimensional CTC include complex or convergent folds, redundant colonic segments with subclinical twisting, and dynamic spasm or collapse, all of which are best appreciated on the three-dimensional endoluminal view. These pitfalls must be distinguished from true flat lesions, which are discussed later.

Diverticular Disease

The prevalence of diverticular disease exceeds 50% in most adult populations, heavily favoring the sigmoid colon, followed by the descending colon.[37]

The pathologic features are characterized by myochosis with elastin deposition, thickening of the circular smooth muscle, shortening of the tenia, decreased compliance, and luminal narrowing. From these pathologic features, and combined with its high prevalence, diverticular disease not surprisingly represents the leading cause of nondiagnostic segmental evaluation at CTC. At two-dimensional evaluation, evaluating segments with advanced diverticular disease can be a daunting task (**Fig. 14**), because diffuse fold thickening combines with luminal narrowing. However, as long as luminal narrowing does not impede three-dimensional endoluminal evaluation (**Fig. 15**), diagnostic performance may not be adversely affected.[37] For cases with persistent complete or near-complete luminal collapse on all views, a pathologic diverticular stricture must be considered (**Fig. 16**).

Unlike barium enema examination, the diverticula themselves cause little problem at CTC

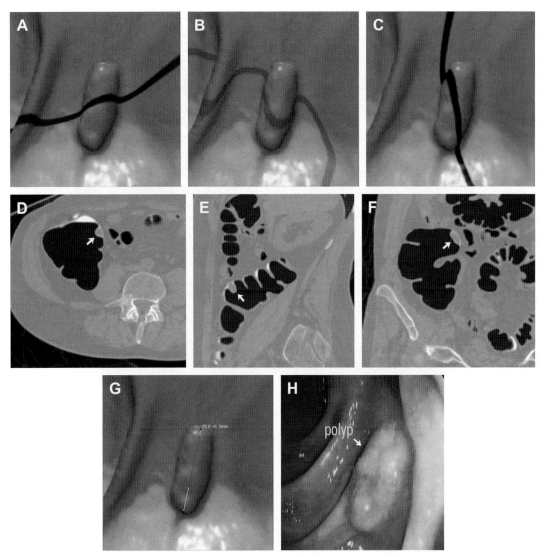

Fig. 12. Two-dimensional versus three-dimensional CTC measurement of an elongated polyp. Three-dimensional endoluminal CTC images show an elongated polyp with the transverse (*A*), sagittal (*B*), and coronal (*C*) two-dimensional planes as colored lines through the polyp, corresponding to the two-dimensional transverse (*D*), sagittal (*E*), and coronal (*F*) images (*arrows*). Even with the "optimized" coronal two-dimensional measurement (*C, F*), the polyp is significantly undersized, whereas the three-dimensional measurement (*G*) corresponds to the actual long axis of the polyp, and correlated best with OC (*H*). (*From* Pickhardt PJ, Kim DH. Potential pitfalls at CTC Interpretation. In: Pickhardt PJ, Kim DH, editors. CT colonography: principles and practice of virtual colonoscopy. Philadelphia: Saunders; 2010; with permission.)

interpretation. However, there are additional pitfalls related to diverticular disease beyond fold thickening and inadequate luminal distention. Stool-filled or "impacted" diverticula, which contain inspissated debris, often bulge or prolapse slightly into the colonic lumen, creating a polypoid appearance on the three-dimensional endoluminal view. Exclusion of a true polyp on the two-dimensional display (or three-dimensional translucency rendering) is straightforward, rendering such "lesions" more of a nuisance than a diagnostic dilemma. Frankly inverted diverticula are rare but represent a related pitfall. Prolapsing mucosal polyps represent redundant colonic mucosa in the setting of sigmoid diverticular disease. These nonneoplastic lesions can be difficult to differentiate from neoplastic disease.[38]

Flat Lesions

Flat lesions represent a subset of sessile polyps that, as the name implies, have a "nonpolypoid"

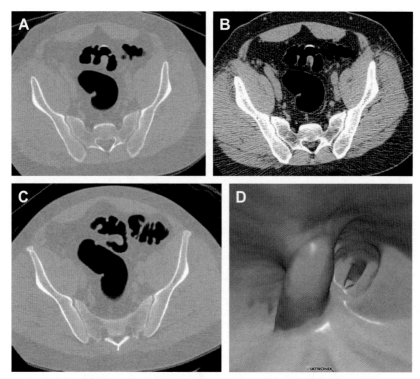

Fig. 13. Persistently thickened fold at CTC. Prone (*A, B*) and supine (*C, D*) CTC images show a thickened sigmoid fold that appears almost mass-like at two-dimensional imaging. The smooth thickening appears to be related to a point of slight twisting or torsion. Note the fat extending into the fold on *B,* which excludes an infiltrating cancer.

plaque-like morphology (see **Fig. 1**). Although the traditional definition was a lesion height that is less than half the width, a preferred definition for flat polyps less than 3 cm in size is an elevation above the mucosal surface that does not exceed 3 mm.[39] Given their intrinsic morphology, flat lesions are less conspicuous and therefore more challenging to initially detect at CTC (and OC). Nonetheless, the sensitivity of combined three-dimensional–two-dimensional polyp detection with contrast tagging seems to be satisfactory.[40] The importance of both contrast tagging for

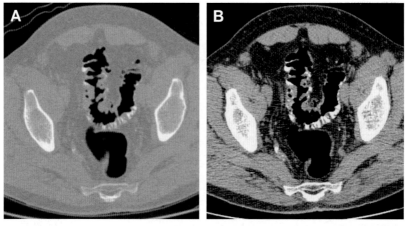

Fig. 14. Sigmoid diverticular disease at CTC. (*A, B*) Supine two-dimensional CTC images show wall thickening and luminal narrowing related to advanced sigmoid diverticulosis. This appearance can make it challenging to exclude superimposed neoplastic pathology. Three-dimensional evaluation can be very valuable in this setting.

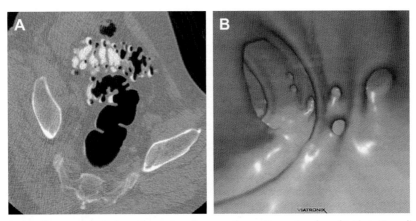

Fig. 15. Diverticular disease at CTC, two-dimensional versus three-dimensional evaluation. Two-dimensional (*A*) and three-dimensional (*B*) CTC images show innumerable sigmoid diverticula. Exclusion of superimposed polyps is a much simpler task on the three-dimensional endoluminal view.

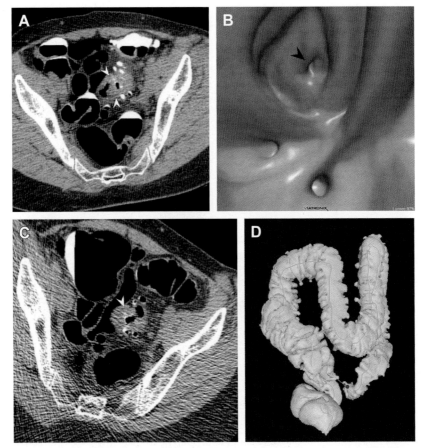

Fig. 16. Nondiagnostic luminal distention related to a diverticular stricture. Supine (*A*, *B*) and decubitus (*C*) CTC images show an area of persistent wall thickening and luminal narrowing (*arrowheads*) in the setting of advanced sigmoid diverticular disease. The prone images had a similar appearance (not shown). (*D*) The three-dimensional colon map shows the site of this persistent stenosis (*arrow* and *red dot*), which proved to be a diverticular stricture.

two-dimensional (given the propensity for flat lesions to coat) and three-dimensional endoluminal evaluation for flat lesion detection cannot be overstated. In the authors' clinical screening experience, more large flat advanced adenomas were detected at primary CTC screening compared with primary OC screening.[41] Of note, histologically advanced or centrally depressed flat lesions are rare in the screening population. Most flat lesions detected (or missed) at CTC are hyperplastic.[42,43] The relative increase in flat hyperplastic lesions is likely caused in part by their tendency to flatten out when the colonic lumen is distended at CTC.[44,45] Most occult polyps at CTC (ie, missed lesions that cannot be identified even retrospectively) represent flat hyperplastic polyps.[43,46,47] Not only do flat lesions constitute an important source of potential false-negatives at CTC, they are a common cause of potential false-positives at CTC (see **Fig. 2**).[48] Although

some of these CTC false-positives could actually represent OC false-negatives, this still underscores the importance of not overcalling flat lesions at CTC.

The prevalence and clinical relevance of flat colonic lesions have been the source of great debate. A clear distinction must be made between relatively flat lesions, and completely flat or depressed lesions, which are quite rare.[49] In general, multiple studies have shown that, for a given size, polypoid lesions greatly outnumber flat lesions and more often harbor aggressive histology.[49–51] For larger flat masses (ie, ≥3 cm), the terms "carpet lesion" and "laterally spreading tumor" are applied (**Fig. 17**).[52] Carpet lesions have a strong predilection for the rectum and cecum.[53] Despite their large linear size, they have a low rate of malignancy but frequently demonstrate villous features, with or without high-grade dysplasia.[52,53] Although classic carpet lesions are

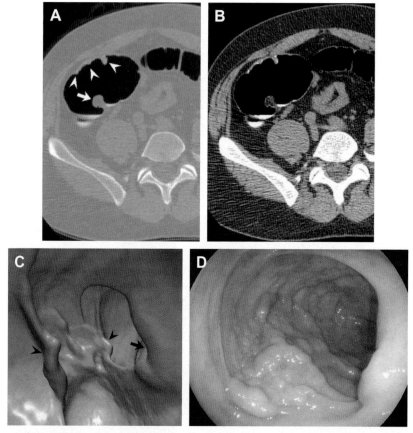

Fig. 17. Large cecal carpet lesion (laterally spreading tumor). Supine transverse two-dimensional (*A, B*) and three-dimensional endoluminal (*C*) CTC images show a large flat soft tissue mass (*arrowheads*) opposite the ileocecal valve (*arrow*) that has a somewhat lobulated appearance and results in fold distortion on three-dimensional imaging. Note the contrast coating portions of the lesion on *B*. This carpet lesion was confirmed at same-day optical colonoscopy (*D*) and proved to be a tubulovillous adenoma. Most nonflat lesions of this large size are malignant.

less conspicuous than obvious polypoid or annular colorectal masses, they are nonetheless detectable at CTC because of the fixed distortion of folds, rolled-up edges, and lobulated appearance (see **Fig. 17**).

Submucosal and Extrinsic Lesions

Broadly speaking, "submucosal" lesions can include anything deep to the mucosal surface, including intramural (**Fig. 18**) and extrinsic lesions (**Fig. 19**). Although a wide variety of neoplastic[54] and nonneoplastic[55] causes for a submucosal luminal impression exist at CTC, only a small subset might potentially be confused for a mucosal-based soft tissue polyp or mass. Two-dimensional correlation at CTC often divulges the nature of an extrinsic impression seen on the three-dimensional endoluminal view, avoiding any potential misdiagnosis. The same cannot be said for luminal examinations, such as barium enema and OC. At CTC, specific definitive diagnosis can be made in the case of submucosal lipomas, pneumatosis, and extrinsic impression from extracolonic structures. The presence of inwardly displaced but uninterrupted folds at three-dimensional endoluminal CTC strongly suggests extrinsic impression (see **Fig. 19**).

Anorectal Pitfalls

There are several findings specific to the anorectum that deserve attention because they are common and can mimic neoplastic disease.[6] Most incidental findings do not require further evaluation, whereas some may require correlation with digital rectal examination, anoscopy, proctoscopy, or flexible sigmoidoscopy. The first key is awareness of anorectal-specific pathology. In many ways, the anorectal region represents the most important source of pitfalls at CTC, because common incidental findings may distract the reader from important underlying pathology, which may be subtle because of its specific location. The anorectal pitfalls that seem to cause the most trouble at CTC interpretation are hypertrophied anal papillae, internal hemorrhoids, the rectal balloon catheter, and low rectal tumors. A variety of other anorectal pathology is much less commonly encountered.[6] Of note, because the anal canal itself is not properly evaluated at CTC, digital rectal examination should still be performed as part of the colorectal screening process.

Hypertrophied anal papillae represent focal fibrous protrusions at the dentate line that essentially represent internal skin tags. These typically have a polypoid sessile appearance and measure 5 to 6 mm or less, but can rarely attain a larger size and become pedunculated. The key to recognition for a typical anal papilla is its constant anatomic location at the anorectal junction, virtually always abutting the rectal catheter at its lowest visualized point. In comparison, low-lying rectal polyps almost always show at least some separation from the anorectal junction.

Internal hemorrhoids are a common finding and represent dilated vascular structures above the dentate line. Internal hemorrhoids may present clinically with bleeding or prolapse. When advanced or thrombosed, internal hemorrhoids may appear polypoid or mass-like at CTC (**Fig. 20**). Circumferential involvement around the rectal catheter is often seen in prominent cases. The soft tissue fullness from internal hemorrhoids often appears prominent on transverse two-dimensional images but is often less mass-like on other two-dimensional planes or the three-dimensional

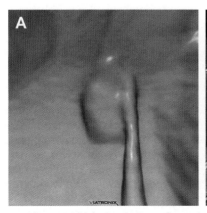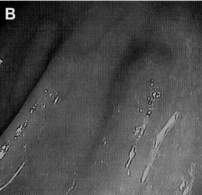

Fig. 18. Submucosal venous bleb simulating a flat polyp at CTC. (*A*) Three-dimensional endoluminal CTC image shows a flat plaque-like lesion adjacent to a colonic fold, which appeared to be soft tissue attenuation on two-dimensional correlation (not shown). (*B*) At subsequent OC, however, the lesion proved to be a submucosal venous bleb.

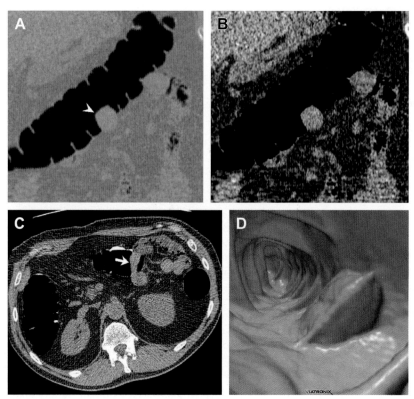

Fig. 19. Extrinsic impression related to an adjacent small bowel loop. (*A, B*) Coronal two-dimensional CTC images show a focal soft tissue "mass" (*arrowhead*) involving the transverse colon. (*C*) Transverse two-dimensional image, however, shows the small bowel loop (*arrow*) extending across the adjacent colon. (*D*) At three-dimensional, the preservation of the overlying colonic fold is a sign that the lesion is caused by extrinsic impression.

endoluminal view, and may change with patient position. In contrast to hemorrhoids, rectal varices have a tubular, serpiginous appearance.

The rectal catheter is a constant finding in the anorectal region at CTC. The associated balloon is nearly invisible except for the mass effect it exerts, often creating pseudolesions through contact with fluid or the rectal wall.

The real issue with the rectal catheter at CTC, however, is its potential for obscuring a pathologic lesion. Although this is of particular concern with the use of large-caliber catheters with large retention cuffs, it remains an issue with the CTC-specific small flexible balloon catheters.[56] To minimize the risk of effacing true pathology in the anorectal region, we advocate the practice of deflating the balloon immediately before obtaining the second CTC series (typically the prone).

Of greatest concern among anorectal pitfalls is the possibility of missing a low rectal tumor or anal cancer. Low rectal polyps and masses can mimic some of the aforementioned incidental anorectal lesions, and can also be effaced by the balloon catheter. Careful attention to this area should be considered a routine part of CTC

interpretation. Additional anorectal pathology that can be encountered at CTC is discussed in more detail elsewhere.[5]

Ileocecal Valve Pitfalls

Given its polypoid or mass-like appearance, confident assessment of the ileocecal valve at CTC seems to be an initial concern for many novice readers.[57] The valve itself is easy to identify given its constant anatomic location relative to the cecum and terminal ileum. However, there is a wide range of normal appearances to the ileocecal valve, ranging from a bulbous papillary or polypoid appearance to a more labial appearance. The overall morphology of the valve is much easier to appreciate on the three-dimensional endoluminal view compared with two-dimensional projections, where it is much more difficult to exclude a superimposed polyp. As with the anorectal region, it is good practice to specifically interrogate the ileocecal valve in each case, assessing its morphology and composition. A diffusely fatty valve or focal fatty projection on three-dimensional translucency rendering or two-dimensional evaluation is

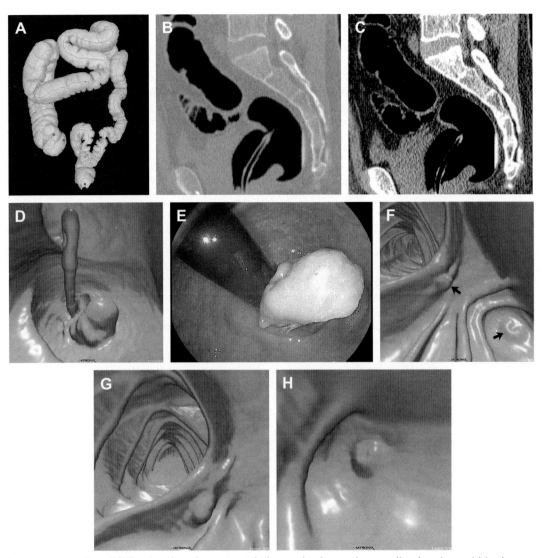

Fig. 20. Interpretive pitfalls related to the anorectal, ileocecal valve, and appendiceal regions within the same case. (*A*) The three-dimensional colon map shows three bookmarks (*red dots*) denoting focal findings in the regions of the anorectum, ileocecal valve, and the appendiceal orifice. Sagittal two-dimensional (*B, C*) and three-dimensional endoluminal (*D*) CTC images show an unusual 3- to 4-cm soft tissue mass extending up from the anorectal region. Note the mass effect on the lesion from the adjacent balloon on the rectal catheter. (*E*) The mass was confirmed at OC but endoscopic biopsies were inconclusive. After transanal excision, a hemorrhoid with organizing thrombosis was confirmed. Focal abnormalities (*arrows*) were also noted at the ileocecal valve (*F, G*) and the appendiceal orifice (*F, H*). At OC, an inflammatory polyp on the ileocecal valve and a small inverted appendiceal stump were confirmed.

reassuring because a focal soft tissue abnormality can be easily excluded. A focal soft tissue protuberance on or adjacent to a fatty valve is suspicious for a true polyp (see **Fig. 20**). A mass involving or replacing the valve itself can present a more challenging problem (see **Fig. 10**). The ileocecal valve is a relatively common location to see a drip of contrast, which can superficially mimic a polyp on the three-dimensional display. With time and experience, recognizing the range of normal and

knowing when to suspect an abnormality on or near the valve eventually become easier tasks.

Appendiceal Pitfalls

As with the ileocecal valve, the vermiform appendix represents another anatomic structure that can give rise to several unique findings at CTC interpretation, most notably false polyps and appendiceal neoplasms. As part of the general intake form, the authors obtain a surgical history on all patients when scheduling the CTC examination. Knowledge of prior appendectomy is useful because an inverted appendiceal stump can mimic a true cecal polyp at CTC, and even at OC (see **Fig. 20**).[58] In some cases, confident distinction between stump and true polyp is not possible and endoscopic evaluation is unavoidable. In patients without a history of appendectomy, partial invagination or rarely even complete intussusception may give rise to an intraluminal polypoid lesion. In these cases, continuity of the remainder of the appendix in its expected location prevents misdiagnosis. The appendiceal orifice is usually easily identified at CTC, allowing for detection of true polyps that are adjacent to but separate from the appendix. The most common primary tumor of the appendix to present as an incidental imaging finding in adults is a benign mucinous adenoma, which manifests as a mucocele from cystic dilatation of the appendix.[59,60] In most cases, OC confirmation of a CTC-detected appendiceal mucocele is not necessary and may even be negative or lead to confusion, given the extraluminal nature of appendiceal tumors. Surgery is indicated for appendiceal mucoceles because almost all lesions are neoplastic (and mucinous) and are considered at least potentially malignant. CTC represents an ideal study for detection and preoperative assessment of these tumors.

SUMMARY

This article covers a wide array of potential pitfalls at CTC interpretation. We have tried to indicate which pitfalls can be avoided altogether, and those that cannot always be avoided but should be recognized as such to prevent mismanagement. In actual practice, the true challenges may come from cases in which more than one pitfall intersects on the same case. Fortunately, the built-in redundancy of two- and three-dimensional CTC interpretation allows for ample opportunity for accurate lesion detection in most cases. With proper attention to technique, including patient preparation, colonic distention, and scanning protocol, in addition to a combined two-dimensional–three-dimensional interpretive strategy, most of these potential pitfalls can be handled appropriately.

REFERENCES

1. Pickhardt PJ, Choi JR, Hwang I, et al. Computed tomographic virtual colonoscopy to screen for colorectal neoplasia in asymptomatic adults. N Engl J Med 2003;349:2191–200.

2. Pickhardt PJ, Hassan C, Halligan S, et al. Colorectal cancer: CT colonography and colonoscopy for detection. Systematic review and meta-analysis. Radiology 2011;259:393–405.

3. Pickhardt PJ. Screening CT colonography: how I do it. AJR Am J Roentgenol 2007;189:290–8.

4. Pickhardt PJ, Kim DH. CT colonography (virtual colonoscopy): a practical approach for population screening. Radiol Clin North Am 2007;45:361–75.

5. Pickhardt PJ, Kim DH. Potential pitfalls at CTC interpretation. In: Pickhardt PJ, Kim DH, editors. CT colonography: principles and practice of virtual colonoscopy. Philadelphia: Saunders; 2010.

6. Pickhardt PJ. Differential diagnosis of polypoid lesions seen at CT colonography (virtual colonoscopy). Radiographics 2004;24:1535–56.

7. Pickhardt PJ, Choi JH. Electronic cleansing and stool tagging in CT colonography: advantages and pitfalls with primary three-dimensional evaluation. AJR Am J Roentgenol 2003;181:799–805.

8. Pickhardt PJ. Translucency rendering in 3D endoluminal CT colonography: a useful tool for increasing polyp specificity and decreasing interpretation time. AJR Am J Roentgenol 2004;183:429–36.

9. Pickhardt PJ. Colonic preparation for computed tomographic colonography: understanding the relative advantages and disadvantages of a noncathartic approach. Mayo Clin Proc 2007;82:659–61.

10. Morrin MM, Farrell RJ, Kruskal JB, et al. Utility of intravenously administered contrast material at CT colonography. Radiology 2000;217:765–71.

11. Zalis ME, Perumpillichira JJ, Magee C, et al. Tagging-based, electronically cleansed CT colonography: evaluation of patient comfort and image readability. Radiology 2006;239:149–59.

12. Pickhardt P, Kim D, Taylor A, et al. Complementary shifting of luminal fluid between supine and prone positioning at CT colonography: implications for 3D mucosal coverage. In: 8th International VC Symposium; 2007. Boston (MA): 2007.

13. Lawrence EM, Pickhardt PJ. Low-volume hybrid bowel preparation combining saline laxatives with oral contrast agents versus standard polyethylene glycol lavage for colonoscopy. Dis Colon Rectum 2010;53:1176–81.

14. Buchach CM, Kim DH, Pickhardt PJ. Performing an additional decubitus series at CT colonography. Abdom Imaging 2011;36:538–44.

15. Choi M, Taylor AJ, VonBerge JL, et al. Can the CT scout reliably assess for adequate colonic distention at CT colonography? Am J Roentgenol 2005;184:21–2.

16. Shinners TJ, Pickhardt PJ, Taylor AJ, et al. Patient-controlled room air insufflation versus automated carbon dioxide delivery for CT colonography. AJR Am J Roentgenol 2006;186:1491–6.

17. Boyce CJ, Vetter JR, Pickhardt PJ. MDCT artifact related to the intra-scan gravitational flow of

opacified luminal fluid (the "Dense Waterfall" sign). Abdom Imaging 2011;37:292–6.

18. Pickhardt PJ. Pictorial review of colonic polyp and mass distortion and recognition with the CT virtual dissection technique (invited commentary). Radiographics 2010;30:e42.

19. Pickhardt PJ, Taylor AJ, Gopal DV. Surface visualization at 3D endoluminal CT colonography: degree of coverage and implications for polyp detection. Gastroenterology 2006;130:1582–7.

20. Pickhardt PJ, Schumacher C, Kim DH. Polyp detection at 3-dimensional endoluminal computed tomography colonography: sensitivity of one-way fly-through at 120 degrees field-of-view angle. J Comput Assist Tomogr 2009;33:631–5.

21. Radiation risk in perspective: position statement of the Health Physics Society: Health Physics Society, Adopted January 1996, revised July 2010.

22. Lubner MG, Pickhardt PJ, Tang J, et al. Reduced image noise at low-dose multidetector CT of the abdomen with prior image constrained compressed sensing algorithm. Radiology 2011;260:248–56.

23. Flicek KT, Hara AK, Silva AC, et al. Reducing the radiation dose for CT colonography using adaptive statistical iterative reconstruction: a pilot study. AJR Am J Roentgenol 2010;195:126–31.

24. O'Connor SD, Summers RM, Choi JR, et al. Oral contrast adherence to polyps on CT colonography. J Comput Assist Tomogr 2006;30:51–7.

25. Cotton PB, Durkalski VL, Benoit PC, et al. Computed tomographic colonography (virtual colonoscopy): a multicenter comparison with standard colonoscopy for detection of colorectal neoplasia. JAMA 2004;291:1713–9.

26. Johnson CD, Harmsen WS, Wilson LA, et al. Prospective blinded evaluation of computed tomographic colonography for screen detection of colorectal polyps. Gastroenterology 2003;125:311–9.

27. Rockey DC, Poulson E, Niedzwiecki D, et al. Analysis of air contrast barium enema, computed tomographic colonography, and colonoscopy: prospective comparison. Lancet 2005;365:305–11.

28. Graser A, Stieber P, Nagel D, et al. Comparison of CT colonography, colonoscopy, sigmoidoscopy and faecal occult blood tests for the detection of advanced adenoma in an average risk population. Gut 2009;58:241–8.

29. Pickhardt PJ, Lee AD, Taylor AJ, et al. Primary 2D versus primary 3D polyp detection at screening CT Colonography. AJR Am J Roentgenol 2007;189: 1451–6.

30. Park SH, Choi EK, Lee SS, et al. Polyp measurement reliability, accuracy, and discrepancy: optical colonoscopy versus CT colonography with pig colonic specimens. Radiology 2007;244:157–64.

31. Barancin C, Pickhardt P, Kim D, et al. Prospective blinded comparison of polyp size on computed tomography colonography and endoscopic colonoscopy. Clin Gastroenterol Hepatol 2011;9:443–5.

32. Pickhardt PJ, Lee AD, McFarland EG, et al. Linear polyp measurement at CT colonography: in vitro and in vivo comparison of two-dimensional and three-dimensional displays. Radiology 2005;236: 872–8.

33. Barancin C, Pickhardt PJ, Kim DH, et al. Prospective Blinded Comparison of Polyp Size on Computed Tomography Colonography and Endoscopic Colonoscopy. Clinical Gastroenterology and Hepatology 2011;9:443–5.

34. Yeshwant SC, Summers RM, Yao JH, et al. Polyps: linear and volumetric measurement at CT colonography. Radiology 2006;241:802–11.

35. Pickhardt PJ, Lehman VT, Winter TC, et al. Polyp volume versus linear size measurements at CT colonography: implications for noninvasive surveillance of unresected colorectal lesions. AJR Am J Roentgenol 2006;186:1605–10.

36. Blake ME, Soto JA, Hayes RA, et al. Automated volumetry at CT colonography: a phantom study. Acad Radiol 2005;12:608–13.

37. Sanford MF, Pickhardt PJ. Diagnostic performance of primary 3-dimensional computed tomography colonography in the setting of colonic diverticular disease. Clin Gastroenterol Hepatol 2006;4:1039–47.

38. Tendler DA, Aboudola S, Zacks JF, et al. Prolapsing mucosal polyps: an underrecognized form of colonic polyp. A clinicopathological study of 15 cases. Am J Gastroenterol 2002;97:370–6.

39. Zalis ME, Barish MA, Choi JR, et al. CT colonography reporting and data system: a consensus proposal. Radiology 2005;236:3–9.

40. Pickhardt PJ, Choi JR, Nugent PA, et al. Flat lesions at virtual and optical colonoscopy: prevalence, histology, and sensitivity for detection in an asymptomatic screening population. Am J Roentgenol 2004;182:74–5.

41. Kim DH, Pickhardt PJ, Taylor AJ, et al. CT colonography versus colonoscopy for the detection of advanced neoplasia. N Engl J Med 2007;357:1403–12.

42. Fidler JL, Johnson CD, MacCarty RL, et al. Detection of flat lesions in the colon with CT colonography. Abdom Imaging 2002;27:292–300.

43. Pickhardt PJ, Choi JR, Hwang I, et al. Nonadenomatous polyps at CT colonography: prevalence, size distribution, and detection rates. Radiology 2004; 232:784–90.

44. Waye JD, Bilotta JJ. Rectal hyperplastic polyps: now you see them, now you don't. A differential point. Am J Gastroenterol 1990;85:1557–9.

45. Summers RM, Liu J, Yao J, et al. Automated measurement of colorectal polyp height at CT colonography: hyperplastic polyps are flatter than adenomatous polyps. AJR Am J Roentgenol 2009; 193:1305–10.

46. Cornett D, Barancin C, Roeder B, et al. Findings on optical colonoscopy after positive CT colonography exam. Am J Gastroenterol 2008;103:2068–74.

47. MacCarty RL, Johnson CD, Fletcher JG, et al. Occult colorectal polyps on CT colonography: implications for surveillance. AJR Am J Roentgenol 2006;186:1380–3.

48. Pickhardt PJ, Wise SM, Kim DH. Positive predictive value for polyps detected at screening CT colonography. Eur Radiol 2010;20:1651–6.

49. Soetikno RM, Kaltenbach T, Rouse RV, et al. Prevalence of nonpolypoid (flat and depressed) colorectal neoplasms in asymptomatic and symptomatic adults. JAMA 2008;299:1027–35.

50. O'Brien MJ, Winawer SJ, Zauber AG, et al. Flat adenomas in the National Polyp Study: is there increased risk for high-grade dysplasia initially or during surveillance? Clin Gastroenterol Hepatol 2004;2:905–11.

51. Pickhardt PJ, Kim DH, Robbins JB. Flat (nonpolypoid) colorectal lesions identified at CT colonography in a US screening population. Acad Radiol 2010;17:784–90.

52. Tanaka S, Haruma K, Oka S, et al. Clinicopathologic features and endoscopic treatment of superficially spreading colorectal neoplasms larger than 20 mm. Gastrointest Endosc 2001;54:62–6.

53. Rubesin S, Saul S, Laufer I, et al. Carpet lesions of the colon. Radiographics 1985;5:537–52.

54. Pickhardt PJ, Kim DH, Menias CO, et al. Evaluation of submucosal lesions of the large intestine. Part 1. Neoplasms. Radiographics 2007;27:1681–92.

55. Pickhardt PJ, Kim DH, Menias CO, et al. Evaluation of submucosal lesions of the large intestine. Part 2. Nonneoplastic causes. Radiographics 2007;27: 1693–703.

56. Pickhardt PJ, Choi JR. Adenomatous polyp obscured by small-caliber rectal catheter at low-dose CT colonography: a rare diagnostic pitfall. AJR Am J Roentgenol 2005;184:1581–3.

57. Iafrate F, Rengo M, Ferrari R, et al. Spectrum of normal findings, anatomic variants and pathology of ileocecal valve: CT colonography appearances and endoscopic correlation. Abdom Imaging 2007; 32:589–95.

58. Prout TM, Taylor AJ, Pickhardt PJ. Inverted appendiceal stumps simulating large pedunculated polyps on screening CT colonography. AJR Am J Roentgenol 2006;186:535–8.

59. Pickhardt PJ, Levy AD, Rohrmann CA, et al. Primary neoplasms of the appendix: radiologic spectrum of disease with pathologic correlation. Radiographics 2003;23:645–62.

60. Pickhardt PJ, Kim DH, Taylor AJ, et al. Extracolonic tumors of the gastrointestinal tract detected incidentally at screening CT colonography. Dis Colon Rectum 2007;50:56–63.

Cost-Effectiveness of CT Colonography

Cesare Hassan, MD[a],*, Perry J. Pickhardt, MD[b]

KEYWORDS

- Colorectal cancer screening • Colonoscopy • CT colonography

KEY POINTS

- Simulation modeling has been extensively applied to CT colonography (CTC) to define its long-term efficacy and cost-effectiveness in the setting of colorectal cancer (CRC) screening.
- Available models indicate that CTC is effective in reducing CRC incidence and mortality, ranging from 40% to 77% for CRC incidence prevention and from 58% to 84% for CRC mortality reduction.
- CTC has been consistently shown to be cost-effective compared with no screening, indicating that it represents, at the very least, an attractive test for individuals who are noncompliant with the available options.
- CTC needs to achieve a higher attendance rate or cost less than colonoscopy to be cost-effective relative to colonoscopy.

INTRODUCTION

There are two main motivations for applying computer microsimulation to colorectal cancer (CRC) screening: to estimate the long-term efficacy of a new test and to extrapolate the results of clinical trials.

Modeling can be exploited to assess the potential long-term efficacy of a new screening technique. Innovative techniques are usually validated through head-to-head comparisons with colonoscopy or other established reference standards. Although such comparisons can define the accuracy of new techniques for relevant targets, such as advanced neoplasia, they fail to assess the potential impact of these tests on the natural history of colorectal neoplasia. Consequently, the actual long-term reductions in incidence and mortality of CRC, which represents the relevant target for society at large, are not addressed by such studies. Ultimate reduction in CRC incidence and mortality can be measured through long-lasting randomized and/or cohort studies, which have already been performed for guaiac-based fecal tests or sigmoidoscopy.[1–5] However, if this were required for every new screening modality, it would significantly delay implementation of a potentially useful new technique for a decade or more while awaiting trial results. Simulation modeling allows for estimation of long-term impact on the natural history of colorectal neoplasia by any new technique by converting the comparison in accuracy with the reference standard technique (ie, colonoscopy) into estimates of long-term CRC incidence or mortality reduction. Although these estimates may be weakened by the incomplete knowledge of the characteristics of the test, the interaction between the test and the natural history of the disease, or the correctness of the model structure, such uncertainty may be fully explored by a proper sensitivity analysis, substantially reducing the risk of error in the decision-making process.

The second reason for using computerized simulation in CRC screening is to project the

[a] Digestive Endoscopy Unit, Nuovo Regina Margherita Hospital, Via Morosini 30, Roma 00153, Italy;
[b] Gastrointestinal Imaging, University of Wisconsin School of Medicine & Public Health, 75D Highland Ave. Madison, WI 53705, USA
* Corresponding author.
E-mail address: cesareh@hotmail.com

Radiol Clin N Am 51 (2013) 89–97
http://dx.doi.org/10.1016/j.rcl.2012.09.006

results of relatively small controlled trials assessing a novel technique onto the general population that would be expected to potentially undergo such a technique. Distinct from the clinical setting for symptomatic conditions, in which only a very small percentage of the population is affected by a technological innovation, novel techniques applied to CRC screening programs may potentially involve millions of individuals in a given country, raising concern for medical and nonmedical issues that are not necessarily addressed within the smaller clinical studies on diagnostic accuracy. The most relevant output of population modeling is represented by the cost-effectiveness ratio, which is the relationship between test efficacy in terms of CRC incidence and mortality reduction, usually expressed as years of life saved (with or without correction for the quality of life), estimated for the new technique and the cost of an eventual screening program based on the same technique. Although this parameter is usually expressed as the amount of money spent to save 1 additional year of life, its meaningfulness is apparently only limited to financial considerations. Indeed, the estimate of cost not only involves the cost of the new test itself, but also takes into account several other economic variables, such as the exploitation of human, technological, and logistic resources, as well as the potential loss of productivity due to the screening test itself or the induced harm.[6]

CT colonography (CTC), also referred to as virtual colonoscopy, is a minimally invasive imaging examination of the entire colon and rectum that is capable of assessing for the presence or absence of structural lesions, most notably large colorectal polyps, and cancer. In clinical studies, CTC has been shown to be highly effective for detecting advanced neoplasia,[7–9] which is the critical target for CRC screening and prevention. Given this high level of performance, CTC has been recommended for CRC screening by the American Cancer Society, working in conjunction with the major gastroenterology and radiology societies.[10] Microsimulation modeling has been extensively applied to CTC to anticipate its potential impact on the CRC screening field. For the remainder of this article, the focus is on the following issues, which have all been systematically addressed in the literature:

1. Can CTC reduce CRC incidence and mortality?
2. Is CTC cost-effective compared with no screening?
3. Is CTC cost-effective compared with previously established tests?

CAN CTC REDUCE CRC INCIDENCE AND MORTALITY?

Colonoscopy has been consistently shown to be effective in reducing CRC incidence and mortality by two main mechanisms. Endoscopic polypectomy has been reported to reduce CRC incidence by 30% to 80% in randomized and cohort studies,[1,2,11–14] whereas the early identification of already developed CRC has been shown to reduce CRC mortality by 20% in randomized studies through the initial use of guaiac-based fecal occult blood testing.[3–5] Comparing CTC accuracy for the different sizes of polyps (ie, diminutive, ≤5 mm; small, 6–9 mm; and large, ≥10 mm) and for the different stages of CRC (ie, localized, regional, and distant) with those of colonoscopy, all the simulation models available in the literature (**Table 1**) consistently indicate the efficacy of CTC in reducing CRC incidence and mortality, ranging from 40% to 77% for reduction in CRC incidence (prevention) and from 58% to 84% for CRC mortality reduction.[6,15–22] Atleast six factors may explain this interstudy variability, as detailed below.

1. The Rate of de novo CRC Versus Benign Polyp Precursor

Assumptions regarding the de novo CRC rate (vs CRC development through a benign precursor polyp) directly affect the percentage of incident CRC that is potentially preventable through polyp detection and removal (via endoscopic polypectomy). The higher the de novo CRC rate, the less effective all techniques that mainly exploit polypectomy to reduce CRC incidence and mortality will be. In theory, such a mechanism should affect both CTC and colonoscopy equally. However, the higher frequency of repetition recommended for CTC screening compared with colonoscopy (5 years vs 10 years, respectively) doubles the opportunity for CTC to down-stage de novo CRC, thereby increasing the relative efficacy of CTC in reducing CRC mortality.

2. The Type and Prevalence of Polyp Size Classes

Because of relatively poor knowledge about the progression of colorectal neoplasia through the different sizes of polyps (ie, diminutive, small, and large), some models assume only two size classes (ie, small and large), while other models simulate all the three classes. Moreover, some models allow only large polyps to progress to early stage CRC, whereas others also simulate the progression of small or diminutive polyps directly to CRC. Presumably, this structural heterogeneity

Table 1
Main characteristics and estimates on CTC long-term efficacy of the simulation models available in the literature

Author, Year[a]	Country	Simulation of de novo Pathogenesis	Polyp Types Simulated	CRC Stages Simulated	Yearly Progression from Large Polyp to CRC	CTC Accuracy for Large Polyps	Frequency of CTC Repetition	CTC-Related CRC Incidence Prevention, %	CTC-Related CRC Mortality Prevention, %
Sonnenberg et al,[15] 1999	US	No	Adenomas[b]	1 stage	NA	80%	10 y	40	NA
Ladabaum et al,[16] 2004	US	Yes	Small Large	Loc Reg Dis	5%	60%–94%[c]	10 y	51–70	58–79
Heitman et al,[17] 2005	Canada	No	Small Large	1 stage	NA	71%	NA	NA	NA
Pickhardt et al,[6] 2007	US	Yes	Dim Small Large	Early Late	3%	85%	10 y	56	NA
Vijan et al,[18] 2007	US	No	Low-risk High-risk	Loc Reg Dis	NA	82%–91%[c]	5–10 y	71–77	76–81
Hassan et al,[19] 2008	US	Yes	Dim Small Large	Loc Reg Dis	3%–4%	90%	10 y	62	NA
Lee et al,[20] 2010	UK	No	Small Large	Dukes A-D	3%	90%	10 y	77[d]	84[d]
Knudsen et al,[21] 2010[e]	US	No	Dim Small Large	AJCC Stages 1–4	NA	84%–92%	5 y	48	NA
Heresbach et al,[22] 2010	France	No	Low-risk High-risk	NA	NA	NA	NA	36–38	42–46

Abbreviations: AJCC, American Joint Committee on Cancer; Dim, diminutive; Dis, distant; Loc, localized; Reg, regional; UK, United Kingdom; US, United States.
[a] In the case of multiple publications, the most recent was included.
[b] Without further classification.
[c] Two different scenarios were simulated.
[d] Compared with colonoscopy, occult blood test.
[e] MISCAN model.

among the different models affects the various colorectal screening tests to the same extent, without generating uncertainty on the model outputs. However, this does not seem to be the case for CTC, mainly because of the different management strategies between CTC and the endoscopic tests. Unlike endoscopy, in which all visualized polyps are generally removed, only polyps 6 mm or larger constitute a positive CTC and trigger referral to endoscopic polypectomy. Furthermore, CTC practice may also allow for in vivo surveillance of small 6 to 9 mm polyps, resulting in a more complex situation to model.[23,24] As such, any variability in polyp size distribution across the models may impact CTC and endoscopy differently, accounting for some of the heterogeneity in results across the studies.

3. The Simulated Stages of CRC

Although the progression of invasive CRC across stages has been clarified in screening studies, different models tend to classify CRC stages in different ways. For instance, some models simplify CRC progression in only two stages (ie, localized and metastatic), other models in three stages (ie, localized, regional, and metastatic), while still other models adopt a tumor, node, metastasis (TNM) or Dukes staging approach. Such variability is at least partially explained by the different sources of data input (eg, the Surveillance Epidemiology and End-Result [SEER] database provides a three-stage classification) among different models. Although such model heterogeneity is unlikely to affect the relative efficacy between CTC and colonoscopy because of the very high CRC sensitivity for each technique,[8] it may affect the yearly rate of progression from curable to incurable CRC, which would affect tests with different frequencies of repetition differently, such as CTC versus colonoscopy.

4. The Rate of Progression Through the Different Types of Polyps and CRC Stages

The rate of progression through the different types of polyps and CRC stages indicates how many lesions transition from one class to the next each year (eg, from diminutive to small adenoma) and it actually represents the real core of the model structure. Indeed, such rates are the main determinant of the natural history of colorectal neoplasia simulated by any model. Unfortunately, because of the poor knowledge of the natural history of colorectal neoplasia, there is a substantial inter-model variability in these transition rates because any difference in assumption in the adenoma-carcinoma sequence will be eventually reflected in these transition rates. For instance, when

assuming the possibility of a de novo CRC pathway (see previous discussion), the transition rates underlying the progression among different classes of polyps should be necessarily decelerated to result in the same incidence of CRC. Similarly, when simulating the possibility of progression through three (diminutive, small, and large) instead of just two classes of polyps, the transition rates should be accelerated to sustain the same CRC incidence. Transition rates may also be changed to simulate different degrees of population risk for CRC. For instance, such rates are usually increased twofold to simulate the CRC incidence in first-degree relatives of CRC patients or the higher incidence of CRC in those with a previous polypectomy. Moreover, models adapted to regions with different CRC risk (eg, Europe vs United States) would have different transition rates to simulate the difference in the natural history of colorectal neoplasia. The impact of this variability on the assumptions of the polyp-transition rates versus the efficacy of screening techniques is large. Any increase in the transition rates will reduce the window of opportunity of CRC screening, exponentially reducing the efficacy of techniques that mainly exploit prevention with polypectomy (CTC, colonoscopy) instead of just CRC detection and down-staging (fecal tests) as the mechanisms of action. On the other hand, any reduction in such transition rates will exponentially increase the efficacy of CRC screening. Although these assumptions should affect both CTC and its reference standard (colonoscopy) to the same extent, the different strategies of the two programs (eg, 5-year vs 10-year interval, non-referral for diminutive lesions) results in divergent estimates when changing these transition rates, explaining the heterogeneity in the estimates of CTC efficacy in the literature.

5. Input Assumptions of CTC Accuracy

The estimate of efficacy of CTC is heavily affected by the assumptions of CTC sensitivity for each of the precancerous and malignant lesions. Because modeling extracts CTC accuracy data from the literature, these estimates could, in theory, be expected to be equal across the different models, reducing the heterogeneity in the model outputs. Unfortunately, this did not occur because different models adopt different accuracy values for the same technique. CTC modeling has evolved over a decade or more, such that some investigators had only the initial studies on CTC available, which may not be representative of what is considered today as state-of-the-art technique (eg, fecal tagging, combined three- and two-dimensional evaluation). Alternatively, some models have been purposely based on just one or a few studies to assess the impact of such a study on CRC screening with CTC. Because of the direct relationship between efficacy in CRC incidence and/or mortality reduction and sensitivity for precancerous lesions, any change in CTC sensitivity may be expected to result in a substantial intermodel variability.

6. The Impact of Extracolonic Findings

Although the potential detection of extracolonic findings has been mainly portrayed as an undesirable outcome of CTC screening, recent evidence supports its efficacy in reducing general mortality by the early detection of abdominal aortic aneurysms (AAA) and extracolonic malignancies. Regarding the former, AAA screening in high-risk subjects (eg, male smokers) has already been shown to be clinically effective and cost-effective in the general population.[25] Therefore, it is likely that, at least in these high-risk subjects, the detection of AAA would increase the overall efficacy of CTC. Regarding the latter, a recent study has shown that most of the extracolonic CTC-detected carcinomas have been detected in early stages, allowing a potentially curable surgical treatment.[26] Although there is no direct evidence that such a down-staging may increase overall survival, this is supported by previously established efficacy seen with other tumors.[27] According to one model, the simultaneous detection of AAA and early extracolonic carcinomas added a substantial advantage to CTC compared with other tests that are unable to visualize extracolonic structures.[19]

Taking all these considerations into account, CTC seems to be able, according to simulation modeling, to substantially reduce CRC incidence and mortality when applied in the CRC screening field at the population level. Although the wide range of variation in model estimates may cause some uncertainty on the exact benefit from CTC screening, it provides a robust interval beyond which it is extremely unlikely such efficacy would not exist.

IS CTC COST-EFFECTIVE COMPARED WITH NO SCREENING?

Nearly half of the eligible American population has not been screened for CRC in the last 10 years, and this figure is likely to be substantially higher in European countries.[28,29] This would indicate that a large part of the eligible population has not been compliant with the tests that were already available to them, such as endoscopy or fecal tests. CTC may be expected to convince at least

part of this noncompliant population to undertake CRC screening because it provides the possibility to image the entire colorectum without the discomfort and risk of colonoscopy. When considering the offer of a new screening test to patients who were noncompliant with the previous tests, it is necessary to assess whether the new test is not only effective but also cost-effective compared with the current no screening scenario of noncompliant patients.

Cost-effectiveness not only depends on efficacy but also on costs. The main cost variables in any screening program are represented by the intrinsic and/or actual cost of the test itself, the cost of any posttest work-up or follow up, and the cost of treatment of CRC (eg, surgery, chemotherapy, and palliative care). It has been customary that any diagnostic, therapeutic, or operative procedure within a given health care system is cost-effective when the amount of money spent to save 1 year of life is inferior to an arbitrary threshold that is usually set between $50,000 and $100,000, according to the financial status of the different health systems.[30] Most of the currently available CRC screening tests, such as fecal tests or endoscopy, have been shown to be extremely cost-effective compared with no screening, with cost-effectiveness ratios much lower than $50,000.[31] Such a favorable profile has been related, on one hand, with the efficacy of CRC screening tests in reducing CRC mortality (ie, gain of life-years) and, on the other, with the substantial reduction of CRC treatment costs related to reduction in CRC incidence. The latter has recently gained even more attention because of the abrupt increase in the cost of metastatic CRC treatment following the introduction of novel but extremely costly chemotherapy agents.[32]

When dealing with CTC, cost-effectiveness not only depends on its efficacy, which is related to CTC sensitivity, but also on CTC-related costs. Such costs are represented by the cost of CTC itself and by the cost of colonoscopies induced by the screening (ie, post-CTC polypectomy) or by the postpolypectomy or postsurgical surveillance program. In contrast to colonoscopy, in which polypectomy is a part of the same diagnostic procedure (albeit with increased costs), the detection of significant lesions at CTC will require the additional cost of the post-CTC colonoscopy. Such cost will not only depend on the sensitivity of the procedure (ie, true positive), but also on the specificity (ie, false positive). A suboptimal CTC specificity would result in the waste of considerable financial and medical resources for overcalls leading to post-CTC colonoscopies, potentially undermining the cost-effectiveness of the technique. A further distinct characteristic of CTC is represented by the cost entailed in the work-up of extracolonic findings, such as renal, ovary, liver, or pancreatic masses or vascular abnormalities (ie, aortic aneurysm). However, such costs have consistently been shown to be quite small, accounting only for a small fraction of the initial cost of CTC.[6,15–22,33–36]

Similar to endoscopic and fecal screening tests, CTC has been consistently shown to be cost-effective compared with no screening by all the available models (**Table 2**).[6,15–22] This would indicate that CTC should be always regarded as an effective and convenient test, at least in all those persons who did not adhere to the competitive options (ie, colonoscopy). For society it would seem prudent to reimburse for CTC screening test instead of having eligible persons noncompliant.

IS CTC COST-EFFECTIVE COMPARED WITH PREVIOUSLY ESTABLISHED TESTS?

Microsimulation allows long-term comparisons of costs and efficacies among multiple competitive options that would require too many resources to be performed within clinical setting. The output of these simulations is usually represented by a rank of the different options according to the overall cost of the program, with the computation of the relative cost-effectiveness ratios between the more costly and effective strategies with the less costly and effective strategies. Similar to the comparison between any screening program with no screening, the relative cost-effectiveness between two tests depends on several characteristics, such as the test accuracy, the frequency of repetition, the assumptions on the natural history of colorectal neoplasia (see previous discussion), the relative cost among the different procedures, and the CRC treatment cost.

When considering the uncertainty surrounding most of these estimates, it is not surprising that different models may lead to different ranking lists of the available options, so that some strategies that seem to be cost-effective using some assumptions on the natural history or cost may not be under different circumstances. However, this does not necessarily indicate that the conclusions of different models are incompatible because

Table 2
Cost-effectiveness of CTC compared with no screening and colonoscopy

Author, Y[a]	CTC Specificity	CTC to Colonoscopy Cost Ratio	CTC Cost-Effective Compared with No Screening	CTC Cost-Effective Compared with Colonoscopy	If Not Cost-Effective vs Colonoscopy, CTC may Reverse when Varying
Sonnenberg et al,[15] 1999	95%	0.65	Yes	No	Cost/adherence
Ladabaum et al,[16] 2004	85%	1	Yes	No	Cost
Heitman et al,[17] 2005	84%	0.8	NA	No	Cost Adherence CTC accuracy Natural history
Pickhardt et al,[6] 2007	86%	0.7	Yes	Yes	Adherence
Vijan et al,[18] 2007	91%	0.8	Yes	No	Accuracy/cost
Hassan et al,[19] 2008	86%	0.8	Yes	Yes	—
Lee et al,[20] 2010	88%	0.3	NA	No	NA
Knudsen et al,[21] 2010[b]	80%–88%	1	Yes	No	Cost Adherence
Heresbach et al,[22] 2010	NA	NA	Yes	NA	NA

[a] In the case of multiple publications, the most recent is used.
[b] MISCAN model.

variations in the model-specific inputs at sensitivity analysis are often able to reproduce similar results across the apparently discordant models.

Regarding CTC, most of the available models have mainly focused on its cost-effectiveness when compared with colonoscopy. Such cost-effectiveness would depend on two main theoretical assumptions:

1. When assuming the same frequency of repetition (ie, every 10 years), the efficacy of CTC is likely to be slightly lower compared with colonoscopy because of the lower sensitivity for smaller polyps and the nonreferral for diminutive lesions. This may also result in a higher expenditure for treatment of unprevented CRC.
2. When assuming the same cost between the two procedures, the cost of CTC screening is likely to be higher than that of colonoscopy, because CTC implies a duplication of cost for the 10% to 20% of CTC-positive subjects who need a post-CTC colonoscopy for true-positive or false-positive results.

In order to reverse this theoretical cost-ineffectiveness for CTC, several possibilities exist:

1. According to official guidelines,[10] CTC needs to be repeated more frequently than colonoscopy. When considering the very high sensitivity of CTC for large polyps and already developed CRC, which represents over 90% of the all advanced neoplasia, it is extremely likely that 5-year CTC is equal, if not more effective, than 10-year colonoscopy in preventing CRC incidence/mortality.
2. When simulating a screening program, the overall efficacy not only depends on the actual detection rate of advanced neoplasia in patients undertaking the screening procedure but also on the actual participation rate. If CTC is able to convince more people to undertake the screening procedure than colonoscopy, the gap of compliance would immediately result in an equivalent increase of the relative efficacy of CTC versus colonoscopy. This has been recently shown to be the case in a randomized study comparing the adherence and detection rate between CTC and colonoscopy.[37-39]
3. CTC cost is substantially less than that of colonoscopy in several health systems. This is related to the reduced exploitation of logistic and medical or nonmedical resources when performing a CTC compared with colonoscopy. CTC also reduces the costs for colonoscopy-related complications (ie, perforation) and productivity loss (ie, working-days lost for CRC screening). By progressively reducing the CTC

cost, virtually any model would indicate the potential efficacy and cost-effectiveness of CTC.[6,15-22] This indicates that the adoption of different reimbursement policies between the clinical and screening settings, as has been widely implemented with endoscopic or fecal tests, will substantially reduce, if not eliminate, the residual uncertainty about the affordability of a CTC screening program.

When considering all these pros and cons of CTC compared with colonoscopy, it is not surprising that models based on different assumptions or structures reach divergent results on the relative cost-effectiveness of CTC compared with colonoscopy, summarized in **Table 2**. Irrespective of the model output with the baseline inputs, however, on sensitivity analysis most of the models also show that the reversed situation may not be excluded when the main input assumptions are changed. Such uncertainty underlines how further clinical research on all the aspects dealing with the relative cost-effectiveness between these two techniques is needed. In particular, a recent article, exploiting modeling to define the priority in clinical research,[40] indicated adherence to screening test is the most influential variable to be addressed in a research setting on the relative cost-effectiveness between the two procedures.

SUMMARY

Microsimulation modeling has been widely applied to CTC to anticipate the potential benefit and costs on the general population. Overall, these simulations suggest that society may expect a substantial benefit when implementing a mass screening program with CTC that would seem affordable compared with other medical procedures within and outside the CRC screening field. This clearly indicates that CTC should at least be immediately offered to all eligible subjects who are not compliant with other screening options, such as colonoscopy or fecal tests. On the other hand, there is a residual uncertainty over the cost-effectiveness of CTC compared with a primary colonoscopy screening that should be addressed by further research.

REFERENCES

1. Atkin WS, Edwards R, Kralj-Hans I, et al. Once-only flexible sigmoidoscopy screening in prevention of colorectal cancer: a multicentre randomised controlled trial. Lancet 2010;375:1624–33.
2. Segnan N, Armaroli P, Bonelli L, et al. Once-only sigmoidoscopy in colorectal cancer screening: follow-up

findings of the Italian randomized controlled trial–SCORE. J Natl Cancer Inst 2011;103:1310–22.

3. Hardcastle JD, Chamberlain JO, Robinson MH, et al. Randomised controlled trial of faecal occult blood screening for colorectal cancer. Lancet 1996;348:1472–7.

4. Kronborg O, Fenger C, Olsen J, et al. Randomised study of screening for colorectal cancer with faecal occult blood test. Lancet 1996;348:1467–71.

5. Mandel JS, Bond JH, Church TR, et al. Reducing mortality from colorectal cancer by screening for fecal occult blood. N Engl J Med 1993;328:1365–71.

6. Pickhardt PJ, Hassan C, Laghi A, et al. Cost-effectiveness of colorectal cancer screening with computed tomography colonography - The impact of not reporting diminutive lesions. Cancer 2007;109:2213–21.

7. Pickhardt PJ, Choi JR, Hwang I, et al. Computed tomographic virtual colonoscopy to screen for colorectal neoplasia in asymptomatic adults. N Engl J Med 2003;349:2191–200.

8. Pickhardt PJ, Hassan C, Halligan S, et al. Colorectal cancer: CT colonography and colonoscopy for detection – systematic review and meta-analysis. Radiology 2011;259:393–405.

9. Kim DH, Pickhardt PJ, Taylor AJ, et al. CT colonography versus colonoscopy for the detection of advanced neoplasia. N Engl J Med 2007;357:1403–12.

10. Levin B, Lieberman DA, McFarland B, et al. Screening and surveillance for the early detection of colorectal cancer and adenomatous polyps, 2008: a joint guideline from the American Cancer Society, the US Multi-Society Task Force on Colorectal Cancer, and the American College of Radiology. Gastroenterology 2008;134:1570–95.

11. Brenner H, Arndt V, Sturmer T, et al. Long-lasting reduction of risk of colorectal cancer following screening endoscopy. Br J Cancer 2001;85:972–6.

12. Winawer SJ, Zauber AG, Ho MN, et al. Prevention of colorectal cancer by colonoscopic polypectomy. The National Polyp Study Workgroup. N Engl J Med 1993;329:1977–81.

13. Baxter NN, Goldwasser MA, Paszat LF, et al. Association of colonoscopy and death from colorectal cancer. Ann Intern Med 2009;150:1–8.

14. Singh H, Turner D, Xue L, et al. Risk of developing colorectal cancer following a negative colonoscopy examination. JAMA 2006;295:2366–73.

15. Sonnenberg A, Delco F, Bauerfeind P. Is virtual colonoscopy a cost-effective option to screen for colorectal cancer? Am J Gastroenterol 1999;94:2268–74.

16. Ladabaum U, Song K, Fendrick AM. Colorectal neoplasia screening with virtual colonoscopy: when, at what cost, and with what national impact. Clin Gastroenterol Hepatol 2004;2:554–63.

17. Heitman SJ, Manns BJ, Hilsden RJ, et al. Cost-effectiveness of computerized tomographic colonography versus colonoscopy for colorectal cancer screening. Can Med Assoc J 2005;173:877–81.

18. Vijan S, Hwang I, Inadomi J, et al. The cost-effectiveness of CT colonography in screening for colorectal neoplasia. Am J Gastroenterol 2007;102:380–90.

19. Hassan C, Pickhardt PJ, Laghi A, et al. Computed tomographic colonography to screen for colorectal cancer, extracolonic cancer, and aortic aneurysm: model simulation with cost-effectiveness analysis. Arch Intern Med 2008;168:696–705.

20. Lee D, Muston D, Sweet A, et al. Cost effectiveness of CT colonography for UK NHS colorectal cancer screening of asymptomatic adults aged 60-69 years. Appl Health Econ Health Policy 2010;8:141–54.

21. Knudsen AB, Lansdorp-Vogelaar I, Rutter CM, et al. Cost-effectiveness of computed tomographic colonography screening for colorectal cancer in the Medicare population. J Natl Cancer Inst 2010;102:1238–52.

22. Heresbach D, Chauvin P, Hess-Migliorretti A, et al. Cost-effectiveness of colorectal cancer screening with computed tomography colonography according to a polyp size threshold for polypectomy. Eur J Gastroenterol Hepatol 2010;22:716–23.

23. Pickhardt PJ, Hassan C, Laghi A, et al. Clinical management of small (6- to 9-mm) polyps detected at screening CT colonography: a cost-effectiveness analysis. AJR Am J Roentgenol 2008;191:1509–16.

24. Pickhardt PJ, Hassan C, Laghi A, et al. Small and diminutive polyps detected at screening CT colonography: a decision analysis for referral to colonoscopy. AJR Am J Roentgenol 2008;190:136–44.

25. Ashton HA, Buxton MJ, Day NE, et al. The Multicentre Aneurysm Screening Study (MASS) into the effect of abdominal aortic aneurysm screening on mortality in men: a randomised controlled trial. Lancet 2002;360:1531–9.

26. Pickhardt PJ, Kim DH, Meiners RJ, et al. Colorectal and extracolonic cancers detected at screening CT colonography in 10,286 asymptomatic adults. Radiology 2010;255:83–8.

27. National Lung Screening Trial Research Team, Aberle DR, Adams AM, et al. Reduced lung-cancer mortality with low-dose computed tomographic screening. N Engl J Med 2011;365:395–409.

28. Stock C, Brenner H, Centers for Disease Control and Prevention (CDC). Vital signs: colorectal cancer screening among adults aged 50-75 years - United States, 2008. MMWR Morb Mortal Wkly Rep 2010;59:808–12.

29. Stock C, Brenner H. Utilization of lower gastrointestinal endoscopy and fecal occult blood test in 11

European countries: evidence from the Survey of Health, Aging and Retirement in Europe (SHARE). Endoscopy 2010;42:546–56.

30. Tengs TO, Wallace A. One thousand health-related quality-of-life estimates. Med Care 2000;38:583–637.

31. Pignone M, Saha S, Hoerger T, et al. Cost-effectiveness analyses of colorectal cancer screening: a systematic review for the U.S. Preventive Services Task Force. Ann Intern Med 2002;137:96–104.

32. Lansdorp-Vogelaar I, van Ballegooijen M, Zauber AG, et al. Effect of rising chemotherapy costs on the cost savings of colorectal cancer screening. J Natl Cancer Inst 2009;101:1412–22.

33. Pickhardt PJ, Taylor AJ. Extracolonic findings identified in asymptomatic adults at screening CT colonography. AJR Am J Roentgenol 2006;186:718–28.

34. Xiong T, Richardson M, Woodroffe R, et al. Incidental lesions found on CT colonography: their nature and frequency. Br J Radiol 2005;78:22–9.

35. Gluecker TM, Johnson CD, Wilson LA, et al. Extracolonic findings at CT colonography: evaluation of prevalence and cost in a screening population. Gastroenterology 2003;124:911–6.

36. Khan KY, Xiong T, McCafferty I, et al. Frequency and impact of extracolonic findings detected at computed tomographic colonography in a symptomatic population. Br J Surg 2007;94:355–61.

37. Stoop EM, de Haan MC, de Wijkerslooth TR, et al. Participation and yield of colonoscopy versus non-cathartic CT colonography in population-based screening for colorectal cancer: a randomised controlled trial. Lancet Oncol 2012;13:55–64.

38. Pickhardt PJ. Strong evidence in support of CT colonography screening. Lancet Oncol 2012;13:6–7.

39. Pooler BD, Baumel MJ, Cash BD, et al. Screening CT colonography: multicenter survey of patient experience, preference, and potential impact on adherence. AJR Am J Roentgenol 2012;198:1361–6.

40. Hassan C, Hunink MG, Laghi A, et al. Value-of-information analysis to guide future research in colorectal cancer screening. Radiology 2009;253:745–52.

Magnetic Resonance Enterography

David J. Grand, MD[a],*, Michael Beland, MD[a],
Adam Harris, MD[b]

KEYWORDS

- Magnetic resonance enterography • Inflammatory bowel disease
- Computed tomography enterography • Crohn's disease

KEY POINTS

- Magnetic resonance (MR) enterography is a targeted examination of the gastrointestinal tract, particularly the small intestine, without nasojejunal intubation (in which case it is referred to as MR enteroclysis).
- MR enterography has been shown to be highly effective in the diagnosis and management of patients with Crohn's disease.
- Additional information, beyond anatomy, available at MR imaging, including T2 signal, diffusion weighting, and dynamic contrast enhancement, will likely be shown to improve our ability to confidently differentiate active inflammation from chronic, fibrostenotic disease.
- MR enterography should be considered a first-line imaging modality for young patients with known or suspected Crohn's disease and, when clinically indicated, to monitor response to potent medical therapies.

INTRODUCTION

Until recently, magnetic resonance (MR) imaging of the small bowel could not reliably compete with the high-quality small bowel images generated by CT. Now, however, MR imaging evaluation of the small bowel, commonly referred to as MR enterography, is not only a feasible alternative to CT, but may provide superior diagnostic information, specifically with regard to differentiating active, inflammatory disease from chronic, fibrostenotic disease. MR enterography is no longer merely adequate and radiation-free; it is an essential part of the imaging armamentarium.

WHAT IS MR ENTEROGRAPHY?

MR enterography is a targeted examination of the gastrointestinal tract, particularly the small intestine, without nasojejunal intubation (in which case it is referred to as MR enteroclysis). The most common indication for MR enterography is known or suspected inflammatory bowel disease (IBD), specifically Crohn's disease. The authors occasionally get requests for MR enterography for anemia or to evaluate for small bowel mass. Despite relishing the technique, one continues to steer these requests to computed tomography (CT) enterography, which is better suited for these indications because of its superior spatial and temporal resolution. But for IBD, and specifically Crohn's disease, MR enterography provides all of the diagnostic information of CT enterography (and possibly more) without exposing patients to ionizing radiation.

WHY PERFORM MR ENTEROGRAPHY?

Despite advances in endoscopic techniques and the ease with which gastroenterologists directly

[a] Department of Diagnostic Imaging, Warren Alpert School of Medicine, Brown University, 593 Eddy Street, Providence, RI 02903, USA; [b] Department of Gastroenterology, Warren Alpert School of Medicine, Brown University, 110 Lockwood Street, Suite 116, Providence, RI 02903, USA
* Corresponding author.
E-mail address: dgrand@lifespan.org

Radiol Clin N Am 51 (2013) 99–112
http://dx.doi.org/10.1016/j.rcl.2012.09.007

visualize the colon, the small bowel remains relatively inaccessible. Capsule endoscopy has been shown to be highly effective in the diagnosis of nonstricturing Crohn's disease[1]; however, it is not ideally suited to IBD patients who may have occult strictures wherein capsule can become lodged, requiring surgical intervention. Capsule endoscopy is therefore contraindicated in any patient suspected of having a stricture, unless a patency capsule is first used.[2] Asymptomatic partial small bowel obstruction, which can lead to capsule retention, has been reported in up to 17% of patients with Crohn's disease.[3] Increasingly complex endoscopic techniques such as double-balloon enteroscopy can directly visualize the mucosa of the entire gastrointestinal tract, but are time consuming and not widely available. In everyday practice, therefore, small bowel imaging remains the domain of the radiologist.

In the past 2 decades, there has been a seismic shift in the use of imaging for Crohn's disease away from small bowel follow-through (SBFT) to cross-sectional techniques, most commonly CT enterography and MR enterography. Because of rapid advances in CT and MR imaging hardware, as well as routine use of oral contrast agents designed to distend the lumen of the small bowel, cross-sectional techniques have become a first-line imaging modality, promising accurate assessment of the mucosa as well as the extraintestinal manifestations of penetrating disease. In most situations, the choice of cross-sectional modality (clinically) is essentially a trade-off between the ease and cost of the study (which favor CT enterography) and the desire to minimize radiation exposure (which favors MR enterography).

CT enterography is an excellent test. It is widely available, relatively inexpensive, well tolerated, and provides the gastroenterologist with a plethora of diagnostic information in a very short period of time. The efficacy of CT enterography has been repeatedly proved in clinical trials, and the technique has gained widespread acceptance. Mayo Clinic, for example, reported a nearly 10-fold increase in its use between 2001 and 2004.[4] This marked increase has occurred in parallel with decreased use of the fluoroscopic SBFT, which CT enterography has largely replaced. As the use of CT for IBD (as well as a myriad of other indications) has expanded, so have concerns regarding the associated radiation exposure.

The potential negative consequences of exposure to diagnostic radiation warrant brief discussion, as they are now in the forefront of the minds of clinicians, radiologists, and patients alike.[5] Two recent studies evaluated the radiation dose associated with commonly ordered CT scans

as well as the potential risk of radiation-induced cancer attributable to CT scans alone.[6,7] The investigators calculated a projected rate of CT-induced cancer of 1 per 250 20-year-old females and 1 per 330 20-year-old males who underwent multiphase CT abdomen/pelvis.

It is critical to remember, though, that these risks are theoretical and are based on principles that are at least questioned, if not rejected, by many medical physicists.[8] However, regardless of whether we can quantify the specific risk(s) of medical radiation, we can all agree that we should strive to limit exposure to the lowest possible dose necessary for diagnosis: the so-called ALARA principle (As Low As Reasonably Achievable).[9]

CT enterography exposes patients to up to 5 times the ionizing radiation dose of the typical SBFT, the test it has largely replaced.[10] That said, the radiation dose from a single CT enterography scan is not high enough to be particularly concerning. Newer CT techniques have demonstrated a significant decrease in radiation dose using modified protocols and reconstruction algorithms.[11,12] One recent study demonstrated that a 50% reduction in dose could be achieved without sacrificing sensitivity for acute inflammation.[13] CT radiation doses will undoubtedly fall even further as advances in scanner hardware and software technology continue to improve.

Despite the uncertainty regarding the true risk of radiation exposure, the IBD population has 2 important characteristics that should alert physicians to use radiation judiciously. First, patients are typically young at the time of initial presentation, and second, will often require numerous examinations throughout their lives. Indeed, the increased lifetime radiation exposure of IBD patients compared with the general population has been well documented; the majority of this exposure is due to repeated CT examinations.[14]

All medical decisions should be informed by analyzing the potential risks and benefits of any course of action as well as the potential risks and benefits of inaction. Coordination between emergency room, primary care, and gastrointestinal physicians is critical to minimize unnecessary radiation exposure in young IBD patients. Radiation exposure should not be a concern in the elderly (in whom the risk is very small) or in patients who are acutely ill (in whom the potential benefit is very high). Overall, CT enterography is too useful clinically, and cost-effective,[15] to avoid based solely on radiation concerns. When used appropriately, it is a powerful tool to aid in the diagnosis and management of Crohn's disease.

Of course, mindful of all the caveats listed, we can all agree that the best radiation dose is no radiation dose. In addition, because MR enterography involves no ionizing radiation, we can use it differently than we use CT enterography. For example:

1. MR enterography is always performed precontrast and with multiple postcontrast phases, allowing contrast enhancement to be evaluated dynamically.
2. MR enterography allows evaluation of each bowel segment at multiple time points, which may facilitate differentiation of stricture from peristalsis as well as small bowel function. (Fig. 1)
3. MR enterography can be used to monitor response to powerful biological therapies without the patient incurring additional risk.[16–18]
4. MR enterography may be a useful, noninvasive, radiation-free method of screening high-risk patients for subclinical intestinal inflammation.[19]

HOW IS MR ENTEROGRAPHY PERFORMED?

There is no single correct way to perform MR enterography although a good, basic MR enterography protocol has common elements, including:

1. Appropriate anatomic coverage
2. Small bowel distension
3. Precontrast imaging: rapid sequences to delineate anatomy without blurring
4. Fluid-sensitive sequence: to evaluate for bowel wall and mesenteric edema
5. Pharmacologic bowel paralysis
6. Dynamic, contrast-enhanced imaging

Appropriate Anatomic Coverage

MR enterography is a targeted examination of the intestinal tract. Perirectal and perianal complications are very common in Crohn's disease, with a lifetime risk of perianal fistula formation ranging from 30% to 50%.[20] While the authors' routine MR enterography protocol does not include high-resolution, small field-of-view imaging to carefully delineate fistulae, it is certainly robust enough to detect or exclude the majority of penetrating complications as long the anatomic coverage is appropriate.

The most common mistake made in this regard is failing to scan inferior enough to visualize perianal disease. Technologists should therefore be instructed to scan until air is visualized between the patient's thighs, ensuring that the perineum is adequately covered. To obtain the entire perineum and the all of the small bowel within a single coronal field of view often requires excluding a portion of the liver and spleen, which is perfectly appropriate for this examination.[21]

Small Bowel Distension

Adequate distension of the small bowel is critical for reliable and reproducible diagnostic enterography, as it facilitates evaluation of both mucosal enhancement and bowel wall thickening. If the lumen is not distended, the mucosa cannot be evaluated accurately. In addition, collapsed bowel segments are too easily mistaken for pathologic thickening of the bowel wall.

Water will not distend the terminal ileum and is therefore not an acceptable oral contrast agent. A hyperosmolar solution is required.

In addition to distending the small bowel, oral contrast agents should be hypointense ("dark") on T1-weighted images to allow evaluation of the adjacent, brightly enhancing mucosa. Contrast agents that are hypointense on both T1-weighted and T2-weighted images may be additionally

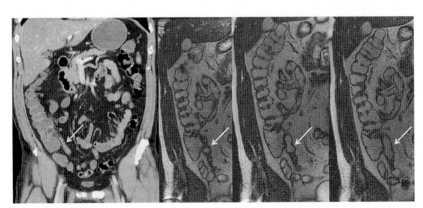

Fig. 1. Value of cine images. Coronal CT image from CT enterography demonstrates a possible terminal ileal stricture (*arrow*). Three sample real-time cine images from follow-up MR enterography demonstrate normal peristalsis of the terminal ileum, indicating that it was simply collapsed.

helpful, but are not in widespread use because of their relatively high cost and poor palatability.

In the literature there is no shortage of effective oral contrast preparations for enterography. As a general rule, as the osmolality of the agent increases, the side effects (nausea, diarrhea, and flatulence) increase and the palatability decreases.[22,23] At the authors' institution, low-density barium sulfate suspension (VoLumen; E-Z-EM, Lake Success, NY) 0.1% is routinely used for both CT enterography and MR enterography, which is reasonably well tolerated and reasonably effective.

The volume and timing of oral contrast also varies among institutions. It is difficult to administer too much oral contrast, keeping in mind that one does not want the patient to be uncomfortable or need to evacuate during the examination. Patients are asked to drink 450 mL VoLumen (1 bottle) over 15 minutes, beginning 45 minutes before imaging; they are then given a second bottle to drink over the next 15 minutes and finally 450 mL of water 15 minutes before imaging begins. Water is used immediately before imaging because it is intended only to distend the proximal small bowel, so the amount of hyperosmolar fluid administered, and its subsequent side effects, can therefore be reduced (Fig. 2).

Unfortunately, in daily practice the distension achieved by oral contrast agents is variable. This variation is in part due to physiologic differences in bowel motility, but successful bowel distension is also dependent on the patients' ability and,

more importantly, their willingness to drink the contrast. (Anecdotally, even a very brief conversation with the patient regarding the utility of oral contrast can go a long way to maximizing the quality of the oral prep.) Overall, however, routine use of oral agents has been shown to be reliable and significantly better tolerated than enteroclysis.[24,25] While enteroclysis (performed with fluoroscopy, CT, or MR) may still have a role for detection of low-grade small bowel obstruction, it is not routinely performed at the authors' institution and is not necessary for routine evaluation of IBD.

In light of the foregoing discussion regarding the importance of oral contrast, it is worth considering the not entirely unusual situation whereby the patient will not or cannot drink any or all of the oral contrast. In this situation, the authors first discuss the value of oral contrast with the patient face to face to inform them that the oral contrast is not simply something given routinely or without thinking but because it genuinely improves the ability to help them. As already mentioned, this "face-time" with the radiologist can be surprisingly effective.

If the patient still cannot or will not drink the contrast, the study is performed without it. Many patients who refuse to drink the oral contrast do so because they are too sick to tolerate it. Anecdotally, the findings in these patients will often be significant enough that they will be detected without the additional sensitivity provided by good bowel distension.

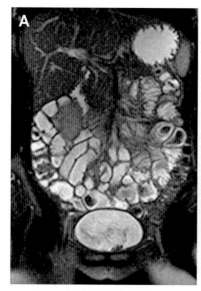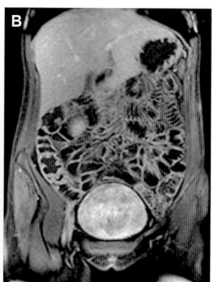

Fig. 2. Excellent bowel distension. Coronal single-shot fast spin-echo (A) and T1-weighted, fat-saturated, postcontrast-enhanced images (B) demonstrate excellent small bowel distension. Note also that coverage includes the entire perineum, even to the exclusion of the superior margins of the liver and spleen.

Precontrast Imaging: Rapid Sequences

Two rapid sequences are routinely performed before the contrast-enhanced images: steady-state free-precession (to be discussed here) and single-shot fast spin-echo, to be discussed in the next section.

Steady-state free-precession sequences are most commonly used for cine imaging during cardiac MR imaging examinations. For MR enterography they are used for 2 reasons: they are fast, essentially eliminating blurring or motion artifacts, and they provide excellent delineation of anatomy.

Having a clear layout of the intestinal anatomy is critical so that one can easily, and definitively, find the terminal ileum, the most commonly affected bowel segment in Crohn's disease. In addition, because the anatomy is so clear on these images, one can search for abnormally kinked or tethered bowel segments that imply entero-entero fistula formation. Finally, many patients have undergone multiple bowel resections for prior bouts of IBD, which can make arduous the seemingly simple task of knowing what portion of the bowel resides where within the abdomen.

Fluid-Sensitive Sequence

A fluid-sensitive (T2-weighted) sequence is critical to good MR enterography and may be responsible for one of MR enterography's advantages over CT enterography. The authors use a fat-saturated, single-shot, fast spin echo.

Single-shot fast spin-echo has the advantage of being quite rapid, effectively eliminating bowel motion (even when performed before administration of bowel paralytics). The trade-off is that, in the authors' experience, it is less fluid-sensitive than a fast spin-echo or inversion recovery sequence, but those more heavily T2-weighted sequences are simply too slow for evaluating the small bowel.

Because this sequence is performed with fat-saturation, the gastrointestinal tract anatomy may be challenging to delineate or follow. Therefore, they are used and interpreted in conjunction with the steady-state free-precession images. This sequence is used simply to detect fluid/edema within or adjacent to the bowel.

Bowel Paralysis

Evaluation of the small bowel with MR enterography faces one major hurdle: bowel motion. Although MR pulse sequences have become increasingly fast, a single series can require greater than 20 seconds of imaging time, during which any bowel motion blurs the resulting image. This issue really only concerns the contrast-enhanced images, as the remainder of the commonly used pulse sequences for MR enterography (single-shot fast spin-echo and steady-state free-precession) are sufficiently rapid. Unfortunately, while the contrast-enhanced images are the most susceptible to motion, they are also the most critical.

Most centers therefore administer pharmacologic bowel paralytics to minimize small bowel motion. Specific techniques vary between institutions; however, in the United States 0.5 to 1 mg of glucagon is most commonly used whether injected intravenously or intramuscularly, in single or split doses. These agents are not necessary for CT enterography, owing to the speed of acquisition of modern multidetector CT scanners. However, just as the radiation dose of CT enterography is certain to decrease, the speed of MR pulse sequences will certainly increase in the near future, which may render this problem irrelevant.

To those who were sensible enough to use pharmacologic agents to minimize small bowel motion from the very beginning, the following will come as no surprise: MR enterography image quality is better and images are easier to interpret when such agents are used. In an effort to simplify the protocol, minimize expense, and maximize patient tolerance, initially a pharmacologic agent to minimize motion was not used. Despite a subjective decrease in image quality, the authors were able not only to achieve diagnostic equivalency to CT enterography but also overall accuracy (compared with endoscopy and pathology) equivalent to that published in the literature.[26,27]

That said, glucagon is now used for all MR enterography scans unless there is a contraindication, most commonly concomitant diabetes or pregnancy. (If there is a contraindication, the study is performed without it.) Why give glucagon if the results were equivalent to CT enterography without it? The job is difficult enough. There is no need make it more difficult by trying to read through bowel motion, nor is avoiding a relatively innocuous dose of glucagon worth potentially missing a subtle finding that could otherwise be obscured.

Similar to the small bowel distension achieved by orally administered contrast agents, the "paralysis" achieved by glucagon (the only such agent available in the United States) is highly variable. Occasionally the images are superlative and occasionally the images appear as though no agent were given. Most often, the result is somewhere in between.

At their institution, the authors currently administer 0.5 mg glucagon intravenously immediately before the contrast-enhanced images. Glucagon is not needed at the beginning of the study, because the precontrast imaging (as already discussed) is sufficiently rapid that it is not compromised by bowel motion.

Glucagon is administered intravenously because the patients already have an IV catheter and the time of onset of glucagon given intravenously is essentially immediate. The technologist administers the glucagon and a subsequent saline flush over the course of 5 full minutes. If the patient vomits, the glucagon (or saline flush) has been administered too quickly. Since switching from 1 mg to 0.5 mg of glucagon, there has been no episode of vomiting.

The patient is then returned to the bore of the scanner, injected with gadolinium, and the postcontrast images are performed.

Contrast-Enhanced Imaging

Contrast-enhanced imaging is a critical part of MR enterography. (If the patient cannot receive gadolinium, most commonly because of pregnancy, the study is performed without it.) The specific gadolinium agent is irrelevant. A standard, "single" dose of gadobutrol injected at 2 mL/s is used, followed by a saline flush and a standard volume interpolated breath-hold gradient-echo pulse sequence. These breath-holds can be relatively long, and the patients should be properly coached by the technologist as to the importance of good breath-holding.

Postcontrast imaging should be performed dynamically and, given that one would wish to cover the entire abdomen and pelvis in a breath-hold, imaging is done in the coronal plane. The first dynamic phase should be in (or near) the "enteric" phase. Imaging is done at 45 seconds, although the exact timing is probably inconsequential.

The abdomen and pelvis are then imaged in the axial plane, which better delineates the anatomy and helps specifically locate and characterize extraintestinal findings. Coronal imaging of the abdomen and pelvis is then repeated, which serves as the "delayed" phase.

Optional Sequences

Diffusion-weighted (DW) imaging is advocated by some investigators as a means of more easily identifying active inflammation and distinguishing it from chronic, fibrotic disease. At least one study demonstrated excellent accuracy and reproducibility using DW imaging to detect active inflammation. Additional studies have shown promising results using DW imaging to detect fistulas and even to grade their inflammatory activity.[28,29] Although the mechanism of restricted diffusion in active inflammatory processes is not known, the apparent efficacy of the technique warrants further investigation.[30]

Chemical shift (in/out of phase) imaging should perhaps be part of all MR imaging examinations of the abdomen/pelvis to help characterize incidentally detected lesions in the solid organs. The authors have recently removed it from their standard MR enterography protocol because of the very low incidence of incidentalomas that have been detected despite a large number of MR enterography scans performed, perhaps because of the relatively young age of the MR enterography patients. The authors view MR enterography as a targeted examination of the small intestine for the detection and evaluation of Crohn's disease. Because chemical shift imaging does not add useful information regarding IBD, it has been eliminated.

Real-time cine imaging of the small bowel is a promising technique used as a problem-solving tool in specific patients. One advantage of MR enterography over CT enterography is the ability to evaluate bowel segments at multiple time point; however, this does not replace the true functional information of SBFT. If a segment of bowel remains decompressed throughout the standard MR enterography examination, and an underlying stricture cannot confidently be excluded, real-time cine imaging is used to evaluate for peristalsis. In addition, at least one small study has shown that routine use of cine imaging may increase detection of abnormal intestinal segments.[31] The investigators believe that altered bowel motility may be an early sign of inflammatory changes within a bowel segment.

The authors have found this technique to be useful in select cases, and it will likely become a standard part of the protocol. However, maximizing its utility requires a radiologist to closely monitor the examination while it is in progress and prescribe the specific slice location where cine information is desired.

Finally, a word on patient positioning. At present, the patient is imaged in the supine position, simply because it is the most comfortable position for most patients, particularly those with abdominal pain. Some investigators have advocated imaging in the prone position, which minimizes patients' anterior-posterior dimension (and therefore may decrease coronal acquisition times), may improve bowel distension, and may minimize bowel motion. However, despite these apparent advantages, investigators to date have been unable to demonstrate improved detection of lesions.[32]

INTERPRETATION OF MR ENTEROGRAPHY

For radiologists accustomed to CT enterography, MR enterography can initially be intimidating because of the number of sequences, some of which may be unfamiliar, as well as the sheer volume of images. Fear not. With experience, interpretation of MR enterography quickly becomes a pleasant part of routine practice. There is no single correct approach. The critical element of interpretation is simply to keep in mind what each sequence adds to the overall value of the examination.

Steady-State Free-Precession

This rapid sequence is used for 2 reasons: first, to get an overall layout of the bowel anatomy including whether the patient has undergone prior bowel resection and, if so, of what segments; and second, to identify bowel wall thickening which, when significant, typically indicates active inflammation.

Single-Shot Fast Spin-Echo

This sequence identifies edema/fluid in the bowel wall and in the mesentery. This finding can be the most difficult to detect, and is often complicated by inhomogeneous fat-saturation and artifacts from intraluminal air and T2 bright oral contrast. These difficulties decrease the sensitivity of abnormally elevated T2 signal, but when it is present, it is highly specific for active inflammation.

Contrast-Enhanced Images

The contrast-enhanced images are the highest-yield sequences in the examination. Precontrast imaging is always obtained in order to be certain that anything that is bright on the postcontrast images is truly enhancement as opposed to some residual T1-bright bowel contents within the bowel lumen.

On the enteric phase images, the first postcontrast acquisition, early enhancement is evaluated. Early enhancement, particularly when it is mucosal or laminar, indicates active inflammation (Fig. 3). One should also evaluate for the "comb sign" or engorgement of the mesenteric vasculature, which is also a fairly reliable indicator of active inflammation (see further discussion below).

Beware of one common potential pitfall: the normal enhancement of the jejunum is greater than that of the remainder of the small bowel. What would be hyperenhancement of the terminal ileum can be normal in the jejunum (Fig. 4). Before reporting jejunal disease, one should look carefully for wall thickening or abnormal T2 signal on the preceding sequences.

Both active inflammation and chronic fibrotic disease will enhance on the delayed images, although typically the enhancement is far more dramatic in active inflammation. In addition, the enhancement in chronic, fibrostenotic disease is typically confined to the bowel wall as opposed to involving the adjacent mesenteric fat (Fig. 5).

Finally, when attempting to distinguish active inflammation from chronic, fibrostenotic disease, it should be remembered that only very rarely does one truly exist without any component of the other. It is therefore more accurate to think of abnormal findings as predominantly active or predominantly chronic.

FINDINGS IN CROHN'S DISEASE

The findings that indicate Crohn's disease on MR enterography include bowel wall thickening, abnormal enhancement, engorgement of the mesenteric vasculature, and elevated T2 signal within or adjacent to the bowel wall.[33] Bowel wall thickening is diagnosed when the small bowel wall exceeds 3 mm in thickness in a well-distended bowel loop.

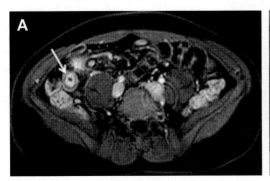 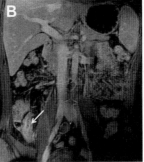

Fig. 3. Active Crohn's disease. Axial and coronal, T1-weighted, fat-saturated, postcontrast images (A, B) demonstrating a laminar enhancement pattern on enteric phase imaging compatible with active inflammation (arrow).

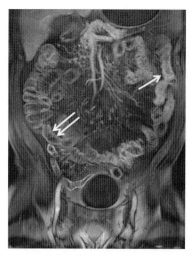

Fig. 4. Normal jejunal enhancement. Coronal T1-weighted, fat-saturated, postcontrast image demonstrates normal enhancement of the jejunum (*single arrow*), which is often more pronounced than the normal enhancement of the terminal ileum (*double arrow*). To avoid "overcalling" jejunal disease, look also for wall thickening and abnormal T2 signal.

The presence of bowel wall thickening in conjunction with asymmetric mural hyperenhancement is essentially pathognomonic for Crohn's disease.[34] The comb sign refers to engorgement of the vasa recta and is highly suggestive of active inflammation.[35] Mesenteric lymphadenopathy and fibrofatty proliferation are also commonly described as findings in Crohn's disease though they are likely less specific and provide less information regarding disease activity.

As discussed previously, elevated T2 signal, though it may be difficult to detect, is caused by the presence of fluid and is a highly specific indicator of an active inflammatory process[36] (**Figs. 6** and **7**). The pattern of abnormal enhancement is also critical for attempting to differentiate active,

inflammatory disease from chronic, fibrostenotic disease. A stratified enhancement pattern on early-phase dynamic, contrast-enhanced images demonstrating brisk enhancement of the mucosa, a dark submucosa, and a bright serosal layer has been shown to be specific for active inflammation.[37–39]

The ability to evaluate the T2 signal of the bowel wall and to evaluate contrast enhancement dynamically is unique to MR enterography. These elements (perhaps in conjunction with DW imaging) will likely allow more confident distinction of active inflammatory disease from chronic fibrostenotic disease; this is the "holy grail" of IBD imaging. If this distinction can be made accurately, gastroenterologists can more effectively triage patients to potent medical therapy versus surgical intervention, and avoid the morbidity inherent in misclassification in either direction. This use of MR enterography as a means of guiding patient therapy has been shown to be highly effective in small studies (**Fig. 8**).[40]

The configuration of the bowel loops should also be carefully evaluated on every MR enterography examination. Abnormally kinked loops or loops that appear tethered suggest entero-entero fistulae. Often a T2-bright, enhancing tract can be seen connecting these loops to one another (**Fig. 9**). MR enterography can also reliably detect intra-abdominal abscesses, which are typically bright on T2-weighted images, with a peripheral rim of enhancement and extraintestinal manifestations of Crohn's disease such as sacroillitis.[41,42]

More recent investigations have gone beyond simply detecting active Crohn's disease to true quantitative assessment of disease severity and activity. Rimola and colleagues[43] have developed one such classification (based on wall thickness, degree of enhancement, T2 signal, and presence of ulceration), which in a study of 48 patients demonstrated excellent correlation with the Crohn's Disease Endoscopic Index of Severity (CDEIS). Another study of 55 patients demonstrated that patients could be classified based on MR imaging findings, which accurately predicted response to medical therapy versus need for surgery.[44] Accurate categorization of disease activity and severity is critical to guide treatment choices and may be helpful in monitoring response to treatment, a powerful and exciting application of this noninvasive, radiation-free technique (**Fig. 10**).

PERFORMANCE OF MR ENTEROGRAPHY

The efficacy of MR enterography has now been repeatedly proved within the radiology and gastroenterology literature. It is important to remember

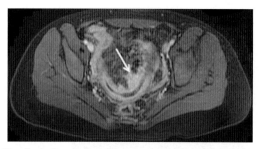

Fig. 5. Active Crohn's disease. Axial T1-weighted, fat-saturated, postcontrast image demonstrating abnormal enhancement that is not particularly mucosal or laminar, but extends through the bowel wall to involve the mesenteric fat (*arrow*). This appearance indicates active disease.

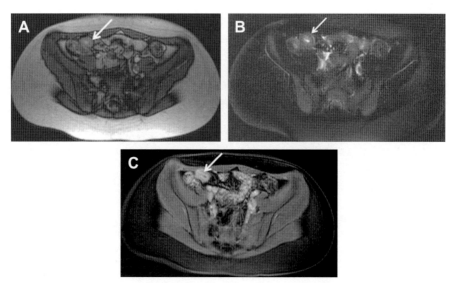

Fig. 6. Active Crohn's disease. Axial steady-state free-precession image (*A*) shows circumferential thickening of the terminal ileum (*arrow*). Axial, single-shot, fast spin-echo image (*B*) demonstrates abnormally elevated T2 signal within and adjacent to the bowel wall (*arrow*). Axial, T1-weighted, fat-saturated, postcontrast image (*C*) shows laminar enhancement of the small bowel (*arrow*). Findings are compatible with mild, active terminal ileitis.

when interpreting the data that MR enterography is most commonly judged against the gold standard of ileocolonoscopy, CT enterography, or both. These standards, however, are far from perfect and are of particular concern in the Crohn population because of the prevalence of stenotic ileocecal valves, disease skipping of the terminal ileum, and intramural Crohn inflammation. In one large series of patients with suspected Crohn's disease and normal endoscopic examination of the terminal ileum, 54% actually had active small

bowel disease when radiologic, serologic, and clinical factors were used as the reference standard.[45] Another endoscopic study reported an inability to adequately evaluate the terminal ileum in nearly 28% of patients.[2]

CT enterography is a natural fit for comparison with MR enterography, as both can evaluate the entire abdominal/pelvic gastrointestinal tract. It is possible, however, that MR enterography may be more sensitive for subtle mucosal and mesenteric changes attributable to superior soft-tissue

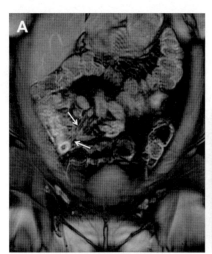

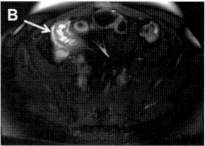

Fig. 7. Active Crohn's disease. Coronal, T1-weighted, fat-saturated, postcontrast image (*A*) demonstrates engorgement of the mesenteric vasculature (*arrows*), often referred to as the Comb sign. Axial, single-shot, fast spin-echo image (*B*) shows abnormally elevated T2 signal within and adjacent to the same loop of small bowel (*arrow*). Findings are compatible with active Crohn's disease.

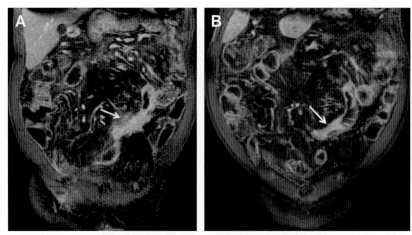

Fig. 8. Response to biological therapy. Coronal, T1-weighted, fat-saturated, postcontrast images of patient with Crohn's disease before (*A*) and after (*B*) initiating therapy with anti–tumor necrosis factor therapy, demonstrating dramatic decrease in enhancement (*arrow*) following treatment, indicating excellent response to therapy.

contrast and therefore, once again, false-positive MR enterography results need to be interpreted in the appropriate context.

Overall, the diagnostic efficacy of MR enterography has been shown to be equivalent to that of CT enterography. Lee and colleagues[46] demonstrated identical accuracies of 87% for CT enterography and MR enterography identification of Crohn's disease within the terminal ileum, compared with colonoscopy, in 30 patients. Diagnostic

equivalence has since been verified by multiple additional investigators with similar reported accuracies.[47,48] It is critical that, although not surprising, MR enterography has been shown to be equally effective in both the adult and pediatric populations.[49,50] Obviously the efficacy of MR enterography is particularly exciting for pediatric patients who are thought to be more sensitive to the potentially deleterious effects of ionizing radiation. In fact, some investigators have suggested

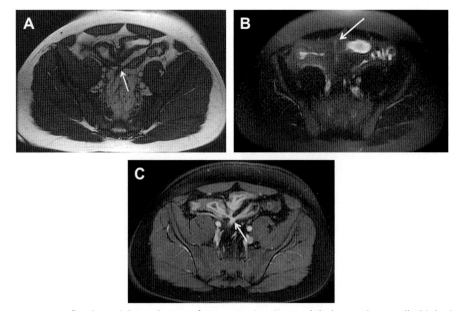

Fig. 9. Entero-entero fistula. Axial steady-state free-precession image (*A*) shows abnormally kinked, tethered bowel loops (*arrow*). Axial single-shot, fast spin-echo image (*B*) demonstrates a T2 bright channel connecting the loops (*arrow*), which enhances on postcontrast image (*C, arrow*). Findings are compatible with actively inflamed, entero-entero fistula.

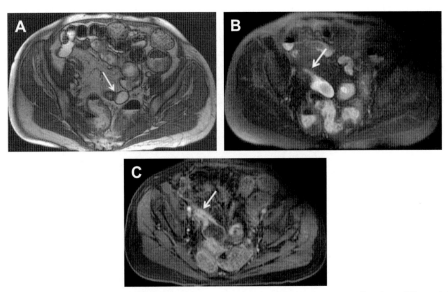

Fig. 10. Chronic stricture. Axial, steady-state free-precession image (A) demonstrates focal small bowel thickening with upstream dilatation (*arrow*). There is no evidence of abnormal T2 signal on single-shot, fast spin-echo image (B, arrow). There is enhancement on postcontrast image (C), but it is mild and does not extend through the bowel wall (*arrow*).

that MR enterography can replace CT enterography as a first-line imaging modality for patients suspected of having Crohn's disease.[51] At the authors' institution, it certainly has.

Because of its inherent, exquisite soft-tissue contrast, MR imaging is the gold standard for detection and characterization of perianal fistulae.

Accurate characterization is critical for surgical planning, and MR enterography easily depicts the relationship of fistulae to the sphincter complexes. MR enterography is clearly superior to CT enterography in this regard, and has also been shown to be more effective than clinical examination and endosonography (**Fig. 11**).[52,53]

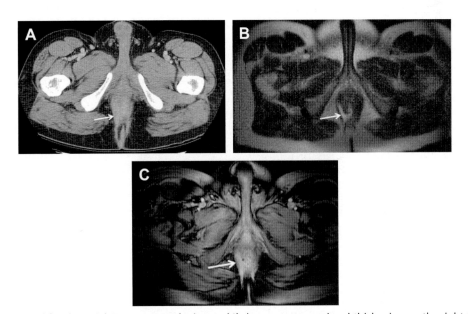

Fig. 11. Perianal fistula. Axial CT enterography image (A) demonstrates perianal thickening on the right (*arrow*), suspicious for perianal fistula formation. This feature is much better seen and characterized on axial single-shot, fast spin-echo image (B, arrow) and axial postcontrast image (C, arrow).

CT ENTEROGRAPHY VERSUS MR ENTEROGRAPHY: HOW TO CHOOSE

The algorithm for deciding between CT enterography or MR enterography to evaluate known or suspected Crohn's disease varies between institutions. As discussed earlier, there is now an abundance of literature demonstrating that the 2 tests are diagnostically equivalent.

CT enterography is more widely available. It is faster and easier for the patient and may be easier to interpret, particularly for the inexperienced.

MR enterography involves no ionizing radiation. It may provide additional information based on T2 signal, DW imaging, dynamic contrast enhancement, and the ability to image bowel segments over time, but it is more expensive and more difficult for the patient because of the increased time in the scanner and breath-holding requirements. At the authors' institution:

> *For young patients with known or suspected IBD, MR enterography is recommended.* The authors do so knowing that if they have IBD they will likely require numerous examinations and that if they later present to the emergency room with abdominal pain they will almost certainly undergo a CT scan.
>
> *When perianal disease is suspected, MR enterography is recommended.* The routine MR enterography protocol allows confident assessment of the entire bowel as well the anus. Small perianal fistulae are simply too difficult to see on CT and too clinically important to miss.
>
> *When the clinical question is active versus chronic disease in a patient with known IBD, MR enterography is recommended.* The authors are more confident assessing disease activity with the additional information of T2 signal and dynamic contrast enhancement than with a single phase of injection.
>
> *In patients older than 50 years or with any indication other than known or suspected IBD, CT enterography is recommended.* CT enterography is fast, reliable, and easy to interpret. In older patients or patients with questionable symptoms, it is the test of choice.

SUMMARY

MR enterography has been shown to be highly effective in the diagnosis and management of patients with Crohn's disease. Multiple studies demonstrate equivalent accuracy to CT without exposing patients to ionizing radiation. Additional information, beyond anatomy, available at MR imaging including T2 signal, diffusion weighting, and dynamic contrast enhancement will likely be shown to improve our ability to confidently differentiate active inflammation from chronic, fibrostenotic disease. For these reasons, MR enterography should be considered a first-line imaging modality for young patients with known or suspected Crohn's disease and, when clinically indicated, to monitor response to potent medical therapies.

REFERENCES

1. Dionisio PM, Gurudu SR, Leighton JA, et al. Capsule endoscopy has a significantly higher diagnostic yield in patients with suspected and established small-bowel Crohn's disease: a meta-analysis. Am J Gastroenterol 2010;105:1240–7.
2. Horsthuis K, Stokkers PC, Stoker J. Detection of inflammatory bowel disease: diagnostic performance of cross-sectional imaging modalities. Abdom Imaging 2008;33:407–16.
3. Solem CA, Loftus EV, Fletcher JG, et al. Small bowel imaging in Crohn's disease: a prospective, blinded, 4-way comparison trial. Gastrointest Endosc 2008; 68(2):255–66.
4. Paulson SR, Huprich JE, Fletcher JG, et al. CT enterography as a diagnostic tool in evaluating small bowel disorders: review of clinical experience with over 700 cases. Radiographics 2006;26:641–62.
5. Brenner DJ, Hall EJ. Computed tomography—an increasing source of radiation exposure. N Engl J Med 2007;357:2277–84.
6. Smith-Bendman R, Lipson J, Marcus R, et al. Radiation dose associated with common computed tomographic examinations and the associated lifetime attributable risk of cancer. Arch Intern Med 2009; 169(22):2078–86.
7. Berrington de Gonzalez A, Mahadevappa M, Kwang-Pyo K, et al. Projected cancer risks from computed tomographic scans performed in the United States in 2007. Arch Intern Med 2009;169(22):2071–7.
8. Tubiana M, Feinendegen LE, Yang C, et al. The linear no-threshold relationship is inconsistent with radiation biologic and experimental data. Radiology 2009;251:13–22.
9. Title 10, Section 20.1003, Code of federal regulations.
10. Jaffe TA, Gaca AM, Delaney S, et al. Radiation doses from small-bowel follow-through and abdominopelvic MDCT in Crohn's disease. AJR Am J Roentgenol 2007;189:1015–22.
11. Silva AC, Lawder HJ, Hara A, et al. Innovations in CT dose reduction strategy: application of the adaptive statistical iterative reconstruction algorithm. AJR Am J Roentgenol 2010;194(1):191–9.

12. Siddiki H, Fletcher JG, Hara AK, et al. Validation of a lower radiation computed tomography enterography imaging protocol to detect Crohn's disease in the small bowel. Inflamm Bowel Dis 2011;17(3): 778–86.

13. Lee SJ, Park SH, Kim AY, et al. A prospective comparison of standard-dose CT enterography and 50% reduced-dose CT enterography with and without noise reduction for evaluating Crohn's disease. AJR Am J Roentgenol 2011;197:50–7.

14. Peloquin JM, Pardi DS, Sandborn WJ, et al. Diagnostic ionizing radiation exposure in a population-based cohort of patients with inflammatory bowel disease. Am J Gastroenterol 2008;103(8):2015–22.

15. Cipriano L, Levesque BG, Zaric GS, et al. Cost-effectiveness of imaging strategies to reduce radiation-induced cancer risk in Crohn's disease. Inflamm Bowel Dis 2012;18(7):1240–8.

16. Loftus E. Using CT and MR enterography to diagnose and monitor IBD. Gastroenterol Hepatol 2010; 6(12):754–6.

17. Gee MS, Harisinghani MG. MRI in patients with inflammatory bowel disease. J Magn Reson Imaging 2011;33(3):527–34.

18. Savoye-Collet C, Savoye G, Koning E, et al. Fistulizing perianal Crohn's disease: contrast-enhanced magnetic resonance imaging assessment at 1 year on maintenance anti-TNF-alpha therapy. Inflamm Bowel Dis 2011;17(8):1751–8.

19. Stoll ML, Patel AS, Punaro M, et al. MR enterography to evaluate sub-clinical intestinal inflammation in children with spondyloarthritis. Pediatr Rheumatol Online J 2012;10:6.

20. Szurowska E, Wypch J, Izycka-Swieszewska E. Perianal fistulas in Crohn's disease: MRI diagnosis and surgical planning. Abdom Imaging 2007;32(6): 705–18.

21. Baker ME, Einstein DM, Veniero JC. Computed tomography enterography and magnetic resonance enterography: the future of small bowel imaging. Clin Colon Rectal Surg 2008;21(3):193–212.

22. Ajaj W, Goyen M, Schneeman, et al. Oral contrast agents for small bowel distension in MRI: influence of the osmolarity for small bowel distension. Eur Radiol 2005;15:1400–6.

23. Borthne AS, Abdelnoor M, Hellund JC, et al. MR imaging of the small bowel with increasing concentrations of an oral osmotic agent. Eur Radiol 2005; 15:667–71.

24. Negaard A, Sandivik L, Berstad AE, et al. A prospective randomized comparison between two MRI studies of the small bowel in Crohn's disease, the oral contrast method and MRE enteroclysis. Eur Radiol 2007;17:2294–301.

25. Negaard A, Sandvik L, Berstad AE, et al. MRI of the small bowel with oral contrast or nasojejunal intubation in Crohn's disease: randomized comparison of patient acceptance. Scand J Gastroenterol 2008; 43:44–51.

26. Grand DJ, Beland MD, Machan JT, et al. Detection of Crohn's disease: comparison of CT and MR enterography without anti-peristaltic agents performed on the same day. Eur J Radiol 2012;81(8):1735–41.

27. Grand DJ, Kampalath V, Harris A, et al. MR enterography correlates highly with colonoscopy and histology for both distal ileal and colonic Crohn's disease in 310 patients. Eur J Radiol 2012;81(5): e763–9.

28. Scmid-Tannwald C, Agrawal G, Dahi F, et al. Diffusion-weighted MRI: role in detecting abdominopelvic internal fistulas and sinus tracts. J Magn Reson Imaging 2012;35:125–31.

29. Yoshizako T, Wada A, Takahara T, et al. Diffusion-weighted MRI for evaluating perianal fistula activity: feasibility study. Eur J Radiol 2011. http://dx.doi.org/10.1016/j.ejrad.2011.06.052.

30. Oto A, Zhu F, Kulkarni K, et al. Evaluation of diffusion-weighted MR imaging for detection of bowel inflammation in patients with Crohn's disease. Acad Radiol 2009;16(5):597–603.

31. Froehlich JM, Waldherr C, Stoupis C, et al. MR motility imaging in Crohn's disease improves lesion detection compared with standard MR imaging. Eur Radiol 2010;20(8):1945–51.

32. Cronin CG, Lohan DG, Mhuircheartaigh JN. MRI small-bowel follow-through: prone versus supine patient positioning for best small-bowel distension and lesion detection. AJR Am J Roentgenol 2008; 191:502–6.

33. Siddiki H, Fidler J. MR imaging of the small bowel in Crohn's disease. Eur J Radiol 2009;69:409–17.

34. Fletcher JG, Fidler JL, Bruining DH, et al. New concepts in intestinal imaging for inflammatory bowel diseases. Gastroenterology 2011;140:1795–806.

35. Lee S, Ha H, Yang S, et al. CT of prominent pericolic or perienteric vasculature in patients with Crohn's disease: correlation with clinical disease activity and findings on barium studies. AJR Am J Roentgenol 2002;179:1029–36.

36. Maccioni F, Bruni A, Viscido A, et al. MR imaging in patients with Crohn disease: value of T2-versus T1-weighted gadolinium-enhanced MR sequences with use of an oral superparamagnetic contrast agent. Radiology 2006;238(2):517–30.

37. Koh DM, Miao Y, Chinn RJ. MR imaging evaluation of the activity of Crohn's disease. AJR Am J Roentgenol 2001;177:1325–32.

38. Sempere GAJ, Sanjuan VM, Chulia EM, et al. MRI evaluation of inflammatory activity in Crohn's disease. AJR Am J Roentgenol 2005;184:1829–35.

39. Rimola J, Rodriguez S, Garcia-Bosch O, et al. Magnetic resonance for assessment of disease activity and severity in ileocolonic Crohn's disease. Gut 2009;58:1113–20.

40. Messaris E, Chandolias N, Grand DJ, et al. Role of magnetic resonance enterography in the management of Crohn disease. Arch Surg 2010;145(5):471–5.

41. Pozza A, Scarpa M, Lacognata C, et al. Magnetic resonance enterography for Crohn's disease: what the surgeon can take home. J Gastrointest Surg 2011;15:1689–98.

42. Smith EA, Dillman JR, Adler J. MR enterography of extraluminal manifestations of inflammatory bowel disease in children and adolescents: moving beyond the bowel wall. AJR Am J Roentgenol 2012;198:W38–45.

43. Rimola J, Ordas I, Rodriguez S, et al. Magnetic resonance imaging for evaluation of Crohn's disease: validation of parameters of severity and quantitative index of activity. Inflamm Bowel Dis 2011;17:1759–68.

44. Lawrance IC, Welman CJ, Shipman P, et al. Correlation of MRI-determined small bowel Crohn's disease categories with medical response and surgical pathology. World J Gastroenterol 2009;15(27):3367–75.

45. Samuel S, Bruining DH, Loftus EV, et al. Skipping of distal terminal ileum in Crohn's disease. Gastroenterology 2011;140(5 Suppl 1):S-72.

46. Lee SS, Kim AY, Yang SK, et al. Crohn disease of the small bowel: comparison of CT enterography, MR enterography, and small-bowel follow-through as diagnostic techniques. Radiology 2009;251(3):751–61.

47. Siddiki HA, Fidler JL, Fletcher JG. Prospective comparison of state-of-the-art MR enterography and CT enterography in small bowel Crohn's disease. AJR Am J Roentgenol 2009;193:113–21.

48. Jensen MD, Kjeldsen JK, Rafaelsen SR, et al. Diagnostic accuracies of MR enterography and CT enterography in symptomatic Crohn's disease. Scand J Gastroenterol 2011;46:1449–57.

49. Dillman JR, Ladino-Torres MF, Adler J, et al. Comparison of MR enterography and histopathology in the evaluation of pediatric Crohn disease. Pediatr Radiol 2011;41:1552–8.

50. Silverstein J, Grand D, Kawatu D, et al. Feasibility of using MR enterography (MRE) for the assessment of terminal ileitis and inflammatory activity in children with Crohn's disease (Crohn's disease). J Pediatr Grastroenterol Nutr 2012;55(2):173–7.

51. Gee MS, Nimkin K, Hsu M, et al. Prospective evaluation of MR enterography as the primary imaging modality for pediatric Crohn disease assessment. AJR Am J Roentgenol 2011;197:224–31.

52. Buchanan GN, Halligan S, Bartram CI, et al. Clinical examination, endosonography, and MR imaging in preoperative assessment of fistula in ano: comparison with outcome-based reference standard. Radiology 2004;233(3):674–81.

53. Morris A, Spencer JA, Ambrose NS. MR imaging classification of perianal fistulas and its implications for patient management. Radiographics 2000;20:623–35.

Magnetic Resonance Colonography

Anno Graser, MD

KEYWORDS

- Magnetic resonance imaging • Large bowel • Colonography • Colorectal cancer • Screening

KEY POINTS

- Magnetic resonance colonography (MRC) is a relatively new imaging test used to exam the large bowel. It provides imaging of the entire colon after it has been cleansed and distended with water.
- High-field magnetic resonance imaging scanners are needed for higher spatial resolution and fast image acquisition at MRC.
- As MRC is a radiation-free examination, and it is ideally suited for colorectal cancer screening, even in younger individuals.
- MRC requires no sedation, but an intravenous application of gadolinium-containing contrast agent is needed. Contraindications to the application of contrast agent have to be considered.

INTRODUCTION

Since it was first described in 1997, magnetic resonance colonography (MRC) has been recognized as a promising noninvasive technique for examining the colon. Clinical indications for MRC include inflammatory bowel disease (IBD), stenosing colonic masses, postoperative surveillance in colorectal cancer (CRC) patients, and CRC screening. Although most centers will perform MR enterography or MR enteroclysis in IBD patients, specific questions concerning the colon can be ideally answered by MRC.

In most Western countries, CRC represents the second most common cause of cancer-related death in both men and women.[1] Most CRCs develop from adenomatous polyps following the adenoma-carcinoma sequence.[2] Conventional colonoscopic surveillance for polyps together with colonoscopic polypectomy has been shown to significantly decrease the prevalence of CRC.[3,4] However, only a small percentage of eligible adults (eg, approximately 10% in Germany and 20% in the United States) are willing to undergo screening by optical colonoscopy (OC).[5] The search for a more acceptable imaging screening examination for CRC has led to the development of virtual colonoscopy, which includes both computed tomographic (CT) colonography and MRC. CT colonography (CTC) has been more thoroughly evaluated in the literature than MRC and shows sensitivities of 90% or greater in the detection of polyps greater than 10 mm in diameter.[6–8] To date, MRC has mainly been studied in research settings, although at some sites, it has been at least partially integrated into clinical practice to meet growing patient demand, especially in Europe, where public and government awareness of potential negative effects of ionizing radiation is high. Developments in magnetic gradient hardware, coil design, and pulse sequences have recently been optimized for MR body imaging. Importantly for bowel imaging, acquisition times and imaging matrix size have been greatly improved by the introduction of new scanner generations in the last 2 years. CTC has several advantages over MRC, including much shorter image acquisition time leading to reduced motion artifacts, isotropic voxel resolution, wider availability, decreased operator dependency, robust 3D evaluation, lack of a water enema, and lower cost. However, a major

Department of Clinical Radiology, University of Munich, Grosshadern, Marchioninistr. 15, 81377 Munich, Germany
E-mail address: anno.graser@med.lmu.de

Radiol Clin N Am 51 (2013) 113–120
http://dx.doi.org/10.1016/j.rcl.2012.10.001
0033-8389/13/$ – see front matter © 2013 Elsevier Inc. All rights reserved.

advantage of MRC over CTC is the absence of ionizing radiation, a potential limitation that may ultimately prevent the use of CTC in a screening population.

Currently, none of the "virtual" colonoscopy modalities are widely reimbursed in the Western world, and the inherent advantage of CTC is that it is associated with lower costs than MRC. Large prospective multicenter trials only exist for CTC; for MRC, such data are missing and need to be generated to prove the validity of the examination.

TECHNICAL CONSIDERATIONS
Background

MRC generally requires a longer in-room examination time than its CT counterpart. Also, it requires intravenous access for the administration of gadolinium-based intravenous contrast agent, which will render the colonic wall as a high signal intensity structure that can be easily differentiated from the dark colonic lumen. This so-called dark lumen technique should nowadays be considered standard of care because it has been shown to be superior to other approaches that rely on "bright lumen" contrast, mostly based on a gadolinium-spiked rectal water enema or the acquisition of T2-weighted sequences without rectal contrast.

Unless fecal tagging techniques are used, the bowel has to be cleansed before performing MRC. The preparation regimen is similar to that used in conventional colonoscopy, which makes it cumbersome for the patient because it mostly involves polyethylene glycol—based formulas that require the patient to drink large amounts of fluid. Because the colon will be distended with water rather than air or CO_2, residual liquid in the lumen does not cause diagnostic difficulties.

In the author's, MC requires more thorough training and dedication of the MR technologist, the radiologist, and, last but not least, the patient to generate consistent diagnostic image quality. This consistency might be one of the major impediments when moving forward toward routine clinical use of the technology. In the following section, detailed information about patient preparation, image acquisition and pulse sequences, as well as image interpretation is provided.

Clinical Indications for MRC

For MRC, patients must be carefully selected and individuals with MR contraindications like cardiac pacemakers and inner ear implants must be excluded (**Box 1**). Total hip replacements are not generally considered a contraindication to MRC, but can cause significant artifacts in the pelvis that may impede evaluation of the rectosigmoid.[9]

> **Box 1**
> **Checklist: Magnetic resonance colonography**
>
> - Exclude contraindications to MR scanning
> - Make sure patient is able to undergo bowel cleansing and can tolerate water filling of the colon
> - Check that patient does not have an allergy to gadolinium
> - Exclude closed-angle glaucoma if planning to use Buscopan (recommended and preferable over Glucagon)
> - Explain examination to the patient—enhance importance of breath-hold instructions to avoid motion artifacts

---

Because MRC is a contrast-enhanced examination, patients must be screened for impaired renal function, which, if severe, will represent a contraindication to MRC because of the risk of nephrogenic systemic fibrosis.[10] Also, because of rectal water administration, patients unable to control their anal sphincter are excluded from MRC, as will patients with severe claustrophobia. Morbidly obese persons are also difficult to image at MRC and often cannot assume a prone position on the scanner table.

Screening

One potential indication for MRC is CRC screening. Because MRC is a radiation-free examination, it is ideally suited as a screening test that will be performed repeatedly over a patient's lifespan. CRC screening should commence at age 50 and be performed in 10-year intervals if no polyps or masses are detected and the screened individual is at average risk for CRC.[5,11] The ultimate goal of screening for CRC is the detection of clinically relevant polyps. Both the European Society of Gastrointestinal and Abdominal Radiology and the American Cancer Society in conjunction with the American College of Radiology recommend that CTC when used for screening should refrain from reporting so-called diminutive polyps less than 6 mm in size[12,13] to avoid that too many CTC participants need to undergo subsequent OC for the removal of unimportant findings. It is a known limitation of MRC that it is literally unable to detect these diminutive lesions even if the most sophisticated scanner and sequence technology are used[14,15]; also, MRC has a known very low sensitivity for nonadenomatous polyps, which in light of a screening setting can be considered advantageous. Colonoscopy, on the other hand, detects polyps regardless of their histology and thereby tends to overtreat because not all resected lesions represent the target lesion, the advanced adenoma.

Inflammatory bowel disease

Next to screening, MRC may be used as an imaging test in patients with IBD. MRC as a radiation-free modality provides high-resolution images of the large bowel and allows for exact diagnosis of the extent and severity of inflammation of the bowel wall, especially in young adults. Furthermore, it provides information about tissues adjacent to the bowel and visualizes transmural inflammatory processes, abscesses, and fistulae. To assess fibrofatty proliferation, wall edema, and post-inflammatory strictures, T2-weighted images must be acquired in addition to T1-weighted (T1w) fat-suppressed sequences. As opposed to MR enteroclysis, MRC is a well-tolerated, relatively rapid examination that can also be performed in patients with severe clinical disease activity. At the author's institution, a combination of MR enteroclysis and MRC represents the standard imaging procedure in patients with known IBD because it allows for the evaluation of both the small and the large bowel; however, placement of a nasojejunal tube may be problematic in younger patients. In ulcerative colitis, MRC might be a valuable alternative.

Incomplete colonoscopy

Another indication for MRC involves patients after incomplete colonoscopy, which occurs in as many as 10% of cases.[16] Ideally, MRC should be performed on the same day as colonoscopy to avoid the need for repeat bowel cleansing. In patients with stenosing tumors in the left-sided colon, MRC can visualize the entire large bowel lumen, thereby allowing for detection of synchronous polyps and cancers. Also, MRC helps to detect liver metastases and lymphadenopathy, which makes it a true one-stop staging examination.

MRC Imaging Technique

MRC relies on high-resolution imaging of the cleansed and distended large bowel. Although the cleansing protocol follows that used for optical colonoscopy, distention can be achieved by insufflation of the colon with air or CO_2, or by rectal water filling with or without gadolinium.

Colonic distention

Both room air and CO_2, well known from CTC for colonic distention, have been used in MRC.[17–19] Although the authors of the most recent report[19] on the use of CO_2 for MRC at 3.0 T showed promising results, in the author's experience, this technique suffers from greater susceptibility and motion artifacts than MRC after water distension

of the large bowel. The author therefore performs MRC exclusively after water enema, even if this might cause slightly greater patient discomfort and requires evacuation of the colon immediately after the end of the examination. Most patients do not experience significant pain associated with water filling of the large bowel.[14] To achieve good distention, the patient is placed on the MR scanner table in the left lateral decubitus position, and an enema bag with 2.5 L warm tap water is placed about 1 to 1.2 m above the patient. The author uses a flexible rubber catheter without an inflatable balloon as the radiologist or technologist applying the enema will be by the side of the patient to monitor patient discomfort during the filling process. Simultaneously, 20 mg n-butyl-scopolamine (Buscopan; Boehringer Ingelheim, Ingelheim, Germany) will be injected intravenously to minimize bowel spasms and motion artifacts and provide greater bowel distension; another 20 mg will be administered before the administration of contrast agent during the examination. In the author's eyes, this "double dose" of Buscopan is essential to minimize bowel motion during the examination. In the United States, where Buscopan is not Food and Drug Administration approved, Glucagon can be used as an alternative, although its antiperistaltic effect on the large bowel wall is less pronounced than that of Buscopan.

Image acquisition

After colonic distension and intravenous injection of an antiperistaltic agent, the patient is placed in the prone position on the scanner table. In the author's experience, prone positioning of the patient improves distention of the sigmoid and descending colon. A combination of a multielement spine coil and flexible surface coils that have been placed on the upper and lower back of the patient is used to guarantee high signal-to-noise ratio.

First, a set of localizer scans is acquired to ensure correct planning of the image stacks for MRC. At the author's institution, a half Fourier single-shot technique (HASTE) sequence in the coronal plane (**Table 1**) is then acquired, followed by an optional fast imaging with stead-state precession, TrueFISP (Siemens Healthcare, Erlangen, Germany), sequence—this is only acquired in patients with IBD and not part of the screening protocol. These 2 sequences render the colonic lumen with high signal intensity and the colonic wall as a dark line and depict the mesentery and its lymph nodes clearly. Both sequences are relatively robust; the TrueFISP sequence provides fairly high isotropic spatial resolution of 1.8 × 1.8 × 1.8 mm (**Fig. 1**). As the author's protocol mainly relies on the dark lumen technique, these sequences

Table 1
Sequence protocol for magnetic resonance colonography

Sequence Name	Time of Acquisition	Voxel Size [mm]	TR [ms]	TE [ms]	No. of Slices	Distance Factor	Orientation	Phase Enc. Direction	PAT Mode	Accel. Factor PE
T2 HASTE	0:31	1.5 × 1.2 × 10.0	1000	96	25	50%	Transversal	A >> P	GRAPPA	2
TTrueFISP	0:17	1.8 × 1.8 × 1.8	4.02	1.77	104 per slab	20%	Coronal	R >> L	GRAPPA	6
T1 VIBE	0:18	1.6 × 1.6 × 1.6	3.20	1.13	120 per slab	20%	Coronal	R >> L	GRAPPA	3

Sequence details are given for a 3 T scanner (Siemens Magnetom Verio, Siemens Health care, Erlangen, Germany) for T2 HASTE and T1 VIBE sequences, and for a 1.5 T scanner (Siemens Magnetom Avanto) for the TrueFISP sequence.

are immediately followed by high-resolution 3D volume interpolated breath-hold (VIBE) sequences that are acquired before and twice after the intravenous injection of gadolinium-based contrast agent (**Fig. 2**A). The protocol used at the author's institution is optimized for CRC screening; if patients with IBD are examined, additional sequences, including T2-weighted fat-suppressed single-shot sequences for depiction of edema in or adjacent to the bowel wall, are recommended.

As the author's 3 T scanner (Magnetom Verio; Siemens Healthcare, Erlangen, Germany) provides a z-axis field of view of only 35 cm, the VIBE sequence must be divided into a cephalad and a caudal stack of images, which overlap in the middle of the desired z-axis coverage, mostly

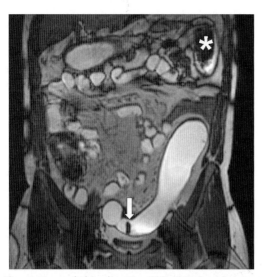

Fig. 1. Coronal thin-slice TrueFISP MRC image in an asymptomatic adult showing a low signal intensity filling defect in the sigmoid colon (*arrow*). To characterize the finding, further information from other sequences is needed. A marked flow artifact is seen at the splenic flexure (*asterisk*).

around the lower edge of the liver. The cranial set of images will cover the upper abdomen and lung bases, while the caudal set will cover the lower abdomen and pelvis. Each set of images can be acquired in a comfortable 18-s breath-hold. The first acquisition is performed before the injection of contrast agent; the second acquisition starts 40 s after contrast injection, and the third acquisition starts immediately after the second (at about 80 s after contrast injection). The author repeats the acquisition of this important sequence to have a backup dataset available in case of motion artifacts or reduced cardiac output. The resulting stacks are combined into one fused image set automatically. In the author's experience, this type of software-based automated image fusion works seamlessly in most cases, even if the inspiratory position is different between the 2 acquisitions. Scanners that provide a larger z-axis field of view (eg, 50 cm) allow for coverage of the entire colon in 1 single acquisition, thereby shortening the examination time. For both types of scanners, higher field strength allows for greater SNR and use of higher parallel imaging acceleration factors, both of which are essential for comfortable short breath-hold times.

For optimal opacification of the bowel wall, the author injects the 1-M contrast agent Gadobutrol (Gadovist, Bayer Healthcare, Berlin, Germany) at a dose of 0.1 mL per kilogram body weight. Compared with 0.5-M agents, it shows superior enhancement characteristics in MR angiography[20] and allows for superior enhancement of the bowel wall at MRC (Graser et al, 2011, personal communication).

Image interpretation

After the image acquisition, all data should be transferred to a dedicated postprocessing workstation or thin-client server postprocessing

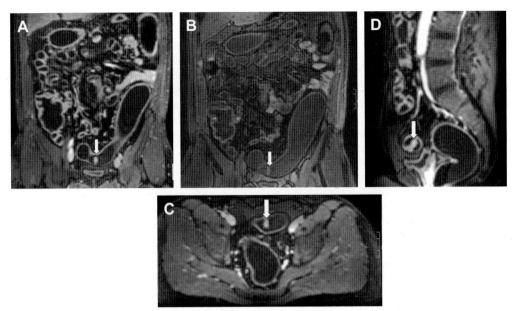

Fig. 2. (A) The coronal T1-weighted VIBE image (same patient as Fig. 1) shows that the lesion enhances with contrast (arrow) when compared with the precontrast image at the same position (B, arrow). (C) The axially reformatted image from the postcontrast T1-weighted VIBE sequence demonstrates the pedunculated morphology of the polypoid filling defect (arrow) that is also seen in the sagittal plane (arrow, D). Endoscopy and histopathology revealed a 1.3-cm pedunculated tubular adenoma.

solution (eg, Siemens Multi Modality Workplace or Siemens Syngo.Via; Siemens Healthcare, Forchheim, Germany). After a quick review of the T2-weighted HASTE sequence, the author recommends that T1w gradient-echo VIBE sequences be used to locate intracolonic abnormalities like polyps and masses in a multiplanar reformation mode (see Fig. 2); the 3D TrueFISP sequence, if available, can be used for problem-solving or in cases with severe motion artifacts on the VIBE images (see Fig. 1). This interpretation mode allows for correlation of findings in every desired plane. To date, MRC software solutions are less advanced than those available for CTC; the latter widely rely on an endoluminal fly-through display that simulates colonoscopy. For MRC, such solutions are not available to date, although several companies are working on them. MPR side-by-side review of the noncontrast and contrast-enhanced T1w data sets enables differentiation of residual stool from colonic lesions because stool never enhances with contrast, whereas true lesions always do. It must be noted that there is a difference in the enhancement characteristics of cancers, adenomas, and nonadenomatous polyps: the enhancement of adenomas is greater than that of cancers, whereas benign hyperplastic lesions do not enhance when they are less than 6 mm in size[21]; larger hyperplastic lesions show enhancement that is similar to the normal bowel wall (own

unpublished data). This enhancement will result in a much greater rate of MRC detection for adenomas than for hyperplastic polyps.[21]

To characterize an intracolonic abnormality, criteria similar to those applied in CTC should be used: morphology and structure of lesions must be analyzed. If a lesion has the morphology of a polyp, which may be flat, sessile, lobulated, or pedunculated, its internal signal intensity on precontrast-enhanced and post-contrast-enhanced T1w images have to be analyzed (compare Fig. 2A and B). Only in the case of significant enhancement can a lesion be confidently called a true polyp, whereas findings that are hyperintense on the noncontrast T1w VIBE sequence must be considered residual stool.

MRC RESULTS AND CLINICAL OUTCOME

Imaging of the large bowel has been a challenge for radiology for decades, and excellent imaging tests that allow for high-resolution morphologic depiction of the colonic wall as well as inflammatory and neoplastic pathologies now exist. Although CTC has been implemented in numerous institutions, MRC is still not routinely used in clinical practice, mainly because of its complexity with regard to patient preparation, positioning, application of rectal water enema and antiperistaltic agents, and data acquisition. However, several high-quality clinical trials have been performed that demonstrate the great potential of this examination technique.

Inflammatory Bowel Disease

MRC studies have mainly focused on 2 areas of interest: IBD and CRC screening. With respect to IBD, it is increasingly recognized that colonoscopy only provides information about mucosal alterations of IBD and MRC is an ideal test that complements or even potentially replaces colonoscopy because it provides information about mucosal, but also about extraluminal, manifestations of IDB, such as abscesses or fistulae. It also depicts a wide spectrum of related lesions like ulcers, wall thickening and edema, and hyperemia. MRC can be used in patients with known colonic manifestations of Crohn's disease and ulcerative colitis (UC), whereas patients with newly diagnosed Crohn or known involvement of the small intestine should be imaged with MR enterography or MR enteroclysis in combination with MRC.[22]

Several studies have investigated the use of MRC in patients with IBD, although endoscopy and biopsy still represent the gold standard in these diseases.[23,24]

The most recent study that was published on the diagnostic accuracy of MRC in patients with UC analyzed the disease activity and severity.[25] In this study, 50 patients with UC underwent colonoscopy and MRC for the evaluation of disease activity, and endoscopic activity was evaluated based on the modified Baron score. The results showed several MR predictors of UC disease activity: relative contrast enhancement, presence of bowel wall edema, enlarged lymph nodes, and the comb sign of the pericolonic fat.[25] Besides these changes, MRC is excellent at demonstrating the extraluminal component of inflammatory fistulae; it also helps to assess disease activity in UC patients, with mild active inflammation showing mild thickening of the colonic wall and reduced ability to distend, whereas moderate to severe disease activity leads to moderate to marked thickening of the hyperenhancing colonic wall with adjacent vascular dilatation.[22] Also, MRC is highly sensitive in the detection of UC-associated CRC in long-standing disease and can be used without bowel purgation.[26] In severe attacks of UC, MRC can be used to assess the whole colon, a great advantage in patients with inflammatory stenoses; also, MRC causes fewer complications in this patient population.[27] Finally, MRC helped to differentiate benign from malignant colonic tumors in a small case series of 14 patients studied by Achiam and colleagues based on rates of washin and washout using fast dynamic gadolinium-enhanced sequences.[28] These promising results show the potential clinical impact of MRC in patients with IBD. At the author's institution, it is increasingly being recognized that a combination of colonoscopy and MRC allows for optimal assessment of a patient's disease activity; furthermore, MRC is superior in treatment monitoring and the demonstration of anti-inflammatory drug effects without the potential side effects of colonoscopy.

Colorectal Cancer Screening

MRC has shown very promising results in the detection of colonic masses early on in its development as a clinical tool. As early as 1997, Luboldt and colleagues reported in a small case series that MRC might be a valuable tool in assessing colonic pathologies.[29] Later on, the same group showed in a population of 132 individuals that, using a bright lumen approach, MRC detected 61% of colonic polyps 5 to 10 mm in size and 94% of polyps greater than 10 mm,[30] whereas another early study reported even higher sensitivities for small polyps less than 10 mm in size.[31] These studies used scanners with lower magnetic field and gradient strengths than more recent publications that used dark lumen techniques that helped to significantly improve the performance of MRC. Lauenstein and his group published several important studies on MRC: a comparison of bright and dark lumen techniques in 37 individuals showed that the intravenous contrast-enhanced dark lumen technique reached a much higher specificity at comparable sensitivity for colonic polyps, and also T1w images were less affected by artifacts.[32] These results were confirmed by another study by the same group[33] in a large population of 122 individuals where MRC was shown to be highly accurate in the detection of clinically relevant colonic lesions less than 5 mm in size. Both studies were performed after rectal water enema and relied on a dark lumen technique.

In 2006, promising results for 1.5 T contrast-enhanced dark lumen MRC were reported by Hartmann and colleagues[34] in a population of 100 study participants with MRC in comparison to colonoscopy being 84% and 100% sensitive in the detection of polyps 6 to 9 and greater than 10 mm in size, respectively. On a per-patient analysis, this trial even reported a 90% sensitivity for relevant colonic masses greater than or equal to 6 mm in size at a very high specificity of 96%. These early studies looked at heterogeneous populations or individuals at increased risk of developing CRC. The first relevant study looking at MRC in an asymptomatic screening population was also performed by Lauenstein's group[21]; as an additional novelty, it was the first larger study to investigate MRC without cathartic bowel cleansing. In this landmark study, 315 individuals over 50 years of age underwent MRC after ingesting a tagging agent composed of 5.0% Gastrografin, 1.0% barium sulfate, and 0.2% locust bean gum with each meal 2 days before their participation in the trial. This trial resulted in 4% of colonic segments being of insufficient image quality because of retained untagged fecal material, whereas 96% of segments were of sufficient quality. Adenomatous polyps greater than 5 mm in size were detected at a sensitivity of 83% and an overall specificity of 90.2%. This trial also showed that MRC is unable to detect diminutive colonic polyps less than 6 mm in size and hyperplastic lesions, of which only 9 of 127 could be visualized. On a lesion basis, MRC was less sensitive for lesions 5 to 10 mm in size (57.6%) than for lesions greater than 10 mm (73.9%), whereas diminutive polyps less than 5 mm were detected at a very low sensitivity of 10.5%.

Patient comfort and preferences were also analyzed in this study population, and although MRC was performed without bowel purgation, overall levels of acceptance and preferences for future examinations (MRC: 46%; colonoscopy: 44%) were comparable. Insertion of the rectal tube was rated most unpleasant for MRC, and bowel purgation was rated most unpleasant for OC.[14]

Box 2, "MRC for CRC screening—Setting up your service," summarizes important strategic and workflow issues that need to be addressed when introducing this modality to a radiologic department; it is of paramount importance to provide optional same-day colonoscopy in the case of a positive MRC result to avoid repeated bowel cleansing.

Box 2
MRC for colorectal cancer screening—Setting up your service

- Train registration office staff and technologists
- Allocate slots to MRC in the morning → enable same-day colonoscopy in case of a positive test result
- Assure immediate read after the examination by experienced abdominal radiologist
- Communicate findings to patient
- Issue recommendation for follow-up examination taking into account the patient's individual CRC risk profile and MRC findings

---

SUMMARY

MRC has evolved significantly since its first description in 1997. Over the last 15 years, it has been shown that MRC can be used to detect and quantify inflammation in patients with IBD, to assess patients with stenosing colorectal masses, and to screen for colonic polyps and masses. The latter indication, especially, seems ideally suited for MRC, as the test is not associated with ionizing radiation. However, controversy remains with regard to patient acceptance and the ideal MRC protocol. Most experts agree that dark lumen techniques using fast T1w pulse sequences acquired after intravenous injection of gadolinium-containing contrast agents provide superior image quality and accuracy in the detection of relevant colonic pathologic abnormalities. T2-weighted sequences and TrueFISP sequences can be used in IBD patients and are useful for the assessment of extracolonic pathologies.

To date, MRC is not used in screening populations on a larger scale; recent results show that it holds great promise in the visualization of relevant colonic polyps and masses, although prospective multicenter trials similar to those performed in CTC are still lacking. In the future, MRC may play an important role in CRC screening programs and be used as an important alternative in patients refusing to undergo colonoscopy. Its importance in imaging patients with IBD has been shown in numerous clinical trials, and MRC has become one of the mainstays in the diagnostic workup of these patients in leading centers around the world.

REFERENCES

1. Amercian Cancer Society. Cancer Facts and Figures 2012. Available at: www.cancer.org/research/cancer factsfigures/acspc-031941. Accessed October 12, 2012.
2. Winawer SJ. Natural history of colorectal cancer. Am J Med 1999;106:3S–6S.
3. Winawer SJ, Zauber AG, Ho MN, et al. Prevention of colorectal cancer by colonoscopic polypectomy. The national polyp study workgroup. N Engl J Med 1993;329:1977–81.
4. Manser CN, Bachmann LM, Brunner J, et al. Colonoscopy screening markedly reduces the occurrence of colon carcinomas and carcinoma-related death: a closed cohort study. Gastrointest Endosc 2012; 76:110–7.
5. Riemann JF. Colonoscopy screening: status in Europe. Dig Dis 2011;29(Suppl 1):53–5.
6. Johnson CD, Chen MH, Toledano AY, et al. Accuracy of CT colonography for detection of large adenomas and cancers. N Engl J Med 2008;359:1207–17.

7. Graser A, Stieber P, Nagel D, et al. Comparison of CT colonography, colonoscopy, sigmoidoscopy and faecal occult blood tests for the detection of advanced adenoma in an average risk population. Gut 2009;58:241–8.

8. Pickhardt PJ, Choi JR, Hwang I, et al. Computed tomographic virtual colonoscopy to screen for colorectal neoplasia in asymptomatic adults. N Engl J Med 2003;349:2191–200.

9. Kinner S, Lauenstein TC. MR colonography. Radiol Clin North Am 2007;45:377–87.

10. Weinreb JC, Kuo PH. Nephrogenic systemic fibrosis. Magn Reson Imaging Clin N Am 2009;17: 159–67.

11. Rex DK, Johnson DA, Anderson JC, et al. American college of gastroenterology guidelines for colorectal cancer screening 2009 [corrected]. Am J Gastroenterol 2009;104:739–50.

12. Taylor SA, Laghi A, Lefere P, et al. European society of gastrointestinal and abdominal radiology (ESGAR): consensus statement on CT colonography. Eur Radiol 2006;17:575–9.

13. Levin B, Lieberman DA, McFarland B, et al. Screening and surveillance for the early detection of colorectal cancer and adenomatous polyps, 2008: a joint guideline from the American Cancer Society, the US Multi-Society Task Force on Colorectal Cancer, and the American College of Radiology. Gastroenterology 2008;134:1570–95.

14. Kinner S, Kuehle CA, Langhorst J, et al. MR colonography vs. optical colonoscopy: comparison of patients' acceptance in a screening population. Eur Radiol 2007;17:2286–93.

15. Zijta FM, Bipat S, Stoker J. Magnetic resonance (MR) colonography in the detection of colorectal lesions: a systematic review of prospective studies. Eur Radiol 2010;20:1031–46.

16. Shah HA, Paszat LF, Saskin R, et al. Factors associated with incomplete colonoscopy: a population-based study. Gastroenterology 2007;132:2297–303.

17. Morrin MM, Hochman MG, Farrell RJ, et al. MR colonography using colonic distention with air as the contrast material: work in progress. AJR Am J Roentgenol 2001;176:144–6.

18. Rodriguez Gomez S, Pages Llinas M, Castells Garangou A, et al. Dark-lumen MR colonography with fecal tagging: a comparison of water enema and air methods of colonic distension for detecting colonic neoplasms. Eur Radiol 2008;18:1396–405.

19. Zijta FM, Nederveen AJ, Jensch S, et al. Feasibility of using automated insufflated carbon dioxide (CO2) for luminal distension in 3.0T MR colonography. Eur J Radiol 2012;81:1128–33.

20. Haneder S, Attenberger UI, Schoenberg SO, et al. Comparison of 0.5M gadoterate and 1.0M gadobutrol in peripheral MRA: a prospective, single-center, randomized, crossover, double-blind study. J Magn Reson Imaging 2012. http://dx.doi.org/10.1002/jmri.23760.

21. Kuehle CA, Langhorst J, Ladd SC, et al. Magnetic resonance colonography without bowel cleansing: a prospective cross-sectional study in a screening population. Gut 2007;56(8):1079–85.

22. Rimola J, Rodriguez S, Garcia-Bosch O, et al. Role of 3.0-T MR colonography in the evaluation of inflammatory bowel disease. Radiographics 2009;29:701–19.

23. Fiocca R, Ceppa P. Endoscopic biopsies. J Clin Pathol 2003;56:321–2.

24. Ajaj WM, Lauenstein TC, Pelster G, et al. Magnetic resonance colonography for the detection of inflammatory diseases of the large bowel: quantifying the inflammatory activity. Gut 2005;54:257–63.

25. Ordas I, Rimola J, Garcia-Bosch O, et al. Diagnostic accuracy of magnetic resonance colonography for the evaluation of disease activity and severity in ulcerative colitis: a prospective study. Gut 2012. [Epub ahead of print].

26. Langhorst J, Kuhle CA, Ajaj W, et al. MR colonography without bowel purgation for the assessment of inflammatory bowel Disease: diagnostic accuracy and patient acceptance. Inflamm Bowel Dis 2007; 13(8):1001–8.

27. Savoye-Collet C, Roset JB, Koning E, et al. Magnetic resonance colonography in severe attacks of ulcerative colitis. Eur Radiol 2012;22:1963–71.

28. Achiam MP, Andersen LP, Klein M, et al. Differentiation between benign and malignant colon tumors using fast dynamic gadolinium-enhanced MR colonography; a feasibility study. Eur J Radiol 2010;74: e45–50.

29. Luboldt W, Bauerfeind P, Steiner P, et al. Preliminary assessment of three-dimensional magnetic resonance imaging for various colonic disorders. Lancet 1997;349:1288–91.

30. Luboldt W, Bauerfeind P, Wildermuth S, et al. Colonic masses: detection with MR colonography. Radiology 2000;216:383–8.

31. Pappalardo G, Polettini E, Frattaroli FM, et al. Magnetic resonance colonography versus conventional colonoscopy for the detection of colonic endoluminal lesions. Gastroenterology 2000;119:300–4.

32. Lauenstein TC, Ajaj W, Kuehle CA, et al. Magnetic resonance colonography: comparison of contrast-enhanced three-dimensional vibe with two-dimensional FISP sequences: preliminary experience. Invest Radiol 2005;40:89–96.

33. Ajaj W, Pelster G, Treichel U, et al. Dark lumen magnetic resonance colonography: comparison with conventional colonoscopy for the detection of colorectal pathology. Gut 2003;52:1738–43.

34. Hartmann D, Bassler B, Schilling D, et al. Colorectal polyps: detection with dark-lumen MR colonography versus conventional colonoscopy. Radiology 2006; 238:143–9.

Magnetic Resonance Imaging of Rectal Cancer

Catherine E. Dewhurst, MB, BCh, BAO, BMedSc[a],
Koenraad J. Mortele, MD[b,c],*

KEYWORDS

- Rectal cancer • Circumferential resection margin • Magnetic resonance imaging

KEY POINTS

- Rectal cancer can be accurately staged using preoperative magnetic resonance imaging if the technique and sequence parameters are optimized, and the reader is familiar with the anatomy, limitations of the technique, and features of the disease.
- Many centers currently perform only noncontrast imaging owing to the fact that gadolinium does not significantly aid in the T staging or differentiation of benign from malignant lymph nodes.
- The circumferential resection margin, as well as presence of extramuscular vascular invasion, is currently not part of the TNM staging but should be incorporated into all reports, as it has both treatment and prognostic implications.

INTRODUCTION

It is estimated that 40,290 new cases of rectal cancer will be diagnosed in the United States in 2012.[1] After lung cancer, colorectal cancer is the second most common cause of cancer mortality in the United States and is the most common gastrointestinal cancer.[2] Rectal cancer comprises a third of all colorectal cancer cases, and of these, approximately 30% arise within 6 cm from the anal verge.[3,4]

The preoperative staging assessment of rectal carcinoma has significant implications in terms of the patient's management and subsequent therapy. Patients with rectal carcinomas that have not breached the rectal wall and are node-negative may be adequately treated by immediate surgery or radiation therapy alone.[5] On the other hand, clinical trials combining neoadjuvant chemoradiation therapy followed by primary resection have shown improved survival in patients who present with transmural invasion or those who are lymph node positive.[6] Therefore, for accurate local staging of rectal cancer, preoperative imaging, by means of endoscopic ultrasound or magnetic resonance imaging (MRI), is used routinely in clinical practice.[6–8]

Nowadays, MRI is considered a robust technique in the detection, characterization, and staging of rectal tumors. It demonstrates superior soft tissue resolution and multiplanar imaging capacity, and has no associated radiation risk. It has become one of the standard imaging modalities in the preoperative assessment of rectal tumors.[9] With the more recent addition of diffusion-weighted imaging (DWI), it has also emerged as a reliable indicator for assessing early response following neoadjuvant chemoradiation.

This article aims to discuss the anatomy of the anorectum, the MRI protocol parameters required

[a] Divisions of Abdominal Imaging and Body MRI, Department of Radiology, Beth Israel Deaconess Medical Center, 330 Brookline Avenue, Boston, MA 02115, USA; [b] Division of Clinical MRI, Beth Israel Deaconess Medical Center, Harvard Medical School, 330 Brookline Avenue, Ansin 224, Boston, MA 02115, USA; [c] Divisions of Abdominal Imaging and Body MRI, Beth Israel Deaconess Medical Center, Harvard Medical School, 330 Brookline Avenue, Ansin 224, Boston, MA 02115, USA
* Corresponding author. Divisions of Abdominal Imaging and Body MRI, Beth Israel Deaconess Medical Center, Harvard Medical School, 330 Brookline Avenue, Ansin 224, Boston, MA 02115.
E-mail address: kmortele@bidmc.harvard.edu

Radiol Clin N Am 51 (2013) 121–131
http://dx.doi.org/10.1016/j.rcl.2012.09.012
0033-8389/13/$ – see front matter © 2013 Elsevier Inc. All rights reserved.

to optimize diagnosis of rectal cancer, and the diagnostic MRI criteria essential to stage rectal cancer accurately, using the TNM staging classification. A brief review of more emerging important aspects of rectal cancer staging, such as the circumferential resection margin, extramural vascular invasion, and the staging of low rectal cancers, will also be provided. Finally, the authors will touch upon the evaluation of tumor response to neoadjuvant chemoradiation therapy in the setting of locally advanced rectal cancer.

ANORECTAL ANATOMY

The rectum extends cranially over a distance of approximately 16 cm from the anocutaneous line (anal verge) and is divided into upper (12–16 cm), middle (6–12 cm), and lower thirds (<6 cm).[4] The lower two-thirds form the rectal ampulla. The rectum is divided into thirds by the valves of Houston, which are transverse folds 12 mm in thickness composed of the circular layer of the rectal wall. Their function is to support the weight of fecal matter and prevent the urge to defecate. The rectum shows 3 lateral curvatures on MRI that correspond anatomically to these transverse folds.

The upper third of the rectum is bordered by the visceral peritoneum anterolaterally, known as the anterior peritoneal reflection. The point of attachment is variable, particularly in women, and may be as low as 5 cm from the anal verge. On axial images, it has the appearance of a seagull, hence the coined term seagull sign. The middle third is covered by the peritoneum anteriorly. The lower third of the rectum is extraperitoneal and is bordered anteriorly by the rectoprostatic fascia or Denonvilliers fascia, which is a membranous partition that separates the prostate and urinary bladder from the rectum in males and follows the course of the vagina posteriorly in females. Posteriorly, the presacral fascia is continuous with the posterior part of the mesorectal fascia or Waldeneyer fascia.

There are 3 layers to the rectal wall, which are best depicted on T2-weighted images: an inner hyperintense layer corresponding to the mucosa and submucosa, an intermediate hypointense layer corresponding to the muscularis propia, and an outer hyperintense layer that consists of the mesorectal fat.[10,11] The rectum has no true serosa.

The mesorectal fascia (MRF) is an important landmark for evaluating the local extent of disease and is characterized as a thin low-signal intensity structure on T2-weighted imaging (**Fig. 1**).[4,7] It is made up of the perirectal fascia, which is a connective tissue sheath enclosing the rectum (posterolaterally), the

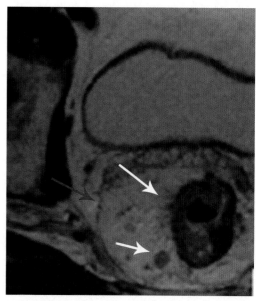

Fig. 1. MRF. Axial T2-weighted image through the lower rectum demonstrates the thin hypointense margin of the MRF (*red arrow*). Tumor is seen along the right lateral wall of the rectum (Extending into the muscularis propria), with associated stranding within the mesorectal fat compatible with desmoplastic reaction (*long white arrow*). There is, however, a single enlarged lymph node (*short white arrow*) noted at the level of the tumor consistent with N1 disease.

perirectal fat, lymph nodes, and lymphatic vessels, and acts as an important natural barrier to tumor spread.[9] The MRF also represents the circumferential resection margin (CRM), a pathology term denoting the plane of surgery during total mesorectal excision.[10] Anteriorly, the MRF fuses with the peritoneum at its reflection off the rectum. At the level of the anorectal junction, the mesorectum thins out.

The lower rectum merges with the anal sphincter complex inferiorly (**Fig. 2**).[4,11] The external sphincter is a striated muscle about 8 to 10 cm in length and is composed of superficial and deep components. The superficial component arises from the anococcygeal raphe, which stretches from the tip of the coccyx to the posterior margin of the anus. These muscles encircle the anus and join with the levator ani muscles anteriorly. The deep component is formed by the puborectalis muscle superiorly. The external sphincter is hypointense on all sequences and enhances poorly postgadolinium administration, like other striated muscles. It is bordered laterally by the ischioanal fossa. The upper end of the anal canal is identified by the insertion of the levator ani complex, which forms the ceiling of the ischiorectal fossa as it joins the rectal muscular wall.[10,11] The internal sphincter is the continuation of the

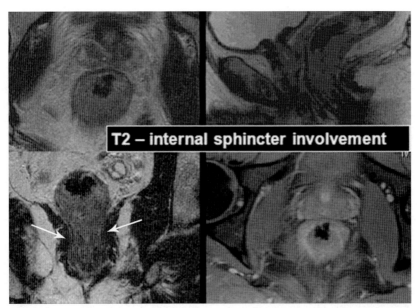

Fig. 2. Low rectal cancer. Multiplanar T2-weighted images and postgadolinium T1-weighted image shows extension of tumor into the internal sphincter complex inferiorly (*white arrows*) indicating T2 disease.

circular layer of the muscularis propria of the rectum but is composed of smooth muscle and innervated by the pudendal nerve. It lies between the intersphincteric space (containing fat and the longitudinal muscle) and the anal canal. It is intermediate in signal intensity on both T1- and T2-weighted images and enhances homogeneously postcontrast administration.[11]

MRI TECHNIQUES
Patient Preparation

Before the MRI examination, the patient is asked to prepare the rectum by a sodium biphosphonate and sodium-phosphate enema. Thereafter, a 16 F Foley catheter is inserted into the rectum, and 60 cc of a mixture of a 8:1 dilution of barium sulfate suspension 15% weight per volume (200 cc) and ferumoxsil (25 cc) (are injected. If the study is being completed on a 3T magnet, then the recommended dilution is 16:1. The Foley catheter is left in place for the remainder of the examination. The rectal solution acts as a negative contrast agent on T2-weighted images relative to the adjacent rectal wall and rectal mass. Alternatively, some authors advocate the use of rectal insertion of 100 cc of ultrasound transmission gel, as this acts as a positive contrast agent and is bright on T2-weighted images compared with the rectal wall and tumor.

Following the rectal contrast administration, the authors administer 1 mg of intramuscular glucagon (Eli Lilly and Company Indianapolis, USA) to reduce bowel motion. If this is contraindicated, as in patients with diabetes or phaeochromocytoma,

hyoscyamine is administered. Outside of the United States, 20 mg of scopolamine butylbromide can also be used as an anti-spasmodic agent in this setting.

MRI Sequences

Rectal MRI examinations can be performed routinely on a 1.5T or a 3.0T system with the patient in the supine position and with an 8- to 32-channel body phased-array coil. Anatomic coverage is usually from the top of the iliac crests to the pubic symphysis for the three plane localizer sequences. For the higher tissue resolution MRI sequences, a smaller field of view (FOV) is employed centered over the rectum. Total MRI room time is approximately 45 minutes.

T2-weighted Half-Fourier single-shot fast spin-echo (SSFSE) images are initially used for anatomic localization of the rectum in the axial, sagittal and oblique coronal plane. In addition, high-resolution oblique axial T2-weighted SSFSE images are obtained perpendicular to the rectal wall at the level of the rectal mass. If the tumor is in the low rectum and if there is concern for anal sphincter involvement, then an additional high-resolution coronal oblique sequence can be performed parallel to the anal canal. The Half-Fourier strategy provides the opportunity for very fast SSFSE acquisitions, with each image obtained in approximately 1 second. Moreover, because SSFSE images are acquired sequentially, they are relatively motion insensitive compared with standard spin echo T2-weighted imaging.

Diffusion-weighted MRI (DW-MRI) with quantitative measurements of apparent diffusion coefficient (ADC) values is an increasingly applied technique in rectal cancer imaging due to its ability to: depict areas of neoplasm without the need for intravenous contrast administration,[12] detect lymph nodes, and assess for early tumor response after neoadjuvant chemoradiation.[13–16] At the authors' institution, an axial, single-shot echo-planar DW sequence with B-value of 0, 600, and 1000 sec/mm^2 is used. The parameters of all sequences employed are detailed in **Table 1**.

Despite recent evidence that intravenous gadolinium-enhanced sequences rarely provide added benefits in the staging of rectal cancer, the authors currently still obtain 3-dimensional axial fast spoiled gradient echo (FSPGR) sequences before and after gadolinium chelate administration.[12,13]

There is also no consensus in the literature as to whether an endorectal coil MRI is superior to a standard phased-array coil MRI in the evaluation of rectal cancers.[2] However, endorectal coils have inherent limitations in assessing upper and stenotic rectal tumors and detection of lateral pelvic and inferior mesenteric lymph nodes. Moreover, the technique is semi-invasive, and there is an extra cost of approximately $120 per patient associated with the examination.

LOCAL STAGING OF RECTAL CANCER WITH MRI
T Stage

T (tumor) stage stands for depth of rectal wall invasion by tumor. In general, rectal tumors are minimally

hyperintense on T2-weighted imaging relative to the adjacent bowel wall. This is why a positive contrast agent can help when distending the rectum, as it allows for better delineation of the mass. The rectal tumor can present as a polypoid, flat or carpet-like, semicircumferential, or fully circumferential lesion. Rectal cancers typically demonstrate avid enhancement after contrast administration and demonstrate restricted diffusion.

A T1 tumor demonstrates invasion through the mucosa and submucosa without extension into the muscularis propria. T2 tumors demonstrate invasion into the muscularis propria (**Fig. 3**). T3 disease is determined by direct extension of the mass outside of the muscularis propria into the mesorectal fat (**Fig. 4**). T4 disease implies spread of tumor into the visceral peritoneum (T4a) or adjacent organs (T4b), including, but not limited to, the prostate gland, uterus, pelvic side wall, and bladder (**Fig. 5**).[17,18] While invasion of the external sphincter is T3 disease, invasion of the levator ani muscles indicates T4 disease. **Table 2** lists the TNM staging of rectal carcinoma.

Mesorectal Fascia

Another important component of staging is assessment of the distance of the tumor to the mesorectal fascia, as this represents the circumferential resection margin (CRM) at the time of total mesorectal excision (TME). MRI has an accuracy of 86% in predicting CRM involvement.[2,19–23] Any extension of tumor through the wall of the rectum and into the MRF that is considered to be

Table 1
MRI sequence parameters

	Sagital T2 FSE	Axial Single-Shot FSE	Oblique Axial T2 FSE	Oblique Coronal T2 FSE	DWI-MRI	Ax 3D FSPGR
Sequence Type	Single shot	Single shot	Single shot	Single shot		SPGR
Repetition Time (ms)	4184.0	6050.0	5868.0	6217.0	8675.0	
Echo Time (ms)	102.0	102.0	102.0	102.0	min	min
2-dimensional (2D) or 3-dimensional (3D)	2D	2D	2D	2D	2D	3D
Section Thickness (mm)	4	4	3.0	4	5.0	3
Interslice Gap (mm)	0	0	0	0	2	0
Field of View (mm)	24	22.0	18.0	24.0	36.0	24.0
Phase x Frequency Steps	256 × 320	256 × 384	256 × 256	256 × 384	192 × 192	256 × 256
Fat Suppression	No	No	No	No	No	No
Single or Multiple Shots	Single	Single	Single	Single	Single	Single
Bandwidth (kHz)	25.0	25.0	25.0	25.0		62.5
B-Value (mm/sec^2)					1000	

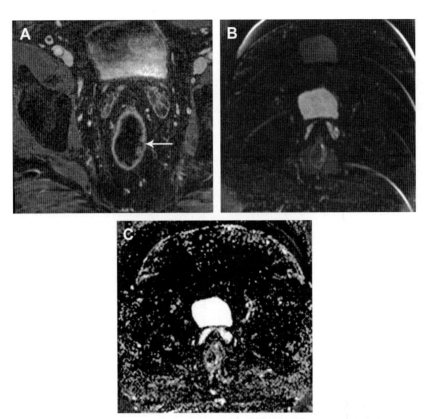

Fig. 3. T2 rectal cancer. (*A*) Flat polypoid lesion (*arrow*) arising from the lower third of the rectum, at approximately 12 to 6 o'clock in the supine position. It is confined to the rectal wall with no definite invasion through the muscularis propria. DWI and the corresponding ADC map confirmed the findings (*B, C*).

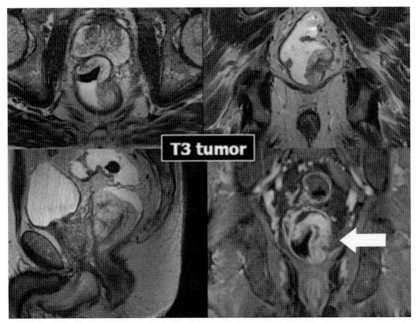

Fig. 4. T3 rectal cancer. Axial, coronal and sagital T2-weighted images of the rectum demonstrating a large lesion involving the left lateral wall of the rectum with extension through the wall consistent with T3 disease. The tumor enhances after contrast (*white arrow*).

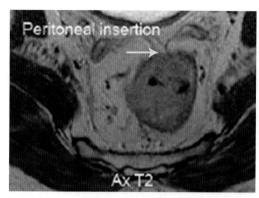

Fig. 5. T4 rectal cancer. On the axial T2-weighted image, there is extension of tumor through the MRF, which has extended anteriorly and has invaded the anterior peritoneal reflection giving the appearance of the term coined seagull sign consistent with stage T4a (*yellow arrow*).

in direct continuity with the tumor is consistent with T3 disease.[24–26]

In addition, there may be separate extramural tumor deposits noted in the mesorectum, which are discontinuous with the primary tumor. They are usually irregular in shape and can de differentiated from the smooth lobular contour of adjacent lymph nodes.[27] These are also considered to represent T3 disease. Tumor infiltration of the MRF should be differentiated from the desmoplastic reaction that occurs as a response to inflammation in the area (**Fig. 6**). These are seen as linear dark structures on T2-weighted imaging extending from the wall of the rectum. Intravenous gadolinium is not useful in differentiating between these entities[28] and, similarly, DWI has not been proven to be helpful in this regard either.[29]

Circumferential Resection Margin

Although the T stage is a stronger predictor for overall prognosis, CRM is probably a more important prognostic indicator in detecting the proximity of the tumor extension to the resection margin and, therefore, local recurrence.[10,21,22,30] When correlated with pathologic specimens, it has been shown that the risk of local recurrence is significantly increased with clearances of 1 mm or less; therefore a clearance of 1 mm or less on MRI is considered a positive CRM.[25,26,31] Using this 1 mm cut-off, large multicenter studies have shown a specificity of 92% and a negative predictive value of 94% for predicting involvement of the CRM by MRI.[18,31–38]

Another published criterion for prediction of CRM infiltration, different and more conservative than that described previously, is to use a cut-off

Table 2	
TNM staging of rectal cancer	
TX	Primary tumor cannot be assessed
T0	No evidence of primary tumor
Tis	Carcinoma in situ
T1	Tumor invades submucosa
T2	Tumor invades muscularis propria
T3	Tumor invades through the muscularis propria into perirectal fat
T4a	Tumor penetrates to the surface of the visceral peritoneum
T4b	Tumor directly invades or is adherent to other organs or structures
NX	Regional lymph nodes cannot be assessed
N0	No regional lymph node metastasis
N1	Metastases in 1–3 regional lymph nodes
N1a	Metastasis in 1 regional lymph node
N1b	Metastases in 2–3 regional lymph nodes
N1c	Tumor deposit(s) in the subserosa, mesentery, or pericolic or perirectal tissues without regional nodal metastases.
N2	Metastases in ≥4 regional lymph nodes.
N2a	Metastases in 4–6 regional lymph nodes.
N2b	Metastases in ≥7 regional lymph nodes
M0	No distant metastasis
M1	Distant metastasis
M1a	Metastasis confined to 1 organ or site (eg, liver, lung, ovary, nonregional node, external iliac lymph node)
M1b	Metastases in >1 organ/site or the peritoneum

Adapted from the American Joint Commission of Cancer 7th edition.

distance of 5 mm between the tumor and the adjacent mesorectal fascia. This criterion was established by Beets-Tan and colleagues,[39] who observed that it was highly accurate in predicting CRM involvement and that a distance of at least 5 mm between a tumor and the mesorectal fascia, MRI helped to predict an uninvolved CRM at histologic analysis with 97% confidence.[40]

The CRM is still not part of the official TNM classification for rectal tumors but should be incorporated into all MRI reports as it is, as mentioned before, an important prognostic indicator. Limitations of assessment of the CRM can be seen in thin patients with minimal perirectal fat, and in patients with low rectal and anterior rectal wall tumors. Important to note is that CRM involvement is only applicable to the nonperitonealized portions of the rectum.

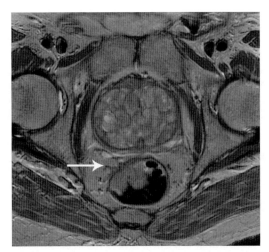

Fig. 6. Desmoplastic reaction. Desmoplasia induced by the tumor should not be confused with tumor infiltration. Desmoplasia (*white arrow*) appears as linear thin speculations within the mesorectal fat, which course along vessels. Desmoplasia typically does not enhance, nor does it demonstrate restricted diffusion.

Nodal Staging

Nodal involvement in rectal cancer is a strong independent predictor of both survival and local recurrence. Nodal spread occurs via the mesorectal lymph nodes and along the superior rectal vessels as well as laterally along the internal and external iliac chains. Detection of lymph node involvement in rectal cancer is difficult, as some lymph nodes measuring less than 5 mm in diameter can be tumor-positive while larger ones can be reactive.[2,41] Using 5 mm (any axis) as a cutoff for an abnormal size lymph node has proven to provide a sensitivity of 66% and a specificity of 76% to predict malignant involvement.[42]

Irregular contour of and heterogeneous signal intensity in lymph nodes on precontrast imaging when correlated with histology have been shown to be greater predictors of malignancy then size alone.[43,44] If suspicious nodes are deemed to be present, then the number of nodes is important as well, since this will differentiate N1 from N2 disease (**Fig. 7** and **Table 2**). Any pelvic side wall lymph nodes are also important to detect.[44]

It should be noted that involved lymph nodes are typically at the level of the primary tumor or above as they aim to drain the tumor cranially. Internal iliac lymph nodes are still considered nodal staging N disease as per the TNM staging criteria, whereas external iliac lymph nodes, obturator lymph nodes, and retroperitoneal adenopathy are considered nonregional lymphadenopathy and therefore consistent with M (metastasis) disease.

Currently, because of lack of an established ADC cut-off value, DWI, although helpful in detecting

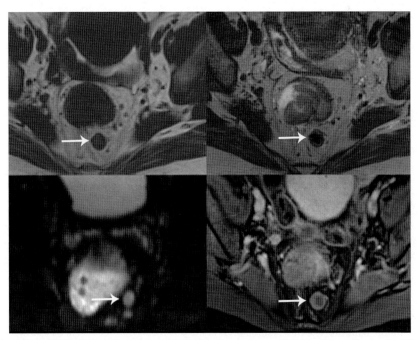

Fig. 7. Nodal staging. Multiple lymph nodes are noted in the mesorectal fat in this patient with T3 rectal cancer. The largest one (*white arrow*) is seen posterior to the rectum measuring greater than 5 mm, consistent with metastatic involvement. Note its heterogeneous signal intensity on T1- and T2-weighted imaging. Of note, all lymph nodes show restricted diffusion and enhancement after contrast. Findings are consistent with N1 disease.

lymph nodes, cannot accurately differentiate benign nodal hyperplasia from metastatic lymph nodes.[10]

Extramuscular Vascular Invasion

EMVI is invasion of large vessels directly by tumor, which are located deep to the muscularis propria. EMVI is an important independent negative prognostic indicator of metastatic disease and survival.[45] On MRI, it is assessed whether EMVI is present, and if so, it is termed positive or negative. EMVI is present if tumor is seen to be growing along a recognizable vessel, typically dilating the involved vessel. If present, assessment of how close the EMVI is to the MRF is also important.[17] Reportedly, MRI has a sensitivity of 62% and a specificity of 88% in detecting EMVI (**Fig. 8**).[18]

Low Rectal Tumors

Low rectal adenocarcinomas occur within 5 cm of the anal verge. Among those, rectal cancers that lie at or below the level of the puborectalis muscle should be evaluated with special attention with regards to their relationship to the anal sphincter complex. Internal sphincter involvement is considered T2 disease; advancement into the intersphincteric space is considered T2 disease, and extension into the external sphincter is considered T3 disease. Adjacent organ involvement is considered T4 disease. Low rectal cancers are also at increased risk of recurrence, due to their close relationship to the CRM. Therefore, many of these patients with low rectal cancer who require an abdomino-peroneal resection (APR) for this tumor often will receive neoadjuvant chemotherapy.[4]

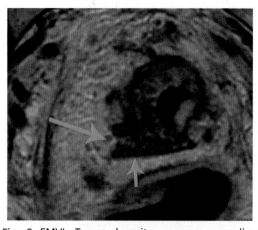

Fig. 8. EMVI. Tumor deposits are seen spreading directly from the wall of the rectum and are seen to be coursing along the lateral rectal vessels, consistent with a positive EMVI (*green arrows*). Of note the tumor deposit is more than 1 mm from the MRF.

Overall Staging Accuracy of MRI

Al-Sukhni and colleagues[36] recently published a meta-analysis in 2012 outlining the diagnostic accuracy of MRI in terms of T staging, CRM, and nodal staging. They compiled data from several studies performed between the years 2000 and 2010. In their analysis, it was shown that MRI had an overall sensitivity of 77% and specificity of 94% for CRM involvement, 87% sensitivity and 75% specificity for T stage assessment, and 77% sensitivity and 71% specificity for nodal staging. The overall range of accuracies for MRI was reported as 92% to 95% for CRM involvement, 85% for T stage determination and 43% to 85% for nodal stage assessment.[46]

MRI of Rectal Cancer After Neoadjuvant Therapies

The goal of neoadjuvant chemotherapy and radiation therapy is to downstage and downsize the tumor before surgery. This improves resectability of the primary tumor at TME, helps to preserve sphincter function if the tumor is low, improves survival, and decreases the risk of local recurrence.[47–49]

However, the overall accuracy of MRI in rectal cancer staging after neoadjuvant treatment is only 50% for T staging, 65% for nodal staging, and 66% for predicting CRM involvement.[46,49] DWI has shown to be important in determining local treatment response,[14] as residual tumors after therapy have higher ADC values than tumors before therapy. DWI after neoadjuvant therapy has been shown to predict therapy response but as yet cannot determine complete response.[50]

MRI Reporting

As the official TNM staging system currently does not incorporate the CRM or EMVI into the protocol, having a standardzed reporting template in one's department gives a complete report to the surgeon or oncologist and helps to determine treatment options. As outlined above, these have been shown to be important predictors for margin clearance, patient survival, and risk of local recurrence. **Table 3** outlines the standard reporting template the authors use in their institution.

SUMMARY

Rectal cancer can be accurately staged using preoperative MRI if the technique and sequence parameters are optimized and the reader is familiar with the anatomy, limitations of the technique, and features of the disease. Many centers currently only perform noncontrast imaging owing to the

Table 3
Standardized reporting template for dictation MRI studies for rectal cancer

Size	_×_×_ cm
Appearance	Circumferential? Ulcerating?
Signal intensity	T1, T2, fat-suppressed images
Distance of lower edge of tumor from anal verge and superior aspect of internal sphincter	cm
T stage	T1, T2, T3, T4a, T4b
Lymph node involvement	Describe all regional and nonregional lymph nodes if present; designate N stage as described in TNM
Minimum distance of tumor/nodes from CRM	mm
Relationship of the tumor to the anterior peritoneal reflection	For upper and middle third tumors
Is the mesorectum intact?	
Evidence for EMVI	Positive or negative
Distant metastases	M0, M1, MX

fact that gadolinium does not significantly aid in the T staging or differentiation of benign from malignant lymph nodes. The CRM, as well as presence of EMVI, is currently not part of the TNM staging but should be incorporated into all reports, as it has both treatment and prognostic implications.

REFERENCES

1. National Cancer Institute. Comprehensive cancer information. Available at: http://seer.cancer.gov/stat facts/html/colorect.html.

2. Dewhurst C, Rosen M, Blake MA, et al. ACR appropriateness Criteria: pretreatment staging of colorectal cancer. J Am Coll Radiol 2012, in press.

3. Salerno G, Daniels I, Brown G, et al. Variations in pelvic dimensions does not predict the risk of circumferential resection margin (CRM) involvement in rectal cancer. World J Surg 2007;31:1315–22.

4. Shihab OC, Moran BJ, Heald R, et al. MRI staging of low rectal cancer. Eur Radiol 2009;19:643–50.

5. Gerard JP, Ayzac L, Coquard R, et al. Endocavitary irradiation for early rectal carcinomas T1 (T2). A series of 101 patients treated with the Papillon's technique. Int J Radiat Oncol Biol Phys 1996;34(4):775–83.

6. Bernini A, Deen KI, Madoff RD, et al. Preoperative adjuvant radiation with chemotherapy for rectal cancer: its impact on stage of disease and the role of endorectal ultrasound. Ann Surg Oncol 1996; 3(2):131–5.

7. Barbaro B, Fiorucci C, Tebala C, et al. Locally advanced rectal cancer: MR imaging in prediction of response after preoperative chemotherapy and radiation therapy. Radiology 2009;250(3):730–9.

8. Perez RO, Pereira DD, Proscurshim I, et al. Lymph node size in rectal cancer following neoadjuvant chemoradiation–can we rely on radiologic nodal staging after chemoradiation? Dis Colon Rectum 2009;52(7):1278–84.

9. Raghunathan G, Mortele KJ. MR imaging of anorectal neoplasms. Clin Gastroenterol Hepatol 2009;7(4): 379–88.

10. Iafrate F, Laghi A, Paolantonio P, et al. Pre-operative staging of rectal cancer with MR imaging: correlation with surgical and histopathologic findings. Radiographics 2006;26:701–14.

11. Laghi A, Iafrate F, Paolantonio P, et al. Magnetic resonance imaging of the anal canal using high resolution sequences and phased array coil: visualization of anal sphincter complex. Radiol Med 2002; 103:353–9 [In English, Italian].

12. Jiao SY, Yang BY, Wing H, et al. Evaluation of gadolinium-enhanced T1-weighted MRI in the preoperative assessment of local staging in rectal cancer. Colorectal Dis 2010;12:1139–48.

13. Vliegen RF, Beets GL, Von Meyenfeldt MF, et al. Rectal cancer: MR imaging in local staging —is gadolinium-based contrast material helpful? Radiology 2005;234:179–88.

14. Kim SH, Lee YJ, Lee JM, et al. Apparent diffusion coefficient for evaluating tumor response to neo-adjuvant chemoradiation therapy for locally advanced rectal cancer. Eur J Radiol 2011;21:987–95.

15. Rosenkrantz A, Oei M, Babb J, et al. Diffusion-weighted imaging of the abdomen at 3.0T: image quality and apparent diffusion coefficient reproducibility compared with 1.5T. J Magn Reson Imaging 2011;33:128–35.

16. Curvo-Semedo L, Lambregts DM, Mass M, et al. Rectal cancer: assessment of complete response

to pre-operative combined radiation therapy with chemotherapy – conventional MR volumetry versus diffusion-weighted imaging. Radiology 2011;260: 734–43.

17. Taylor FG, Swift RI, Blomqvist L, et al. A systematic approach to the interpretation of preoperative staging MRI for rectal cancer. AJR Am J Roentgenol 2008;191(6):1827–35.

18. MERCURY Study Group. Diagnostic accuracy of pre-operative magnetic resonance imaging in predicting curative resection of rectal cancer: prospective observational study. BMJ 2006;333:779.

19. Videhult P, Smedh K, Lundin P, et al. Magnetic resonance imaging for preoperative staging of rectal cancer in clinical practice: high accuracy in predicting circumferential margin with clinical benefit. Colorectal Dis 2007;9(5):412–9.

20. Purkayastha S, Tekkis PP, Athanasiou T, et al. Diagnostic precision of magnetic resonance imaging for preoperative prediction of the circumferential margin involvement in patients with rectal cancer. Colorectal Dis 2007;9(5):402–11.

21. Brown G, Kirkham A, Williams GT, et al. High-resolution MRI of the anatomy important in total mesorectal excision of the rectum. AJR Am J Roentgenol 2004;182(2): 431–9.

22. Heald RJ, Ryall RD. Recurrence and survival after total mesorectal excision for rectal cancer. Lancet 1986;1:1479–82.

23. Reynolds JV, Joyce WP, Dolan J, et al. Pathological evidence in support of total mesorectal excision in the management of rectal cancer. Br J Surg 1996; 83:1112–5.

24. Brown G, Richards C, Newcombe RG, et al. Rectal carcinoma: thin section MR imaging for staging in 28 patients. Radiology 1999;211:215–22.

25. Bissett IP, Fernando CC, Hough DM, et al. Identification of the fascia propria by magnetic resonance imaging and its relevance to preoperative assessment of rectal cancer. Dis Colon Rectum 2001;44: 259–65.

26. Rao SX, Zeng MS, Xu JM, et al. Assessment of T staging and mesorectal fascia status using high resolution MRI in rectal cancer with rectal distension. World J Gastroenterol 2007;13(30):4141–6.

27. Compton CC, Greene FL. The staging of colorectal cancer: 2004 and beyond. CA Cancer J Clin 2004; 54:295–308.

28. Soyer P, Lagadec M, Sirol M, et al. Free breathing diffusion-weighted single-shot echo-planar MR imaging using parallel imaging (GRAPPA2) and high b value for the detection of primary rectal adenocarcinoma. Cancer Imaging 2010;10(1):32.

29. Curvo-Semedo L, Lambregts DM, Maas M, et al. Diffusion-weighted imaging in rectal cancer: apparent diffusion coefficient as a potential noninvasive marker of tumor aggressiveness. J Magn Reson Imaging 2012;35(6):1365–71.

30. Chan TW, Kressel HY, Milestone B, et al. Rectal carcinoma staging at MR imaging with endorectal surface coil – work in progress. Radiology 1991;181:461–7.

31. Landmann RG, Wong WD, Hoepfl J, et al. Limitations of early rectal cancer nodal staging may explain failure after local excision. Dis Colon Rectum 2007;50(10):1520–5.

32. Schnall MD, Furth EE, Rosato EF, et al. Rectal tumor stage: correlation of endorectal MR imaging and pathologic findings. Radiology 1994;190:709–14.

33. Birbeck KF, Macklin CP, Tiffin NJ, et al. Rates of circumferential resection margin involvement varies between surgeons and predicts outcomes in rectal cancer surgery. Ann Surg 2002;235:449–57.

34. Beets-Tan RG, Beets GL. Local staging of rectal cancer: a review of imaging. J Magn Reson Imaging 2011;33:1012–29.

35. Torksad MR, Hansson KA, Lindholm J, et al. Significance of mesorectal volume in staging of rectal cancer with magnetic resonance imaging and the assessment of involvement of the mesorectal fascia. Eur Radiol 2007;17:1694–9.

36. Al-Sukhni E, Milot L, Fruitman M, et al. Diagnostic accuracy of MRI for assessment of T category, lymph node metastases, and circumferential resection margin involvement in patients with rectal cancer: a systematic review and meta-analysis. Ann Surg Oncol 2012;19(7):2212–23.

37. Brown G. Local radiological staging of rectal cancer. Clin Radiol 2004;59:213–4.

38. Hall NR, Finan PJ, al-Jaberi T, et al. Circumferential margin involvement after mesorectal excision of rectal cancer with curative intent: predictor of survival but not local recurrence? Dis Colon Rectum 1998;41: 979–83.

39. Beets Tan RG, Beets GL, Vliegen RF, et al. Accuracy of magnetic resonance imaging in prediction of tumor-free resection margin in rectal cancer surgery. Lancet 2001;357:497–504.

40. Nagtegaal ID, Marijnen CA, Kranenbarg EK, et al. Circumferential margin involvement is still an important predictor of local recurrence in rectal carcinoma: not one millimeter but two millimeters is the limit. Am J Surg Pathol 2002;26:350–7.

41. Koh DM, Brown G, Husband JE. Nodal staging in rectal cancer. Abdom Imaging 2006;31(6):652–9.

42. Brown G, Richards CJ, Bourne MW, et al. Morphologic predictors of lymph node status in rectal cancer with use of high-spatial-resolution MR imaging with histopathologic comparison. Radiology 2003;227(2):371–7.

43. Klessen C, Rogalla P, Taupitz M. Local staging of rectal cancer: the current role of MRI. Eur Radiol 2007;17(2):379–89.

44. Sugihara K, Kobayashi H, Kato T, et al. Indication and benefit of pelvic sidewall dissection for rectal cancer. Dis Colon Rectum 2006;49:1663–72.

45. Smith NJ, Shihab O, Arnaout A, et al. MRI for detection of extramural invasion in rectal cancer. AJR Am J Roentgenol 2008;191(5):1517–22.

46. Vliegen RF, Beets GL, Lammering G, et al. Mesorectal fascia invasion after neoadjuvent chemoradiotherapy and radiation therapy for locally advanced cancer: accuracy of MRI for prediction. Radiology 2008;246(2):454–62.

47. Kim DJ, Kim HJ, Lim JS, et al. Restaging of rectal cancer with MR imaging after concurrent chemotherapy and radiation therapy. Radiographics 2010;30:503–16.

48. Sauer R, Becker H, Hohenberger W, et al. Preoperative versus postoperative chemoradiotherapy for rectal cancer. N Engl J Med 2004;351(17): 1731–40.

49. Janjan NA, Crane C, Feig BW, et al. Improved overall survival among responders to preoperative chemoradiation for locally advanced rectal cancer. Am J Clin Oncol 2001;24(2):107–12.

50. Enqin G, Sharifov R, Gural Z, et al. Can diffusion-weighted MRI determine complete responders after neoadjuvant chemoradiation for locally advanced rectal cancer? Diagn Interv Radiol 2012 Jul 13. http://dx.doi.org/10.4261/1305-3825.DIR.5755-12.1. [Epub ahead of print].

Transabdominal Ultrasound for Bowel Evaluation

Peter M. Rodgers, FRCR[a],*, Ratan Verma, FRCR[b]

KEYWORDS

- Ultrasound • Sonography • Bowel • Diverticulitis • Appendicitis • Crohn's disease • Strategy

KEY POINTS

- Transabdominal ultrasound (TAUS) of the bowel has the potential to play a significant role in imaging strategies directed at managing acute and elective gastrointestinal disorders and their mimics.
- However, this potential cannot be achieved without the systematic provision of adequate numbers of specifically trained personnel to match the clinical need. Imaging in acute and elective scenarios is most effective when the prevalence of the suspected conditions is high.
- Provision of an appendicitis scanning service within limited hours or for a population largely expected not to have appendicitis or performed by operators who seldom identify a normal appendix, is unlikely to perform to standards that justify continued provision of the service.
- Similarly, TAUS for Crohn's disease needs to be a strategically supported part of a multimodality imaging service within a multidisciplinary inflammatory bowel disease team to achieve results justifying clinical confidence in referring clinicians and patients.

INTRODUCTION

Since the late 1970s, there have been many original publications and review articles documenting the transabdominal ultrasound (TAUS) appearances of a broad range of common and uncommon gastrointestinal (GI) diseases.[1–3] In earlier decades these investigators presented their evidence, experience, and commentary in the context of the ubiquitous availability, affordability, and speed of ultrasound (US) imaging. The context has shifted with technological advances in imaging. CT and MRI scanning are widely available on a 24-7, 365, basis. Fast volume acquisition and multiplanar reconstruction have improved accuracy and confidence in CT imaging. In contrast, the high level of operator skills and experience required for TAUS to compete with CT diagnostically in GI imaging are rarely available outside office hours. US is notoriously operator-dependent, requiring not only excellent general and specific technical training and aptitude but also considerable experience of a case-mix appropriate to the clinical differential being considered.

US TECHNIQUE

In the authors' practice, TAUS of the bowel begins with a complete examination of the abdomen and pelvis, including the solid and hollow extraintestinal viscera. The complications of bowel disease often extend to involve adjacent organs, the mesentery, and peritoneal recesses (eg, subdiaphragmatic and pelvic collections), or spread hematogenously, particularly via the portal vein to the liver. Using a lower frequency curvilinear probe, particular

Funding: Dr Rodgers, Dr Verma: Nil.
Competing Interest: Dr Rodgers, Dr Verma: Nil.
[a] Radiology Department, Leicester Royal Infirmary, University Hospitals of Leicester, Infirmary Square, Leicester LE1 5WW, United Kingdom; [b] Radiology Department, Leicester General Hospital, University Hospitals of Leicester, Gwendolen Road, Leicester LE5 4PW, United Kingdom
* Corresponding author.
E-mail address: peter.rodgers@uhl-tr.nhs.uk

Radiol Clin N Am 51 (2013) 133–148
http://dx.doi.org/10.1016/j.rcl.2012.09.008
0033-8389/13/$ – see front matter © 2013 Elsevier Inc. All rights reserved.

attention should be paid to those areas beyond the reach of the higher frequency probes needed for detailed interrogation of the bowel wall. This also provides an opportunity to map the layout of the large bowel, identified by its typical haustral pattern, and the distribution and motility of the small bowel. Fortunately, most bowel pathologic findings displace bowel gas and feces, making them stand out against normal bowel segments (**Fig. 1**).

Focal bowel masses, segments of wall thickening, and dilated loops may be apparent even at lower frequencies, but high-frequency probes are essential to identify and characterize changes in the layers of the bowel wall.

GRADED COMPRESSION

Puylaert[4] introduced the term "graded compression" to describe the gradual progressive increase in the pressure the operator applies to the probe while making gentle sweeping movements. Done carefully to avoid causing pain, this is an essential technique in bowel scanning. Overlying soft tissues are compressed, bringing the probe closer to the bowel, gas is displaced from bowel loops to reveal the posterior bowel wall, overlying bowel loops are displaced from those beneath, and the compressibility and/or rigidity of normal and abnormal bowel loops and mesenteric fat can be assessed.

MOWING THE LAWN

A systematic technique is required to survey the entire intestine within the abdominal cavity. Puylaert[5] promoted the use of overlapping vertical sweeps of a high-frequency probe up and down the abdomen in the manner of a lawnmower. Additional operator techniques have been described to examine difficult recesses, including posterior manual compression and scanning in the left lateral decubitus position to assess the retrocecal area.[6]

It is the authors' practice to commence the focused examination of the bowel in the left iliac fossa where the sigmoid colon easily may be identified crossing in front of the left psoas muscle and over the iliac vessels (**Fig. 2**). This is an opportunity to optimize scanning parameters so that the bowel wall layers can be clearly identified while allowing crisp observation of often brisk small bowel peristalsis.

The relationship between the terminal ileum, caecum, appendix, and the right iliac fossa is less constant. The terminal ileum should only be specified as such if seen in continuity with the ileocecal valve. It is often advantageous to reexamine the right iliac fossa with the patient in a left decubitus position that allows movement of mobile small-bowel and caecum into a different position and often reduces the amount of soft tissue between probe and target loops. In adult female patients transvaginal scanning may give excellent views of pelvic small bowel loops.

If a suspicious bowel segment is identified, it should be specifically examined for bowel thickening and alteration in individual bowel layers (see later discussion). Extraintestinal abnormalities, such as thickened mesenteric fat, interloop fluid, exudates, lymphadenopathy, and so forth, should be sought. The vascularity of the abnormal segment should be assessed with color and power Doppler.

NORMAL BOWEL WALL "GUT SIGNATURE"

At higher frequencies, TAUS images the bowel wall as five alternating bands of high and low echogenicity to produce a characteristic sonographic

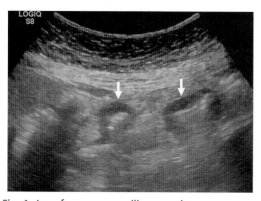

Fig. 1. Low-frequency curvilinear probe sweep across the upper abdomen immediately identifies abnormal target signs of thickened small bowel (*short white arrows*).

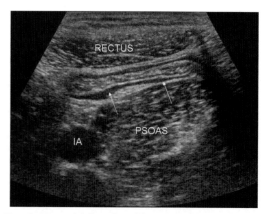

Fig. 2. Normal left colon (*short white arrows*) compressed between rectus and psoas muscles with a high frequency probe. Bowel wall layers clearly shown. IA, Iliac Artery.

signature approximating to the concentric layered histologic structure (**Box 1**).[7]

Visualization of the fine inner and outer bright layers (interface echoes) is highly dependent on the echogenicity of adjacent structures and is most easily seen where there is fluid in the bowel lumen or ascites between bowel loops.

Even at lower diagnostic frequencies in loops further from the probe, at least the two most prominent layers are evident due to their relative thickness and high contrast: the bright submucosa (third layer) and the dark muscularis propria (fourth layer). The deep mucosa is of similar thickness but, being of intermediate echogenicity, is more easily lost against the luminal contents (**Fig. 3**).

The normal bowel wall is up to 2 to 3 mm thick, varying with the state of contraction or relaxation as do the composite layers. Small bowel folds extend into the lumen. Jejunal folds are taller, slightly thicker and more numerous than in the ileum where folds are absent or sparse; in the collapsed state at fasting US examination jejunal folds fill the lumen.

Peristaltic waves pass along small bowel segments at a frequency determined by multiple factors, such as gastric distension. Because elective US examinations are usually performed after a period of fasting, the intestines are generally observed in a quiescent state, but some peristalsis should be seen in healthy bowel segments.

Slung in the peritoneal cavity on a long mesentery, the small bowel is mobile and adjacent loops are easily displaced by compression, as are the mesenteric segments of colon. Healthy small bowel and gas-filled colonic segments are easily compressed.

Doppler scanning demonstrates no signal in normal bowel wall.[8]

SONOGRAPHY OF ABNORMAL BOWEL

The most common and striking feature of bowel disease is wall thickening, which may be focal or diffuse, or circumferential or segmental (**Box 2**). Thickening may be due to the presence of edema,

---

Box 1
Sonographic gut signature
Layer 1: superficial mucosa (fine bright line)
Layer 2: deep mucosa including the lamina propria (gray)
Layer 3: submucosa (bright)
Layer 4: muscularis propria (dark)
Layer 5: serosa (fine bright line)

---

hemorrhage, inflammation, tumor growth, or infiltration. Any of these may result in the classic US feature of an hypoechoic circumferential thickening around a strong echogenic center (lumen),- variously referred to as the target sign, ring sign, or pseudokidney sign (**Fig. 4**).

ALTERED GUT SIGNATURE

In diseased segments, the normal bowel layer pattern may be preserved, exaggerated, distorted, diminished, or obliterated. While there is overlap between the changes produced by various pathologic processes, high-resolution TAUS provides a unique opportunity to identify the specific bowel layers affected, to characterize the lesions, and to diagnose the underlying process.

BOWEL LUMEN

When the bowel wall is thickened, the bowel lumen is usually narrowed or strictured. An uncommon exception to this is aneurysmal dilatation in which the lumen in the diseased segment enlarges. This is most commonly seen in intestinal lymphoma.

Dilatation of the bowel lumen is seen proximal to an obstructing lesion, where it may initially be accompanied by increased peristalsis. Dilatation with no peristalsis may be due to late-stage obstruction or "paralytic" ileus (most commonly seen after abdominal surgery).

BOWEL PLASTICITY AND/OR MOBILITY AND/OR PERISTALSIS

Most disease processes result in stiffening of the affected bowel segments uniquely observed in real-time TAUS as more rigid, less compressible, less easily displaced loops, or segments with reduced or absent peristalsis.

ALTERED BLOOD FLOW

Normal bowel wall perfusion cannot be demonstrated by color or power Doppler techniques, so the identification of flow indicates pathologic perfusion (eg, hyperemia in actively inflamed segments).

EXTRAMURAL CHANGES

Bowel wall disease may extend out to involve adjacent loops or solid organs, or be the result of external disease involving the bowel loop. Identification of peri-intestinal fluid, collections or abscesses or fistulous tracks, and altered mesenteric fat are important features to characterize processes and assess local complications.

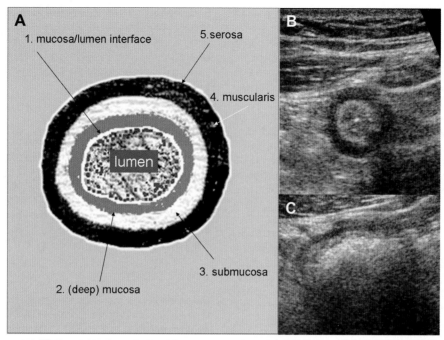

Fig. 3. Normal small bowel ultrasound. Graphic representation of a transverse US view of distal small bowel (A) demonstrating the five layer structure (gut signature). Transverse US images of normal distal small bowel in contracted (B) and distended (C) states. Only the bright submucosa and dark muscularis propria are easily discernible. (*Adapted from* Rodgers PM. Small intestine. In: Allan PL, Baxter GM, Weston MJ, eds. Clinical Ultrasound, 3rd ed. Edinburgh: Churchill Livingstone, 2011; with permission.)

MESENTERIC LYMPHADENOPATHY

Lymph node size, shape (oval or round), echotexture (hyperechoic or hypoechoic, heterogeneous), smooth or irregular surface, conglomeration or matting, should be documented because these may aid in narrowing the diagnosis.

ACUTE APPENDICITIS

Acute appendicitis is the most common indication for urgent abdominal surgery and one of the most common causes of acute abdominal pain. It is more prevalent in older children and young adults.

Box 2
A useful checklist for TAUS bowel examinations

- Bowel wall thickness
- Altered gut signature
- Bowel lumen
- Bowel plasticity and/or mobility and/or peristalsis
- Altered blood flow
- Mesenteric and/or interloop changes

In most cases, this is the result of luminal obstruction usually by a fecalith or appendicolith. A variety of less common causes include lymphoid hyperplasia, parasites, and primary and secondary tumors. Continued secretion in the presence of obstruction results in lumen distension, mucosal ischemia, and necrosis. Consequences may include bacterial invasion, transmural inflammation, full-thickness infarction, and perforation (in about 20% of cases).

The high mortality and morbidity rate associated with appendiceal perforation in the pre-antibiotic era produced a policy of early surgical intervention based on clinical assessment. The "typical" clinical presentation is of vague central or epigastric abdominal pain with anorexia progressing to nausea and vomiting, followed by migration of the pain to the right lower quadrant, and accompanied by fever, leukocytosis and rebound tenderness. Atypical presentations are not infrequent, so symptoms, signs, and laboratory tests only have a moderate accuracy in predicting appendicitis.

This policy is still widely practiced even though between one in five and one in three of the removed appendices will be healthy[9,10] and despite more than 20-years evidence of the potential for diagnostic imaging to reduce the number of unnecessary appendectomies.[11,12]

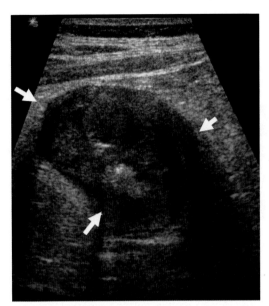

Fig. 4. Pseudokidney appearance of a right colon cancer (*white arrows*) in an 80-year-old male with abdominal pain and anemia.

SONOGRAPHY OF THE APPENDIX

Using the graded compression technique, the appendix is identified as a thin, blind-ending tube, with the typical gut wall sonographic signature, in continuity with the cecal pole, rising a couple of centimeters below the ileocecal valve (**Fig. 5**). The appendix varies greatly in size (average 8 cm; range 1–24 cm) and position (pelvic or descending and retrocecal being the most common).[13] US visualization of the normal appendix is difficult and often only partial (**Fig. 6**). Identification rates for the normal appendix in a population not presenting with suspected appendicitis varies widely and is related to numerous factors including technique, operator experience, examination time, and patient body habitus.

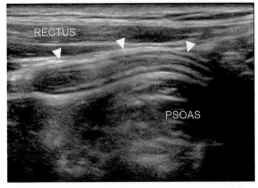

Fig. 5. Long section of normal appendix; a thin, blind-ending tube with clear gut signature (*white arrows*) compressed between rectus and psoas muscles.

SONOGRAPHY OF ACUTE APPENDICITIS

In early publications, the dominant sonographic criterion for the diagnosis of acute appendicitis was the identification of a noncompressible blind-ending tube with a maximum outside diameter (MOD) greater than 6 mm. More recent studies have shown a wide range of normal appendiceal diameters extending above 6 mm and demonstrated lumen distension by impacted feces and/or air, such that this threshold diameter is unreliable unless included with other sonographic signs of appendiceal or extra-appendiceal inflammation (**Box 3**, **Fig. 7**).[14,15]

Requiring at least two of these criteria to be present together with significant clinical evidence of acute appendicitis reduces the number of false positive diagnoses (**Fig. 8**A, B and **Fig. 9**).

Early reports identified the presence of an appendicolith as a reliable indicator of inflammation. This is not the authors experience; we see appendicoliths frequently in asymptomatic patients (**Fig. 10**).

In a minority of cases, the appendiceal inflammation will be focal and may be overlooked if the entire appendix is not visualized.[16] In focal appendicitis the appendix may not exceed the 6 mm threshold.[17]

The performance of US in identifying the perforated appendix is reduced but may most reliably be identified by loss of the hyperechoic appendiceal wall layer (indicating transmural inflammation) and loculated periappendiceal or pelvic fluid collections[18] (**Fig. 11**).

The negative predictive value of a scan in which the appendix is not identified differs widely across studies but is more reliable when the operator regularly identifies a normal or abnormal appendix.[17]

STRATEGIC APPROACH TO IMAGING APPENDICITIS

It is still common practice in the United Kingdom for patients presenting with "typical" features of acute appendicitis to be taken directly for laparoscopic appendectomy. The only adult patients routinely referred for preoperative imaging are those with atypical features (ie, patients who are less likely to have appendicitis and younger women referred for exclusion of a gynecological basis for their presentation because there can be considerable cross-over of the clinical presentation of this patient group). However, an excellent gynecological sonographer may have no training in bowel US. This strategy provides a poor case-mix for training sonographers to identify all confidently excluded appendicitis.

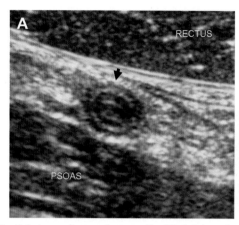

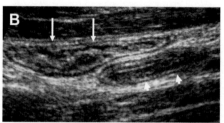

Fig. 6. Partial views of normal appendix. (*A*) Axial section showing normal gut signature (*black arrowhead*). (*B*) Long oblique section showing appendix (*white arrowheads*) deep to an adjacent ileal loop (*long white arrows*).

Prospective comparative studies of the performance of CT and US in acute appendicitis favor CT. The diagnostic value of graded compression US has a summary sensitivity of 0.78 and summary specificity of 0.83. The diagnostic value of CT has a summary sensitivity of 0.91 and summary specificity of 0.90.[19]

The investigators of this meta-analysis and many others relegate US to the first-line test for children and younger or pregnant women to avoid ionizing radiation.[20,21] However, equivocal CT findings are a significant problem with up to one-third of these having acute appendicitis.[22] TAUS can usefully be used as an adjunct to CT in equivocal cases.[23]

A key difficulty with any US-based strategy is the availability of sufficiently skilled operatives to offer reliable results within an acceptable timeframe. Imaging to reduce the negative appendectomy rate should not be bought at the expense of increasing perforation rates, which relate to the time since onset of symptoms. A potential solution is specific TAUS training of personnel who are not radiologists, such as emergency department personnel, but other studies demonstrate that these high-performance values for US and CT are not being matched in day-to-day use in a mixture of clinical settings.[24,25] Valid concerns are also raised about potential delays to surgery that need addressing in strategic planning.

Factors in "underperformance" issues include training and experience, particularly of staff scanning after office hours. This problem may have been underestimated by retrospective studies in which out-of-office-hours cases were managed without imaging and prospective studies in which similar exclusions were made.

A stratified approach commencing with US using a high-frequency probe and proceeding to CT for inconclusive cases has been recommended.[26–28] Low-dose CT techniques and/or limited scan areas have been demonstrated as effective while reducing radiation.[29]

Box 3
Sonographic criteria for appendicitis

Noncompressible blind-ending tube

Lumen distension (MOD >6 mm)

Wall thickness greater than 3 mm

Loss of gut signature

Hyperemia on Doppler scanning

Hyperechoic periappendiceal fat-thickening

Local transducer tenderness

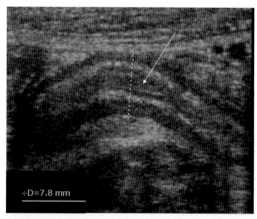

÷D=7.8 mm

Fig. 7. Appendicitis: false positive sonography. A 53-year-old female with right iliac fossa (RIF) pain. TAUS-identified appendix in region of pain. Maximum outer diameter 7.8 mm. Echogenic fluid in lumen (*long arrow*). Gut signature intact. No other cause for symptoms. Appendectomy within 24 hours. Normal appendix at histology.

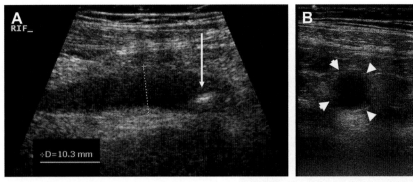

Fig. 8. Acute appendicitis. (A) Long section distended (10 mm MOD), noncompressible appendix with tip appendicolith (*long arrow*). (B) Wall thinned with no gut signature indicating ischemic necrosis. Acute suppurative appendicitis confirmed post-resection within 24 hours.

A consensus seems to be forming around a selective, combined US, or low-dose CT approach. Local solutions will vary but, although the chosen imaging strategy is driven by the primary objective of surgical removal of every inflamed appendix (to reduce the rate of perforation), it needs to be benchmarked against performance indicators, including the negative appendectomy rate and the perforation rate.

A current meta-analysis of randomized controlled trials supports a paradigm shift to antibiotic treatment of uncomplicated appendicitis.[30] This would shift the burden of imaging from identifying a normal appendix to identifying those cases in which complications had already risen.

MIMICS OF ACUTE APPENDICITIS

When imaging is applied to patients with suspected acute appendicitis, identification of alternative diagnoses is an essential outcome. The most common differentials are acute diverticulitis, gynecological causes, and mesenteric adenitis (in children). However, prospective studies identify a wide range of less frequent mimics (**Table 1**) and their US features have been well documented.[31] These include a variety of conditions, such as epiploic appendagitis, in which surgery is to be avoided and where the advantage of having an US operator is that he or she may be guided to the pathologic finding by local tenderness (**Fig. 12**).

ACUTE DIVERTICULITIS

Acute colonic diverticulitis is a common reason for acute hospital admission. Clinical differentiation from nonspecific abdominal pain and a range of acute abdominopelvic pathologic findings is inexact (**Table 2**) and imaging is used in most cases although 85% will recover with nonoperative

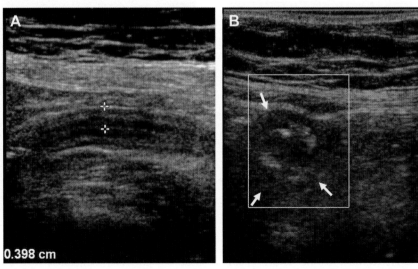

Fig. 9. Acute appendicitis. (A) Long section showing appendiceal wall thickening with gut signature intact. (B) Axial section of thickened enlarged appendix tip with loss of signature and hyperemia on power Doppler.

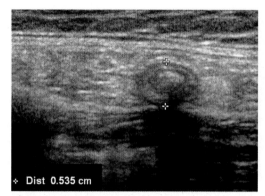

Fig. 10. Appendicolith. Axial image showing the appendix lumen distended by echogenic material with an acoustic shadow. An incidental finding in a man with no related symptoms.

treatment.[32] Heavy reliance is placed on CT for reasons considered previously and with less constraint by concerns about radiation. However, TAUS is highly sensitive and specific for uncomplicated acute diverticulitis and for the primary complication of pericolic abscess.[33]

PATHOGENESIS

Most colonic diverticula are "false diverticula" containing no muscularis propria. The diverticula wall consists of mucosa-submucosa blown out through defects in the muscularis propria. These occur at weak points in the colonic wall, generally at the site of entry of a blood vessel. Diverticula are most commonly seen in sigmoid colon where they are often associated with other typical features of

Table 1
Alternative diagnoses made by US in the absence of acute appendicitis

Diagnosis	Frequency
Ovarian or paraovarian cyst	17
Gastroenteritis	14
Cystitis	9
Hemorrhagic ovarian cyst	6
Inflammatory bowel disease	5
Pyelonephritis	4
Nephrolithiasis	3
Obstructing ureteric calculus	3
Ruptured ovarian follicle	3
Colitis	3
Intussusception	1
Hydrosalpinx	1
Hip effusion	1
Transplant pyelonephritis	1
Small bowel obstruction	1
Constipation	1
Cholelithiasis	1

Data from Trout AT, Sanchez R, Ladino-Torres MF. A critical evaluation of US for the diagnosis of pediatric acute appendicitis in a real-life setting: how can we improve the diagnostic value of sonography? Pediatr Radiol 2012;42:813–23.

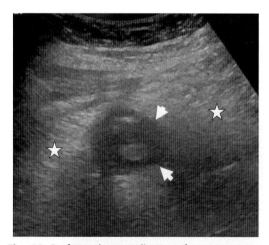

Fig. 11. Perforated appendix. Low-frequency sonogram showing axial sections of the appendix surrounded by loculated fluid (*white arrow heads*) contained by increased hyperechoic mesenteric fat (*stars*).

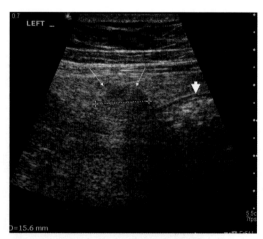

Fig. 12. Epiploic appendagitis. A 24-year-old male presenting with acute left iliac fossa (LIF) pain. Blood normal. TAUS showed the focus of tenderness to be a noncompressible, moderately hyperechoic 15 mm mass (*white arrows*) adjacent to the left colon (*arrowhead*). No intervention was required.

Table 2 Alternative diagnosis in 47 of 175 patients clinically suspected of having diverticulitis	
Epiploic appendagitis	8
Ureterolithiasis	6
Urinary tract infection	4
Pelvic Inflammatory disease	4
Ischemic colitis	3
Infectious enterocolitis	3
Perforated carcinoma	3
Small bowel obstruction	2
Ulcerative colitis	2
Hemorrhagic ovarian cyst	2
Musculoskeletal pain	2
Appendicitis	2
Crohn's disease	1
Nonspecific colitis	1
Small bowel infarction	1
Cholecystitis	1

Data from Hollerweger A, Macheiner P, Rettenbacher T, et al. Colonic diverticulitis: diagnostic value and appearance of inflamed diverticula-sonographic evaluation. Eur Radiol 2001;11:1956–63.

diverticular disease (eg, muscularis propria thickening, shortening, and narrowing of the lumen). Diverticula vary in size from tiny intramural and transient phenomena to permanent protrusions up to several centimeters in diameter, and rarely much greater. The prevalence of diverticula increases with age, affecting 50% of patients over 70 years old.

Retention of fecal matter within a diverticulum may produce mucosal abrasion resulting in infection or inflammation of the diverticulum wall (diverticulitis). The process may produce a focal intramural inflammatory mass or abscess, infiltrate along the bowel wall to produce an inflammatory bowel segment, and perforate into sigmoid mesentery where the process is usually contained. However, perforation can cause intraperitoneal contamination that is associated with a much higher morbidity and mortality. The incidence of diverticulitis increases with the duration of diverticulosis.

CLINICAL FEATURES

Compared with patients with nonspecific abdominal pain, those with diverticulitis are more likely to have subacute onset of pain (>1 hr), tenderness to palpation only in the left lower quadrant, and

raised inflammatory markers; and are less likely to have nausea and vomiting.[32]

SONOGRAPHIC FEATURES OF DIVERTICULOSIS

Sonographic features of diverticulosis include

- Diverticula appear as bright "ears" out with the bowel wall with acoustic shadowing due to the presence of gas or inspissated feces
- A thinned diverticular wall may be demonstrated at higher probe frequencies with a reduced gut signature due to the absence of muscularis propria (**Fig. 13**).
- The neck of a diverticulum may be identified as an echogenic band traversing hypoechoic muscularis propria that is often thickened.

SONOGRAPHIC FEATURES OF DIVERTICULITIS

An isolated inflamed diverticulum is identified as an enlarged echo-poor protrusion from the colon wall, with an ill-defined margin surrounded by echogenic noncompressible fat. The diverticulum wall signature is lost. A central shadowing echogenicity may indicate the presence of fecalith.[34]

Often the inflammation will have extended into the bowel producing asymmetrical or circumferential hypoechoic mural thickening that may demonstrate hyperemia on Doppler scanning. Diverticulitis may progress to an intramural or pericolic abscess indicated by an anechoic collection that may contain pockets of air or debris (**Fig. 14**).

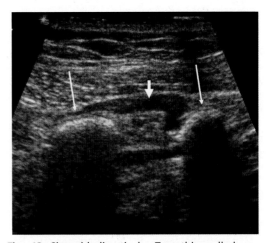

Fig. 13. Sigmoid diverticula. Two thin-walled, gas-filled, reduced gut signature outpouchings (*long arrows*) through the thickened muscularis propria of the sigmoid colon (*short arrow*).

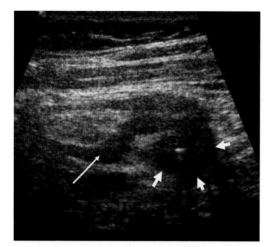

Fig. 14. Acute diverticulitis: pericolic abscess. Echo-poor pericolic collection (*short arrows*) containing central bright gas echo. Asymmetrical thickening of muscularis propria (*long arrow*).

STRATEGIC APPROACH TO IMAGING DIVERTICULITIS

CT scanning is essential for investigating complicated diverticular disease especially where there are diffuse signs and clinical suspicion of secondary peritonitis. CT has advantages when the diagnosis is wide open and patient factors, including age, preclude serious concerns about radiation exposure. However, in most uncomplicated cases the experienced sonographer may quickly confirm a diagnosis guided by the clinical signs. If TAUS is to be recommended in premenopausal women, a place in the general strategic approach to acute diverticulitis should be considered.

CROHN'S DISEASE

Crohn's disease (CD) is a lifelong inflammatory GI condition of uncertain cause characterized by episodes of remission and relapse. The inflammatory process may extend through all the bowel layers and beyond, resulting in intraperitoneal disease and involvement of adjacent bowel loops and/or organs.

CD may involve any part of the GI tract and may involve multiple segments at the same or different times. Large bowel, ileocolic, and terminal ileal disease are most common patterns with the terminal ileum being involved in up to 75% of cases at presentation. Proximal small bowel CD without terminal ileal involvement is seen in only 3% of cases.

Management depends on characterizing the behavior of lesions into the subtypes inflammatory, stenosing, fistulating, and/or penetrating. The disease course may be modified by medical therapy but 90% of patients will require surgery within 10 years of diagnosis.[35]

CD: IMAGING STRATEGY

There are about 87,000 people with CD in the United Kingdom and most are referred to hospital for evaluation.[35] In the authors' practice, the investigation of new suspected cases of inflammatory bowel disease, known cases with complications, or cases at critical therapeutic decision points are decisions made and reviewed within a multidisciplinary team of gastroenterologists, surgeons, radiologists, and clinical specialist nurses. Acute cases, often critically ill and presenting out-of-office hours, almost invariably undergo CT scanning. Given the increasing concern about lifetime radiation exposure to these patients, it is the authors' practice to minimize the use of CT at all elective presentations. The authors use focused bowel US as the primary imaging modality in new presenters and for assessment of known cases of small bowel CD with symptomatic relapse. When there is a mismatch between the US findings and the clinical indicators, the MR enterography or small bowel barium studies have a useful additional role.

CLINICAL FEATURES OF CD

Patients with CD may present at any age but most commonly present in their late teens and early adulthood. Diarrhea of more than 6 weeks duration, abdominal pain, and weight loss are the most common presenting symptoms. The young patient with right iliac fossa pain and a mass may easily be misdiagnosed as having acute appendicitis. Blood and/or mucus in the stool generally indicate colonic involvement. Perianal fistulas are present in 10% of patients at presentation.

ULTRASOUND FEATURES OF CROHN'S DISEASE

US has a well-documented role in diagnosing CD, assessing and monitoring disease, and identifying complications.[36–38]

BOWEL WALL THICKENING

The primary imaging feature of CD is thickening of the bowel wall and US has shown to identify wall thickening in patients with suspected CD with a sensitivity of 75% to 94% and a specificity of 67% to 100%.[39]

Most studies have used a 4-mm threshold for thickening in nondistended bowel. Moving this threshold affects the sensitivity and specificity; however, any thickening must be interpreted in the context of other changes.

ALTERATION IN GUT SIGNATURE

Inflammatory lesions may be confined to the mucosa, or mucosa and submucosa, resulting in thickening of these layers alone. Thickening of these layers may be judged in comparison with the muscularis propria, which, in health, is the thickest layer in all states of contraction.

Isolated thickening of the mucosa may be accompanied by interruption of the lumen-interface echo (layer 1), due to sloughing of the mucosal surface, and/or tiny bright echoes, due to gas in mucosal ulcers (**Fig. 15**).

The dark-bright strata may be preserved, blurred, or obliterated. The latter usually indicates transmural inflammation and may be accompanied by irregular mixed hypoechoic inflammatory exudate on the serosal bowel surface. These changes may be circumferential or focal (**Fig. 16**). Inflamed and normal bowel may be identified on the same axial circumference (skip lesion) and strongly indicates CD (**Fig. 17**).

These patterns indicate the progress of the disease through the bowel wall[40]; pattern 3, indicating transmural inflammation, may be accompanied by complications.[38]

FAT-WRAPPING

Transmural inflammation stimulates proliferation of mesenteric or subserosal fat, which "creeps" around the inflamed bowel segment, a distinguishing characteristic of transmural CD (**Fig. 18**).

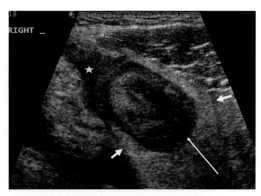

Fig. 16. CD transmural inflammation. 26-year-old male with known ileo-colic CD presenting with increasing right iliac fossa pain worse on leg extension. TAUS demonstrates ileal wall thickening with a focal segment of hypoechoic transmural inflammation (*long arrow*), creeping hyperechoic mesenteric fat (*short arrows*) and inflammatory exudate on the serosal surface (*star*).

Fat-wrapping correlates with histologic evidence of transmural inflammation and associated complications such as fistulation.[38]

VASCULAR CHANGES

Actively inflamed bowel segments have an increased blood flow that may be demonstrated with color Doppler or power Doppler imaging (**Fig. 19**). Studies have shown this phenomenon to be helpful in distinguishing active inflammatory lesions from fibrotic strictures and in monitoring response to medical therapies. The use of US contrast media may further increase the diagnostic confidence by quantifying this phenomenon.[41]

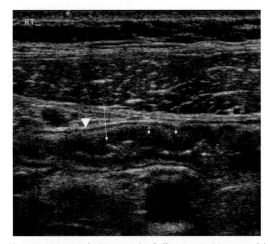

Fig. 15. Mucosal CD terminal ileum. A 22-year-old female presenting with alternating bowel habit with bright red rectal bleeding and abdominal pain. TAUS showed thickening of the terminal ileal mucosa and blurring of the submucosa (*short arrows*) with mucosal ulceration (*long arrow*). The muscularis propria appears normal (*arrowhead*). Ileocolonoscopy showed mild ileitis and a few small ileal ulcers.

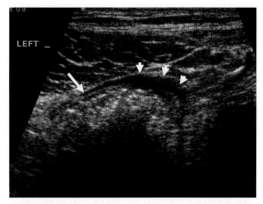

Fig. 17. CD colon skip lesion. Young male presenting with several months rectal bleeding and weight loss. Axial US image of colon in LIF showing a transmural inflammatory skip lesion (*arrow heads*) adjacent to normal thin bowel wall with normal gut signature (*long arrow*).

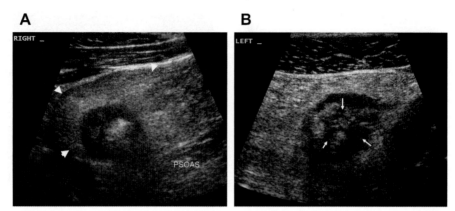

Fig. 18. (A and B) Ileocecal and sigmoid CD: the 24-year-old male presenting with RIF pain, blood mixed with stool and raised inflammatory markers. (A) Transmural hypoechoic thickening of the terminal ileum with creeping fat (*arrowheads*). (B) LIF axial image showing a thickened, contracted large bowel with hypoechoic disruptions of the submucosa (*short arrows*). Subsequent colonoscopy was limited by Crohn stricture in the left colon.

LOCOREGIONAL LYMPHADENOPATHY

Active intestinal CD is usually accompanied by lymphadenopathy in the mesentery.

LOCAL COMPLICATIONS OF CD

Transmural inflammation is a hallmark of CD, resulting in the local complications of stricture, abscess, and fistula. US is useful in detecting these complications but, as with all imaging modalities, may miss subtle enteroenteric fistulas.[42]

STRICTURE

Narrowing of the bowel lumen sufficient to produce impaired intestinal function and obstructive symptoms may be seen both in active

inflammatory segments (hot strictures) and in segments where fibrosis dominates (cold strictures) (see **Fig. 18**B). Spasm and edema contribute to the narrowing of active disease segments and may rapidly respond to medical therapy. Persistent symptomatic stricture is the most common indication for surgery. In addition to clinical assessment, laboratory results, and

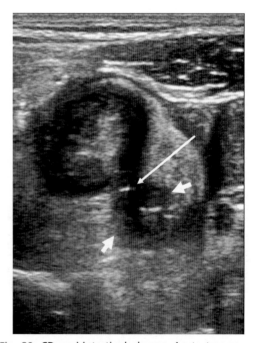

Fig. 20. CD peri-intestinal abscess. Acute transmural ileal inflammation with echopoor fluid and bright gas bubbles passing through a wall defect (*long arrow*) into an adjacent collection (*arrow heads*) contained within creeping fat.

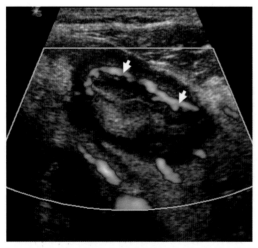

Fig. 19. CD TI power Doppler: power Doppler indicates hyperemia with flow seen clearly in a vessel running within the submucosa (*short arrows*).

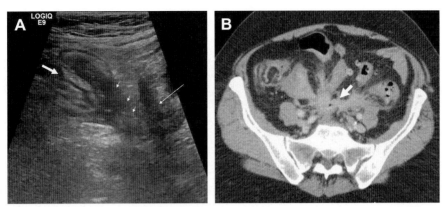

Fig. 21. (*A*) CD enterocolic fistula: US. Angulated ileal (*short arrow*) and colon (*long arrow*) loops connected by echo-poor fistula (*arrow heads*) with moving, bright, gas echoes in real-time. (*B*) CD enterocolic fistula: CT. Same-day CT scan confirms an inflammatory mass involving small and large bowel extending onto the posterior pelvic brim. A tiny gas bubble marks the fistula.

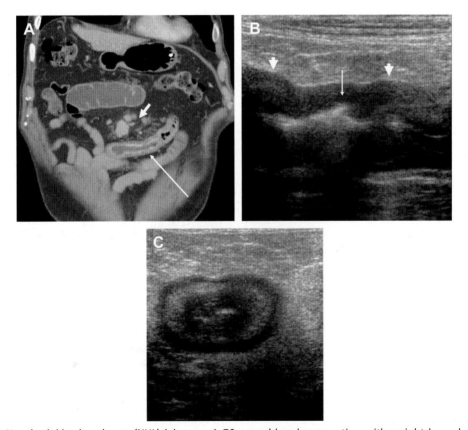

Fig. 22. Non hodgkins lymphoma (NHL) jejunum. A 76-year-old male presenting with weight loss, abdominal pain and vomiting. (*A*) Coronal CT image showing a greater than 10 cm segment of continuous thickening of proximal small bowel (*long arrow*) with local lymphadenopathy (*short arrow*). Malignant or inflammatory differentials were considered and US was performed to characterize the lesion. (*B*) Long image from the middle of the lesion shows low/mixed echo circumferential thickening (*arrowheads*) and bright gas in a deep ulcer (*long arrow*). (*C*) Axial image showing preservation of the gut signature with mucosal and submucosal thickening and blurring. Doppler showed vascular flow in the submucosa. At endoscopy the mixed features of raised edges and complex ulcers left the diagnosis unclear. However, biopsy and subsequent resection showed enteropathy-associated T-cell lymphoma.

endoscopic findings, imaging makes a significant contribution in distinguishing between the two.

Active inflammatory strictures are hyperemic compared with normal bowel and with fibrotic strictures. Color and power Doppler demonstrate no vascular activity in healthy bowel wall but both demonstrate the increased flow in inflamed bowel wall and inflammatory masses.

FISTULATING OR PENETRATING DISEASE
Abscess

Transmural inflammation extending out to and beyond the serosal bowel surface may be seen at US as irregular mixed low-echo inflammatory exudate on the serosal surface, a mixed low-echo inflammatory mass between bowel loops, or an irregularly thick and walled collection with a liquid center (abscess). Abscesses may form between bowel loops or in adjacent structures such as the abdominal wall (**Fig. 20**).

Fistula

In up to one-third of patients, penetrating fissures can extend to create an abnormal communication between the lumen of the diseased bowel segment and adjacent bowel loops or any adjacent hollow organ (eg, uterus, bladder).

The communication between adherent bowel loops may be difficult to identify and underestimated by all imaging modalities. At US fistula are identified as irregular tubular hypoechoic tracks (**Fig. 21**) and, occasionally, may demonstrate small hyperreflective air bubbles within.[43] However, the presence of adjacent indrawn, angulated bowel loops connected by mixed hypoechoic inflammatory exudate is highly suspicious of fistulation.

Disease Activity

Management decisions in CD depend on estimates of disease activity. Clinical assessment and laboratory results are central and are commonly used to monitor therapeutic responses. However, symptoms may be due to factors other than active inflammation (eg, cold strictures, bacterial overgrowth) and US may usefully contribute to assessment of disease activity by documenting the vascularity of lesions with color or power Doppler. Current research suggests accuracy may be improved by the use of intravenous contrast agents.[44]

Differential Diagnosis

Caution is required in interpreting any of the above imaging findings because there is considerable overlap with other intestinal pathologic findings (**Fig. 22**). It is strongly recommended that imaging in inflammatory bowel disease be practiced in the setting of a multidisciplinary team in which clinical events, laboratory results, endoscopy, and histology can inform the selection of the appropriate imaging modality and interpretation of the imaging findings.

SUMMARY

TAUS of the bowel has the potential to play a significant role in imaging strategies directed at managing acute and elective GI disorders and their mimics.

However, this potential cannot be achieved without the systematic provision of adequate numbers of specifically trained personnel to match the clinical need. Imaging in acute and elective scenarios is most effective when the prevalence of the suspected conditions is high.

Provision of an appendicitis scanning service within limited hours or for a population largely expected not to have appendicitis or performed by operators who seldom identify a normal appendix, is unlikely to perform to standards that justify continued provision of the service.

Similarly, TAUS for Crohn's disease needs to be a strategically supported part of a multimodality imaging service within a multidisciplinary irritable bowel disease team to achieve results justifying clinical confidence in the referring clinicians and patients.

REFERENCES

1. Ledermann HP, Börner N, Strunk H, et al. Bowel wall thickening on transabdominal sonography. AJR Am J Roentgenol 2000;174(1):107–17.
2. O'Malley ME, Wilson SR. US of gastrointestinal tract abnormalities with CT correlation. Radiographics 2003;23(1):59–72.
3. Puylaert JB. Ultrasonography of the acute abdomen: gastrointestinal conditions. Radiol Clin North Am 2003;41(6):1227–42.
4. Puylaert JB. Acute appendicitis: US evaluation using graded compression. Radiology 1986;158(2):355–60.
5. Puylaert JB. Ultrasound of acute GI tract conditions. Eur Radiol 2001;11(10):1867–77.
6. Lee JH, Jeong YK, Hwang JC, et al. Graded compression sonography with adjuvant use of a posterior manual compression technique in the sonographic diagnosis of acute appendicitis. AJR Am J Roentgenol 2002;178(4):863–8.
7. Kimmey MB, Martin RW, Haggitt RC, et al. Histologic correlates of gastrointestinal ultrasound images. Gastroenterology 1989;96(2 Pt 1):433–41.

8. Esteban JM, Maldonado L, Sanchiz V, et al. Activity of Crohn's disease assessed by colour Doppler ultrasound analysis of the affected loops. Eur Radiol 2001;11(8):1423–8.

9. Gilmore OJ, Browett JP, Griffin PH, et al. Appendicitis and mimicking conditions. Lancet 1975; 306(7932):421–4.

10. Baigrie RJ, Dehn TC, Fowler SM, et al. Analysis of 8651 appendicectomies in England and Wales during 1992. Br J Surg 1995;82(7):933.

11. Jeffrey RB Jr, Laing FC, Townsend RR. Acute appendicitis: sonographic criteria based on 250 cases. Radiology 1988;167(2):327–9.

12. Puig S, Hörmann M, Rebhandl W, et al. US as a primary diagnostic tool in relation to negative appendectomy: six years experience. Radiology 2003;226(1):101–4.

13. Collins DC. The length and position of the vermiform appendix: a study of 4,680 specimens. Ann Surg 1932;96(6):1044–8.

14. Rettenbacher T, Hollerweger A, Macheiner P, et al. Outer diameter of the vermiform appendix as a sign of acute appendicitis: evaluation at US. Radiology 2001;218(3):757–62.

15. Park NH, Park CS, Lee EJ, et al. Ultrasonographic findings identifying the faecal-impacted appendix: differential findings with acute appendicitis. Br J Radiol 2007;80(959):872–7.

16. Lim HK, Lee WJ, Lee SJ, et al. Focal appendicitis confined to the tip: diagnosis at US. Radiology 1996;200(3):799–801.

17. Kessler N, Cyteval C, Gallix B, et al. Appendicitis: evaluation of sensitivity, specificity, and predictive values of US, Doppler US, and laboratory findings. Radiology 2004;230(2):472–8.

18. Quillin SP, Siegel MJ, Coffin CM. Acute appendicitis in children: value of sonography in detecting perforation. AJR Am J Roentgenol 1992;159(6):1265–8.

19. van Randen A, Bipat S, Zwinderman AH, et al. Acute appendicitis: meta-analysis of diagnostic performance of CT and graded compression US related to prevalence of disease. Radiology 2008;249(1):97–106.

20. Jacobs JE. CT and sonography for suspected acute appendicitis: a commentary. AJR Am J Roentgenol 2006;186(4):1094–6.

21. Rosen MP, Ding A, Blake MA, et al. ACR Appropriateness Criteria® right lower quadrant pain—suspected appendicitis. J Am Coll Radiol 2011;8(11): 749–55.

22. Rhea JT, Halpern EF, Ptak T, et al. The status of appendiceal CT in an urban medical center 5 years after its introduction: experience with 753 patients. AJR Am J Roentgenol 2005;184(6):1802–8.

23. Jang KM, Lee K, Kim M-J, et al. What is the complementary role of ultrasound evaluation in the diagnosis of acute appendicitis after CT? Eur J Radiol 2010;74(1):71–6.

24. Trout AT, Sanchez R, Ladino-Torres MF. A critical evaluation of US for the diagnosis of pediatric acute appendicitis in a real-life setting: how can we improve the diagnostic value of sonography? Pediatr Radiol 2012;42(7):813–23. Available at: http://www.ncbi.nlm.nih.gov/pubmed/22402833. Accessed July 17, 2012.

25. Lee SL, Walsh AJ, Ho HS. Computed tomography and ultrasonography do not improve and may delay the diagnosis and treatment of acute appendicitis. Arch Surg 2001;136(5):556–62.

26. van Breda Vriesman AC, Kole BJ, Puylaert JB. Effect of ultrasonography and optional computed tomography on the outcome of appendectomy. Eur Radiol 2003;13(10):2278–82.

27. Krishnamoorthi R, Ramarajan N, Wang NE, et al. Effectiveness of a staged US and CT protocol for the diagnosis of pediatric appendicitis: reducing radiation exposure in the age of ALARA. Radiology 2011;259(1):231–9.

28. Poortman P, Oostvogel HJ, Bosma E, et al. Improving diagnosis of acute appendicitis: results of a diagnostic pathway with standard use of ultrasonography followed by selective use of CT. J Am Coll Surg 2009;208(3):434–41.

29. Kim K, Kim YH, Kim SY, et al. Low-dose abdominal CT for evaluating suspected appendicitis. N Engl J Med 2012;366(17):1596–605.

30. Varadhan KK, Neal KR, Lobo DN. Safety and efficacy of antibiotics compared with appendicectomy for treatment of uncomplicated acute appendicitis: meta-analysis of randomised controlled trials. BMJ 2012;344(Apr05 1):e2156.

31. van Breda Vriesman AC. Mimics of appendicitis: alternative nonsurgical diagnoses with sonography and CT. Am J Roentgenol 2006;186(4):1103–12.

32. Laméris W, van Randen A, van Gulik TM, et al. A clinical decision rule to establish the diagnosis of acute diverticulitis at the emergency department. Dis Colon Rectum 2010;53(6):896–904.

33. Schwerk WB, Schwarz S, Rothmund M. Sonography in acute colonic diverticulitis. Dis Colon Rectum 1992;35(11):1077–84.

34. Wilson SR, Toi A. The value of sonography in the diagnosis of acute diverticulitis of the colon. Am J Roentgenol 1990;154(6):1199–202.

35. Mowat C, Cole A, Windsor A, et al. Guidelines for the management of inflammatory bowel disease in adults. Gut 2011;60(5):571–607.

36. Sheridan MB, Nicholson DA, Martin DF. Transabdominal ultrasonography as the primary investigation in patients with suspected Crohn's disease or recurrence: a prospective study. Clin Radiol 1993;48(6): 402–4.

37. Parente F, Greco S, Molteni M, et al. Role of early ultrasound in detecting inflammatory intestinal disorders and identifying their anatomical location within

the bowel. Aliment Pharmacol Ther 2003;18(10): 1009–16.

38. Sheehan AL, Warren BF, Gear MW, et al. Fat-wrapping in Crohn's disease: pathological basis and relevance to surgical practice. Br J Surg 1992;79(9):955–8.

39. Fraquelli M, Colli A, Casazza G, et al. Role of US in detection of Crohn disease: meta-analysis. Radiology 2005;236(1):95–101.

40. Hata J, Haruma K, Suenaga K, et al. Ultrasonographic assessment of inflammatory bowel disease. Am J Gastroenterol 1992;87(4):443–7.

41. Kratzer W, Schmidt SA, Mittrach C, et al. Contrast-enhanced wideband harmonic imaging ultrasound (SonoVue): a new technique for quantifying bowel wall vascularity in Crohn's disease. Scand J Gastroenterol 2005;40(8):985–91.

42. Maconi G, Bollani S, Bianchi Porro G. Ultrasonographic detection of intestinal complications in Crohn's disease. Dig Dis Sci 1996;41(8):1643–8.

43. Sarrazin J, Wilson SR. Manifestations of Crohn disease at US. Radiographics 1996;16(3):499–520 [discussion: 520–1].

44. Migaleddu V, Scanu AM, Quaia E, et al. Contrast-enhanced ultrasonographic evaluation of inflammatory activity in Crohn's disease. Gastroenterology 2009;137(1):43–52.

Fluoroscopic and CT Enteroclysis:
Evidence-Based Clinical Update

Dean D.T. Maglinte, MD

KEYWORDS

- Small-bowel obstruction • Small-bowel Crohn's disease • Small-bowel tumors • CT enterography
- Enteroclysis • CT enteroclysis • MR enterography • MR enteroclysis

KEY POINTS

- The clinical investigation of small bowel (SB) diseases requires methods of imaging that have a high negative predictive value and high sensitivity because of the low incidence of disease and clinical presentations that are mimicked by diseases of contiguous or adjacent viscera with higher incidence.
- There are no shortcuts to reliable SB imaging; evidence- and experience-based analyses have shown that examinations that distend the SB diagnose smaller, early lesions and allow confident exclusion of SB disease, the latter an important and misunderstood role when interpreting examinations of the most difficult segment of the alimentary tube to examine.
- Computed tomographic enteroclysis (CTE) is important in the clinical management of the patient with suspected small-bowel obstruction (SBO) in whom (1) orally ingested or nonenteral volume-challenged examinations are not informative or equivocal, (2) additional questions relevant to management are not answered, and (3) intestinal obstruction or distention is present but surgeons prefer nonsurgical management.
- Air (or CO_2) double-contrast (DC) barium enteroclysis and CTE with due considerations for patient care are reproducible and reliable methods of SB investigation, the proper implementation and clinical use of which has long been poorly understood by radiologists and referring physicians.
- SB malignancies are rare and frequently underdiagnosed or diagnosed late and require methods of imaging to improve long-term survival; CTE accurately depicts early-stage disease. DC barium enteroclysis depicts mucosal alterations of early SB Crohn's disease and nonsteroidal antiinflammatory drug (NSAID)-induced enteropathy better than cross-sectional methods of imaging; it can also depict submucosal masses and is complementary to capsule endoscopy (CE).

INTRODUCTION

Insisting that we take only decisions that are grounded in high-quality clinical trials would mean denying patients important expertise on which their health may depend.
— Gunderman and Chou, 2011.[1]

The diagnostic evaluation of SB diseases has changed profoundly during the past few decades.[2] The important role of radiology in the investigation of SB diseases remains poorly understood by both referring physicians who treat the patients and radiologists who perform the examinations. The mesenteric small intestine is the most challenging

Financial disclosure: Consultant, Cook, Inc, Bloomington, IN.
Department of Radiology and Imaging Sciences, IU Health - University Hospital, School of Medicine, Indiana University, 550 North University Boulevard, UH0279, Indianapolis, IN 46202-5253, USA
E-mail address: dmaglint@iupui.edu

Radiol Clin N Am 51 (2013) 149–176
http://dx.doi.org/10.1016/j.rcl.2012.09.009
0033-8389/13/$ – see front matter © 2013 Elsevier Inc. All rights reserved.

segment of the gastrointestinal (GI) tract to examine. It is the longest segment of the alimentary tube and has the widest mucosal surface, yet the incidence of disease is low and the clinical presentations are mimicked by diseases of adjacent visceral organs with higher incidence of abnormalities. The significant role of imaging therefore is to reliably exclude SB disease or diagnose early, small, or localized disease with confidence.[3–18] Methods of imaging that do not distend the SB lumen have historically been shown not to allow reliable exclusion of SB disease or early demonstration of small or early mucosal or submucosal abnormalities. In addition, these examinations do not give the radiologist and the clinician the confidence to exclude small neoplasms and low-grade SBO or depict early mucosal SB Crohn's disease (aphthae) or NSAID enteropathy. SB imaging reports are therefore not infrequently equivocal or not informative, and repeated imaging examinations or performance of more expensive and invasive endoscopic methods are done before a definitive diagnosis or confident exclusion of SB disease is made. The investigation of SB diseases requires methods of examination that have a high negative predictive value and high sensitivity. Intubation-infusion examinations (enteroclysis and its modifications) have been shown to overcome most of the inherent limitations of conventional (peroral ingested or nonenteral volume-challenged) examinations but have inherent limitations.[19] Decades of experience have shown that only examinations that distend the lumen and coat the mucosa fulfill these roles.[3–18,20] Several of these reports are not generated from well-controlled clinical trials. Many are experience based. The enteroclysis technique and its modifications have remained the most accurate methods that reliably exclude SB abnormality and allow early diagnosis of disease.

Results of analyses that are evidence based and the method of how the SB examinations were done as shown in several recent reports should be critically analyzed, as a cursory assessment of only the sensitivity and specificity data will uniformly show high sensitivity and specificity of almost all methods of SB examination because of the low incidence of disease,[20] resulting in an illusion of high SB imaging reliability. Specific attention to the negative predictive values of comparative studies and the reference standard of the particular SB disease are important variables that help understand the role of imaging in confidently ruling out or confirming the presence of SB disease. An example is a recent meta-analysis of prospective studies on inflammatory bowel disease comparing ultrasonography, magnetic resonance (MR) imaging, scintigraphy, and computed tomography (CT), which showed high sensitivity and specificity for all examinations, with no significant statistical differences in diagnostic accuracy among the imaging techniques compared.[21] The small bowel follow-through (SBFT) was part of the gold standard, and the disease phenotype was not categorized. Does the negative result of any of the imaging methods assessed despite the high sensitivity, specificity, and accuracy in this report confidently answer the clinical indication to rule out early SB Crohn's disease in a symptomatic patient and does it give referring physicians confidence in formulating a course of management? What is the negative predictive value of each imaging study evaluated in depicting the early mucosal alterations (aphthoid lesions) of early SB Crohn's disease? In the patient with recurrent abdominal pain with a prior history of abdominal surgery or with unexplained intermittent GI bleeding, do negative nonenteral volume-challenged cross-sectional imaging exclude low-grade adhesive obstruction or small SB tumors despite the reported high sensitivity and specificity of reports from enthusiasts of these methods?

Progress in imaging of the SB during the past few decades is due largely to refinements in the application of orally ingested conventional abdominal and pelvic CT or MR imaging with intravenous (IV) contrast (CT enterography and MR enterography) and conventional barium enteroclysis methods (CTE and magnetic resonance enteroclysis [MRE]) and technical refinements in performing DC barium enteroclysis.[8,22–84] An update on how to perform CTE and its modifications and DC barium enteroclysis, as well as its clinical applications, have been recently described and is beyond the scope of this article. Interested readers are referred to these articles.[53,85–87]

This article presents an update on the current role of DC barium enteroclysis and CTE modifications in the diagnosis and management of SB diseases from evidence- and experience-based analyses and examines factors why enteral volume-challenged examinations despite their reported higher accuracy and reliability in ruling out SB disease are infrequently performed in clinical practice. The roles of these methods of SB examination in practice are discussed. Evidence- and experience-based recommendations are made to improve early diagnosis and influence prognosis, decrease irradiation of the patient, and decrease costs of investigation. An overview of the common technical problems and limitations of DC barium enteroclysis and CTE are briefly discussed.

HISTORICAL PERSPECTIVE

The underlying hypothesis for performing intubation infusion SB examinations (enteroclysis) was the realization by early twentieth century radiologists that the clinical diagnosis of disease in an anatomic structure such as the SB was improved or its absence reliably excluded when the SB lumen is distended rather than when it is collapsed or in its normal state.[88–95] This idea was based on the realization of the inherent limitations of the serial oral SBFT barium examination (also known as barium meal or SB series) (**Fig. 1**).[96]

Enteroclysis was first described by Pesquera in 1929.[88] Several investigators have modified his technique,[89,91–93,95,97,98] but the method did not gain popularity because of technical problems, including issues with enteric tubes and inadequacy of fluoroscopic units. It was not until 1971 that Johan Sellink[94] rejuvenated the technique in Europe and gained notice across the Atlantic Ocean through additional publications by several investigators in the late seventies and early eighties.[13,98,99] His technique was tried by interested radiologists in North America but was not adopted by the majority because of discomfort to patients and the time requirement.

Several enteric tubes have been used by several enthusiasts, but the most commonly used enteroclysis catheters are modifications of the Bilbao Dotter tube[100] originally used for hypotonic duodenography. Maglinte[101] added a balloon attachment proximal to the tip and lengthened it to diminish duodenogastric reflux (Maglinte enteroclysis catheter [MEC], Cook Inc, Bloomington, IN, USA) (**Fig. 2**). Herlinger[98] further modified the tube to a single end hole catheter. Other modifications essentially adopted the balloon attachment of the MEC, which remains in use.

A further modification of the Maglinte catheter was enlargement of the lumen and addition of sump ports (Maglinte Decompression/Enteroclysis Catheter or Maglinte Long Tube, MDEC, Cook Inc), which allowed not only the performance of diagnostic enteroclysis but also had the added benefit of long tube decompression for SBO or ileus before or after the performance of the diagnostic enteroclysis (**Fig. 3**).[102,103] It can also be used for nasogastric (NG) suction. Sump ports were added to keep the lumen and side ports patent for longer periods. This prevented dual intubations (use of MEC for enteroclysis followed by placement of an NG tube after the examination) in patients who had a preexisting NG tube or who would benefit from it after the examination.[102,104] The lumen of the MEC is small and is readily clogged by enteric debris compared with the NG tube. The NG tube cannot be used for enteroclysis because of duodenogastric reflux, the possibility of aspiration, and the short length of the tube.

The choice of enteral contrast agents differed among enthusiasts. Sellink preferred the low-density single-contrast barium mixture followed by a water flush to produce a DC effect if needed; this method was popularized by Nolan and colleagues.[17,18,105–109] Herlinger preferred the DC method using methylcellulose suspension and a small volume of a high-density/viscosity barium mixture,[93,98] reported initially by Trickey and colleagues,[110] whereas Maglinte preferred a biphasic method using a larger volume of medium-density barium mixture and a methylcellulose suspension for DC.[111] Japanese proponents of enteroclysis popularized the use of air DC

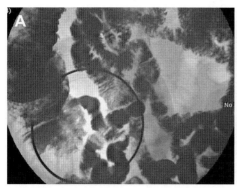
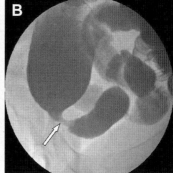

Fig. 1. (*A*) False-negative results of orally ingested SB examination in mechanical SBO. Patient with symptoms of intermittent low-grade SBO from ileal tuberculosis. Compression radiograph of distal SB and ileocecal region during SBFT do not show evidence of mechanical SBO. (*B*) Tuberculous stricture (*arrow*) apparent during fluoroscopic assessment because of exaggerated prestenotic dilatation with continuous infusion providing an enteral volume challenge. (*From* Gollub MJ, Maglinte DD. CT enterography and CT enteroclysis. In: Shirkhoda A, editor. Variants and pitfalls in body imaging. 2nd edition. Philadelphia: Lippincott Williams and Wilkins; 2011; with permission.)

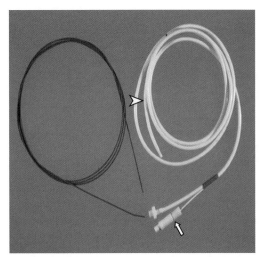

Fig. 2. Maglinte enteroclysis catheter (MEC, Cook Inc). Balloon attachment port (*arrow*) and antireflux balloon proximal to catheter tip (*arrowhead*).

barium enteroclysis using a small volume of high-density barium.[112–116] This method was recently modified by Maglinte and colleagues[85] using a larger amount of medium-density barium and carbon dioxide with conscious sedation using an amnesic and analgesic to improve patient comfort using materials available in North America. This modification was necessary after the results of a survey of outpatients who recently underwent a biphasic enteroclysis using a small amount of a sedative.[117,118]

Kloppel Von modified the Sellink method using a lower density water-soluble enteral contrast and adapted it to monoslice CT.[23] With the development of multislice CT technology, this method was subsequently modified by Maglinte and colleagues[54,86,119,120] into a positive enteral contrast CTE and a neutral enteral contrast with IV contrast CTE in several newer publications. Each modification has distinct strengths and limitations for different clinical indications. An 11% dilution of water-soluble contrast was used for the positive enteral contrast CTE after trials of multiple dilutions of iodinated contrast, and water was used for the neutral enteral with IV contrast CTE. Using a wide-window CT setting for the positive enteral contrast optimizes visualization of the valvulae conniventes from several dilutions that we have tried in the past.[53,86,87,121] The use of methylcellulose suspension, which has been withdrawn from commercial distribution in the United States because of contamination as a neutral enteral contrast, was abandoned and replaced with plain tap water for the neutral CTE with IV contrast modification. Absorption is not an issue with CTE compared with CT enterography because of the volume used, the use of a hypotonic agent (glucagon), and continued infusion during CT acquisition (Fig. 4). An important reason for abandoning the biphasic DC barium enteroclysis method with methylcellulose was based on data from early clinical experience with CE at the Indiana University Hospital. A group of patients with unexplained GI bleeding or anemia who had noninformative SBFT, conventional CT examinations

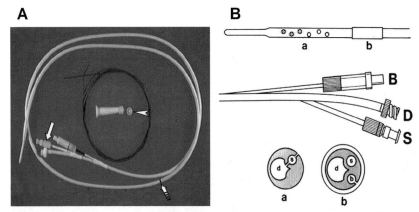

Fig. 3. (*A*) Decompression/enteroclysis catheter (Maglinte Long Tube, MDEC, Cook Inc). Added sump port (*arrow*) to catheter helps prevent obstruction of the decompression lumen by enteric debris. Occlusion cap of sump port (*arrowhead*). Adapter adjacent to cap allows attachment of the suction lumen to wall suction bedside. Black mark in catheter (*broken arrow*) indicates level of catheter tip in the lower body of stomach from nasal entry. (*B*) Line diagram of Maglinte long tube. B, balloon port; D, suction/drainage port (main lumen); S, sump port. The inset figures (*A, B*) show the cross-sectional appearances of the long tube at positions a and b. The tube is 13.5F; it is better tolerated than the smallest nasogastric tube particularly with the routine conscious sedation used for our tube placements.

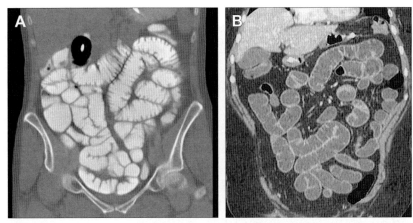

Fig. 4. CTE modifications. Normal examinations. (*A*) Positive enteral contrast CTE. The 11% dilution of water-soluble iodinated contrast with wide window settings used optimizes visualization of the valvulae conniventes. (*B*) Neutral enteral contrast CTE with IV contrast using water. Soft-tissue window settings optimizes evaluation of intestinal wall, mesentery, and solid abdominal organs, a global abdominal examination. Volume (3.5 mL) of neutral enteral contrast used in our protocol includes filling of the colon needed for appropriate staging of Crohn's disease, which includes assessment of the perianal region according to the current report of the working party of the 2005 Montreal World Congress of Gastroenterology for inflammatory bowel disease. (*Data from* Silverberg MS, Satsangi J, Ahmad T, et al. Toward an integrated clinical, molecular and serologic classification of inflammatory bowel disease: Report of a Working Party of the 2005 Montreal World Congress of Gastroenterology. Can J Gastroenterol 2005;19(Suppl A):5A–36A.)

with oral and IV contrast from their local institutions, who were referred to gastroenterologists, underwent CE. After CE, a biphasic barium enteroclysis was performed. Our experience showed that the infusion of methylcellulose to produce DC effaced the surface pattern and minimized the demonstration of mucosal scratches or erosions (**Fig. 5**) and small submucosal defects (**Fig. 6**).[122] This result led us to revisit the DC barium enteroclysis modification popularized by Japanese investigators after adoption of CE in our practice. Our modification of the DC

enteroclysis[69,85,123] has been reported. The modification was necessary, as the Japanese method took longer to perform in our experience and was not tolerated by our patient population despite mild sedation.[117] This also led us to perform a survey and reevaluate our method of conscious sedation.[118] Biscaldi and colleagues[29,124–126] have applied the enteroclysis technique using retrograde infusion for selected indications.

MR imaging to modify the enteroclysis technique was first reported by Holzknecht and colleagues[127] in 1998. The first report on MRE in

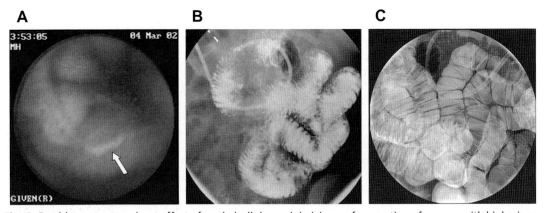

Fig. 5. Double-contrast washout effect of methylcellulose minimizing surface coating of mucosa with biphasic enterolcysis. (*A*) CE image at the level of proximal jejunum shows linear circumferential ulcer (*arrow*) consistent with SB Crohn's disease. (*B*) Single-contrast barium infusion phase of enteroclysis. Hyperperistalsis is seen. (*C*) Establishment of double-contrast effect shows normal jejunum at level seen at CE. ([*A*] *Courtesy of* S. Liangpunsakul, MD.)

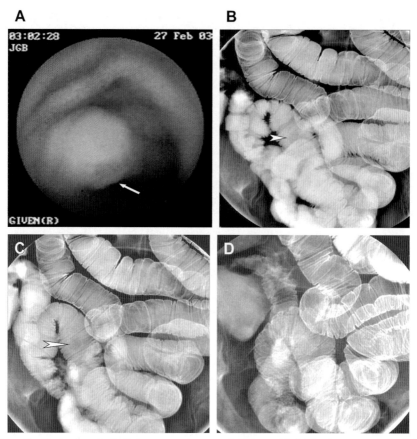

Fig. 6. "Wash out" effect of methylcellulose on submucosal defect with biphasic enteroclysis. (*A*) Submucosal mass (*arrow*) in distal SB at CE. (*B*) Arrowhead indicates submucosal polypoid defect at start of infusion of methylcellulose. Subtle defect seen (*arrowhead*) in single-contrast phase. (*C*) Further infusion with beginning double-contrast effect seen shows gradual diminution of the defect (*arrowhead*) seen in (*B*). (*D*) Subtle defect no longer discernible with full double-contrast of segment involved. ([A] *Courtesy of* S. Liangpunsakul, MD.)

North America was in 2000 by Umschaden and colleagues.[25,76] The potential of MRE was readily recognized by an accompanying editorial[24]; the foremost was the lack of ionizing radiation and the improved soft-tissue contrast resolution. Gourtsoyiannis and colleagues[22,128–133] refined the technique of MRE and popularized its use in Europe. A more recent update has been provided by Masselli and Gualdi.[84] Positive and neutral enteral contrast CTEs, MRE, and DC barium enteroclysis remain in clinical use in referral centers in Europe, North America, and Asia.

Enteroclysis and its cross-sectional modifications, despite the reported accuracy, are mostly performed as a problem-solving tool in tertiary medical centers at present. This method usually follows orally ingested SB examinations (conventional abdominal/pelvic CT with oral and IV contrast, CT enterography or MR enterography) in patients with negative or equivocal findings or with persistent symptoms despite negative findings. In a minority of specialist centers where the various enteroclysis modifications are done regularly, the method is used as a primary diagnostic investigation to confidently exclude or diagnose early SB disease and in patients with high clinical suspicion of SB disease to decrease radiation burden, decrease cost of work-up, and minimize delays in diagnosis of SB diseases.[2,24,85–87,96,123]

EVIDENCE-BASED ANALYSIS: IMAGING IN THE INVESTIGATION OF SB DISEASES

In this century, there are multiple methods of imaging the small intestine (**Table 1**) without updated evidence-based guidelines for appropriate use. The lack of a current evidence-based guideline results in inappropriate use and overuse in clinical practice,[134] wasting expenditures by inappropriate referrals, incorrect interpretation, and duplicative use[134] and resulting in increased cost of investigation, increased radiation burden to patient, and

Table 1	
SB radiology: twenty-first century	
Peroral SB Examinations	**Intubation Infusion Distended SB Examinations**
SB follow-through	Barium enteroclysis Methylcellulose DC enteroclysis, Air (CO_2) DC enteroclysis
CT abdomen/pelvis With oral and IV contrast CT enterography With IV contrast	CT enteroclysis 1. Neutral enteral with IV contrast 2. Positive enteral CTE
MR enterography With IV contrast	MR enteroclysis With IV contrast
Ultrasonography	Sonoenteroclysis

delays in diagnosis, which influence prognosis. Evidence- and experience-based comparisons provide insights on the clinical performance of the different methods of investigation of SB diseases and a rational basis for making recommendations. Although there are limitations in the appraisal of these research studies, they can provide useful guidelines for optimal use of current imaging studies.

The efficacy of imaging procedures in confirming or confidently excluding SB disease is not frequently considered in the investigation of SB diseases by radiologists and referring physicians. The influence on the referring physician's diagnostic confidence in formulating a course of management by the method of SB examination and how it is reported is also infrequently considered by radiologists, which may involve looking beyond reported statistical accuracy.[135] Hence, it is not uncommon to see patients with several imaging examinations previously done before a diagnostic examination is performed or its confident exclusion is established. This situation also explains requests for second reading/opinion on examinations already reported. Imaging is a rapidly growing part of health care spending, and an overall cost consideration in looking at the effectiveness of SB diagnostic procedures are not given serious consideration; what is convenient and revenue producing seem to be the primary considerations. Not infrequently, peroral ingested SB examinations that do not involve direct participation by radiologists are done several times before a diagnosis is made. Available guidelines do not include assessment of the evidence of efficacy of diagnostic imaging on diagnostic confidence and patient management.[135]

Small Bowel Obstruction

This is a common clinical condition, often presenting with signs and symptoms similar to those seen in other acute abdominal disorders. Once suspected based on the patient's clinical history and physical examination, radiologists are charged with the task of verifying or excluding the presence of obstruction and providing cogent information on the site, severity, and probable cause of the obstruction and the presence of strangulation.[104,136–139]

Although initial reports showed high accuracy of CT of the abdomen and pelvis with oral and IV contrasts in the diagnoses of SBO,[140,141] a subsequent evidence-based comparison showed an overall accuracy of 65%.[142–144] In this analysis, however, the accuracy of conventional CT increased to 81% for high-grade and complete obstruction. With low-grade obstruction, accuracy was 48%, statistically similar to the sensitivity of abdominal radiography for SBO.[145] These patients have recurrent symptoms, and multiple additional conventional CT examinations are often obtained until the obstruction becomes severe enough to be diagnosed. In patients with symptoms of recurrent low-grade adhesive obstruction, following an initial negative orally ingested CT examination usually done in the emergency department, a recommendation should be made to the referring physician that if a further investigation is needed, these patients should be referred for enteral volume-challenged examinations. In this subset of patients, similar to patients with suspected SB Crohn's disease or tumor, repeated examinations that are unable to reliably rule out obstruction are done before appropriate imaging is requested. Findings of adhesions are often present in retrospect but are not confidently diagnosed because of the lack of an appreciable transition point; the latter is exaggerated with enteral volume-challenged examinations. This diagnosis should be made even when nonobstructive, as these are known to cause symptoms of recurrent or chronic abdominal pain in patients with prior abdominal surgery (**Figs. 7** and **8**). Dense anterior parietal peritoneal adhesions increase the risk of bowel injury during laparoscopy and may require alternative trocar insertion sites.[146] The number and sites of SBO and the length of the SB proximal to the first point of obstruction assists the surgeon in deciding whether an adequate absorptive surface is available for the formation of either an ostomy or a bypass (generally 125 cm).[104,137,138]

Conventional CT and other nonenteral volume-challenged examinations are not sensitive for lower grades of SBO that present usually in the subacute

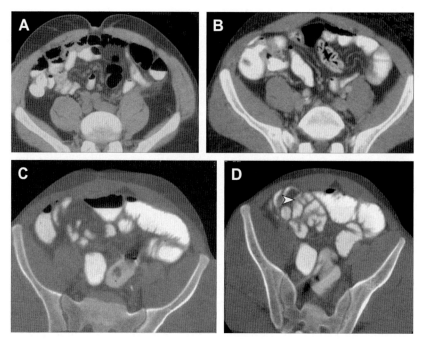

Fig. 7. Conventional CT and CTE in low-grade small-bowel obstruction. (*A, B*) There is no evidence of a gradient or transition point to suggest mechanical obstruction in a patient with symptoms of recurrent SBO. (*C, D*) CTE of the same patient demonstrates the transition point and prestenotic dilatation from anterior peritoneal adhesive obstruction posterior to the right rectus muscle. Interloop (visceral) adhesions (*arrowhead*) noted in segments posterior to parietal adhesive obstruction.

or in the outpatient setting (see **Fig. 7**).[96,142–144,147] CTE is the most accurate method in the further investigation of these patients and in those with SBO diagnosed by conventional CT in whom additional management-relevant questions are not answered.[137–139,142] In the former group of patients, symptoms frequently subside with nonsurgical management. Confirmation of the diagnosis by CTE prevents repeated performance of orally ingested enteral contrast SB CT or MR

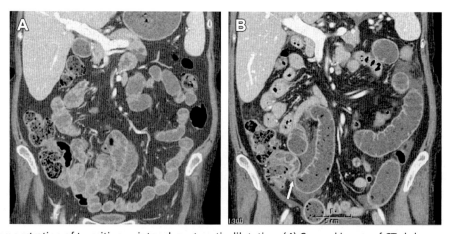

Fig. 8. Demonstration of transition point and prestenotic dilatation. (*A*) Coronal image of CT abdomen and pelvis with orally ingested neutral contrast shows filling loops of the SB including distal loops but no evidence of mechanical obstruction seen in patient with tuberculous stricture (same patient as in **Fig. 1**). (*B*) Stricture now apparent (*arrow*) with prestenotic dilatation during enteral volume challenge. Note the "dirty feces sign" from inspissated debris. (*From* Gollub MJ, Maglinte DD. CT enterography and CT enteroclysis. In: Shirkhoda A, editor. Variants and pitfalls in body imaging. 2nd edition. Philadelphia: Lippincott Williams and Wilkins; 2011; with permission.)

examinations. These examinations neither confidently diagnose nor exclude low-grade obstruction in the appropriate clinical setting. A larger volume of neutral oral contrast may minimize this disadvantage, but patients with this condition experience nausea and sometimes vomit with the volumes given for CT enterography. Not infrequently, they are not able to finish the optimal volume required. By directly infusing contrast into the SB and providing a fluid volume challenge, the presence of an existing low-grade obstruction, the gradient, or prestenotic dilatation is exaggerated and reliably diagnosed; vomiting is avoided by control of infusion rates fluoroscopically and understanding several variables involved in enteroclysis that require fluoroscopic experience (see **Fig. 8**).[104,138] Even when no gradient is observed, demonstration of subtle deformities such as luminal narrowing and fixations are easier to appreciate. Real-time (fluoroscopic) observations add to the confidence in making or excluding the diagnosis. This observation adds to the morphologic details provided by multiplanar CT. Cross-referenced assessment adds to the more precise assessment of the location and characterization of the cause. The positive enteral CTE modification is preferred for this subset of patients, although this condition can be diagnosed also with neutral enteral CTE with IV contrast. The lack of real-time control by the radiologist on the rate of infusion and volume needed for neutral enteral CTE added to the possibility of vomiting in this group of patients makes this modification less ideal. The method can be modified particularly in patients with inflammatory SB disease with low-grade obstructive symptoms with indirect monitoring of the infusion rates; this requires fluoroscopic experience. Determining the optimal infusion rates on either modification is difficult and requires experience, as there are several variables that influence it and each patient is different.[87] In the subset of patients with recurrent symptoms, a subtle gradient or transient stasis may be observed fluoroscopically and may not be shown on the CT image. Correlating the fluoroscopic observation and the anatomic information depicted by multiplanar CT allows a confident report of low-grade adhesive obstruction from a parietal or visceral adhesion or both. Neutral enteral with IV contrast CTE excels in evaluating mural abnormalities in addition to the mesentery and solid viscera. In patients in whom the obstruction has resolved, adhesions are still reliably visualized on CTE.

An added observation obtained during fluoroscopy in the subset of patients with recurrent abdominal pain is that, in some patients with visceral hypersensitivity or irritable bowel syndrome (IBS), the abdominal symptoms are reproduced during contrast infusion and distention of the SB. This confirms the clinical suspicion.[3,148] Lack of reproduction of abdominal symptoms, however, does not exclude the diagnosis, as no scientific validation of this fluoroscopic observation during enteroclysis has been reported to my knowledge; the predictive values are difficult to evaluate scientifically. In our experience, it may coexist with an SB anatomic abnormality and may be important information for management. The primary role of imaging in the investigation of patients suspected of IBS is to exclude morphologic SB abnormality. No guidelines exist for imaging IBS; this awaits further research.[149]

When patients with a history of malignant neoplasm and prior abdominal surgery present with SBO, radiologists are often faced with the difficult task of determining the exact cause of the obstruction. CTE provides the necessary intraluminal and extraluminal information to help differentiate SBO caused by seeded or hematogenous metastases from that caused by radiation exposure or postsurgical adhesions.[7,119,150,151] Thus, in addition to anatomic information regarding tumor size and location, CTE can reliably assess for the presence of associated low-grade obstruction.[152]

There is a subset of patients presenting with SBO in whom surgeons prefer initial conservative management (ie, tube decompression of the distended SB) over surgery.[153,154] These are patients with (1) SBO in the immediate postoperative period, (2) a history of prior abdominal surgery for malignant tumor, (3) a prior history of radiation therapy, and (4) Crohn's disease with prior surgery. Further characterization of the severity and nature of the obstruction are of value for management. The use of the triple lumen long decompression/enteroclysis (MDEC, Cook, Inc) has allowed us to participate in the management of these patients by preliminary decompression of the distended SB, performance of a diagnostic CTE, and further long-tube decompression after the examination.[86,87,102–104,137,138,155] The use of positive enteral CTE allows the assessment of the cause and severity of the obstruction in addition to more efficient long-tube suction (**Fig. 9**).[104,138,156] Participation in the care and management of this subset of patients is important for radiologists to consider changing the low prestige and perception of mediocrity of radiology as a specialty by other physicians.[157,158]

In patients with a prior history of pancreatoduodenectomy (Whipple procedure) who present with symptoms in the subacute or chronic setting unexplained by cross-sectional imaging, which is now the routine examination of the postoperative pancreas,[159,160] when questions relevant to

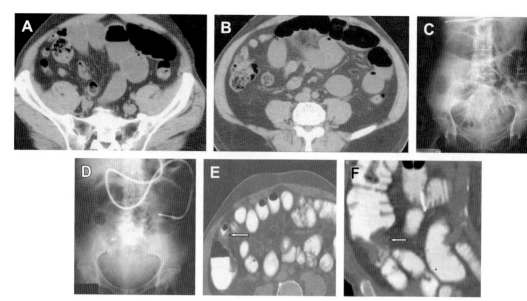

Fig. 9. Use of long tube decompression in postoperative examinations. (*A, B*) Axial images of CT of abdomen and pelvis in a patient with symptoms of SBO, taken in an outside institution, show findings consistent with mechanical SBO. Laparoscopic exploration did not show a point of mechanical obstruction. (*C*) Abdominal radiograph obtained following initial NG suction with long tube (note catheter tip in gastric antrum) at the Indiana University Hospital. (*D*) Overnight suction after long tube advanced to proximal jejunum shows decrease in distention of SB loops. (*E*) Axial CT section of positive enteral CTE shows mural thickening and narrowed lumen at the level of proximal ascending colon (*arrow*). (*F*) Coronal image of CTE shows an annular lesion, raising the possibility of carcinoma. Colonoscopy and biopsy showed tuberculous colitis simulating malignancy (patient had a false-negative result from an incomplete colonoscopy at the outside institution).

management require the need to evaluate the hepaticojejunal, pancreatojejunal, and gastro/pylorojejunal anastomoses, our technique of examination is modified.[161–167] The catheter tip and balloon are positioned immediately distal to the gastroesophageal junction and retracted until mild resistance is met to prevent gastroesophageal reflux during controlled infusion. This modification allows evaluation of the pylorojejunal anastomosis and the hepaticojejunal and pancreatojejunal as well as distal segments of the SB in real-time and cross-sectional images. I have called this modification the "CT Whipplegram" for lack of a better name (**Fig. 10**). It simplifies the evaluation of all the anastomoses as well as the distal SB when partial obstruction enters the differential diagnosis to explain postoperative symptoms in those with prior lower abdominal surgical procedures. We also use this modification in patients with prior Billroth procedures or prior partial or total removal of the upper GI tract and a Roux-en-Y anastomosis (**Fig. 11**). The balloon and catheter tip are positioned immediately distal to the anastomosis. The esophageal anastomosis is evaluated initially using the enteral contrast with the catheter tip above it before advancement of the catheter. This simplifies

the examination of this subset of postsurgical patients in whom examination is difficult with orally ingested contrast with conventional fluoroscopic or cross-sectional imaging.

The timing of surgical intervention as well as the optimal method of radiological investigation in patients with incomplete, open-loop SBO has changed during the past 2 decades.[49,138,168] Evidence-based analysis has shown the added value of CTE over other methods of examination.[96,142–144,147] Reliable exclusion or confirmation of the diagnosis, detection of multiple levels of obstruction, and objective classification of severity and cause are useful information provided by CTE in the evaluation of these patients. Advances in imaging techniques have changed the way in which workups are planned for patients with suspected SBO. Conventional CT has high sensitivity in diagnosing high-grade obstruction and is of value in confirming the presence or absence of strangulation; several reports confirm the value of CT for this indication (**Fig. 12**).[104,136–144,156,169–173] Although the specificity of contrast-enhanced CT for intestinal ischemia has been reported to be as low as 44%, its high sensitivity (90%) and negative predictive

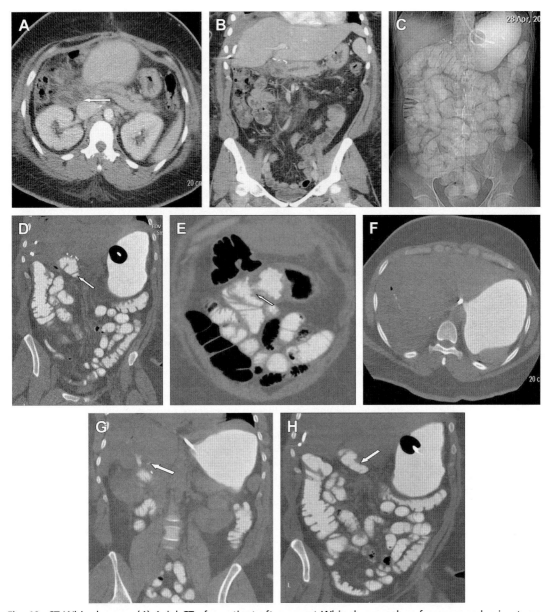

Fig. 10. CT Whipplegram. (*A*) Axial CT of a patient after recent Whipple procedure for neuroendocrine tumor with persistent vomiting and nonresolving fluid collection in perihepatic space referred for CTE to exclude distal SBO and leak at the level of pancreatojejunostomy. Note reactive inflammatory changes to the right of the dilated pancreatic duct (*arrow*). (*B*) Coronal image shows fluid collection and drainage catheter in the right peri-hepatic space. (*C*) Scannogram showing uniform distention of the SB with antireflux balloon of enteroclysis cath-eter immediately distal to the gastroesophageal junction. (*D*) Coronal CTE image shows normal caliber of biliopancreatic limb (*arrow*). (*E*) Coronal image shows a patent pyloroduodenal anastomosis (*arrow*) without evidence of a leak. (*F*) Axial image shows small amount of pneumobilia and contrast in intrahepatic tributary (*arrow*). (*G*) Coronal image of CTE shows small amount of leak to the left of the hepaticojejunostomy (*arrow*). (*H*) Coronal image of CTE shows no evidence of distal mechanical SBO. Arrow points to well-delineated bilio-pancreatic limb.

value (89%) are helpful in making decisions con-cerning continued nonoperative management versus surgery.[169,174–179] The dictum "never let the sun rise or set on small-bowel obstruction," once popular among general surgeons because of the feared complication of strangulation and the clinical difficulty associated with its preopera-tive recognition, is now outdated.[180,181]

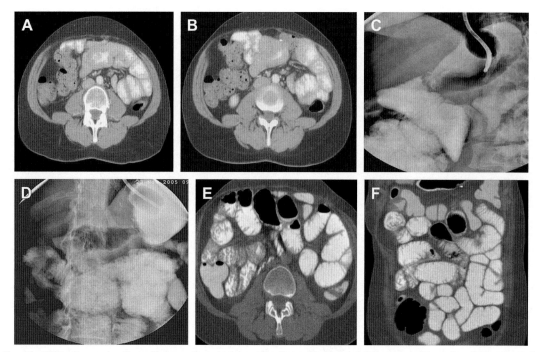

Fig. 11. CTE in the evaluation of late postsurgical complications. (*A, B*) Axial CT images with oral and IV contrast in a patient with abdominal distention, nausea, and vomiting and a history of prior ulcer surgery. Apparent abnormality is seen in proximal SB. The possibility of intussusception and a mass were reported. (*C*) Image during fluoroscopic phase of positive enteral CTE shows the balloon distal to the gastroesophageal junction. (*D*) Frontal radiograph shows dilated gas and fluid-filled proximal SB without evidence of a mass or intussusception. Stasis was seen at fluoroscopy at this level, suggesting postsurgical dysmotility. (*E, F*) Axial and coronal images of CTE show dilated proximal SB loop compatible with dysmotility noted on real-time (fluoroscopic) evaluation without evidence of a mass or intussusception. Abnormality noted is secondary to admixture defects secondary to stasis related to dysmotility from prior Bilroth 1 procedure done with vagotomy. (*Data from* Gollub MJ, Maglinte DD. CT enterography and CT enteroclysis. In: Shirkhoda A, editor. Variants and pitfalls in body imaging. 2nd edition. Philadelphia: Lippincott Williams and Wilkins; 2011.)

SB Crohn's Disease

The optimal radiological approach to the patient with suspected early SB Crohn's disease or when the clinical indication is to rule out SB Crohn's disease compared with the patient with established SB Crohn's disease is poorly understood. Although phenotype classification is required when disease is diagnosed, the latter

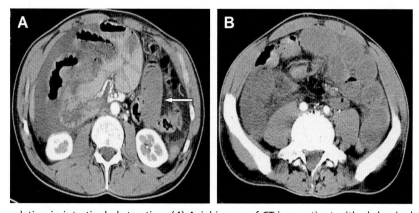

Fig. 12. Strangulation in intestinal obstruction. (*A*) Axial image of CT in a patient with abdominal pain, nausea, and vomiting. Arrow shows a nonperfused segment of the proximal jejunum in late arterial-phase CT acquisition. Note the abnormal superior mesenteric vascular course that suggests midgut volvulus. (*B*) Axial image below Fig. 12A shows the absence of perfusion of mesenteric SB consistent with infarction confirmed at surgery.

requires staging details for therapeutic decision making, whereas the former requires reliable exclusion of disease. The lag time from the onset of symptoms to confirmation of the diagnosis of SB Crohn's disease has been approximately 36 months.[182] Transmural and penetrating phenotypes are usually manifest at the time of diagnosis; it is no longer early SB disease. There has been no recent update on this information since the more common use of CT enterography, CE, and recent modifications of barium and cross-sectional enteroclysis hybrids. It is likely that the lag time will shorten with these newer albeit more expensive innovations. The use of conventional SBFT as the initial method of examination because of its low cost seems misguided, as this likely contributes to the long lag time; it does not reliably exclude early disease and when an abnormality is suspected requires additional imaging to confirm the finding.[16,96] This is one of the reasons for repeated SB imaging with orally ingested methods of investigation before a diagnosis is made.

In the United States, CT enterography has recently replaced the SBFT as the most frequently used method of SB imaging particularly for SB Crohn's disease in most practices.[19,20,28,83,183] With advances in multidetector CT technology, there is validity in this shift.[20,184] Multidetector CT has simplified evaluation of the small intestine and mesentery compared with the SBFT. The term CT enterography was first introduced by Raptopoulos and colleagues[12,20,184] in 1997 in reference to a modified abdominal CT technique to address SB Crohn's disease. A large volume of a 2% barium-based or 2% to 5% water-soluble iodine-based oral contrast material was administered 1 to 2 hours before scanning. A high dose of IV contrast material and a biphasic injection rate regimen of IV contrast were used. Another orally ingested SB-focused CT method was subsequently described in which a neutral enteric contrast material (polyethylene glycol [PEG] solution and whole milk) and an isotonic oral solution were used.[185,186] It was not until 2006 when the Mayo Clinic, Rochester group, reported their experience initially using water and water-methylcellulose solution, replaced by PEG electrolyte solution and subsequently by low-concentration barium (0.1% w/v ultra-low-dose barium with sorbitol [VoLumen, Bracco Diagnostics, Princeton, NJ, USA]) that CT enterography caught the attention of the radiology and gastroenterology community.[187,188] Invited commentaries that accompanied the reports by Bodily and colleagues[189] and Paulsen and colleagues[190] by Maglinte[20,189,190] predicted that CT enterography will replace the traditional SBFT as the initial radiological method of investigation for SB Crohn's disease and other SB diseases in practices in which expertise in DC barium enteroclysis/CTE is not available; enteroclysis is used as a problem-solving tool in referral centers when questions relevant to management are not fully answered by CT enterography.

Evidence-based analysis has shown that the negative predictive value of CT enterography is 67% (compared with 48% for SBFT or 63% for MR enterography); these were in cases with aphthoid manifestations of the disease.[191] Complementing the SBFT with peroral pneumocolon, recently revisited[192] to evaluate the ileocecal region as was done in the past,[193–196] is of value in practices in which expertise in performing DC barium enteroclysis is not available. Another option to improve the SBFT is with the use of an oral effervescent agent.[197,198] These modifications unfamiliar to younger radiologists allow demonstration of early mucosal lesions of more proximal segments; CT enterography excels with diagnosis of transmural disease, complications, and extraintestinal manifestations. A well-performed fluoroscopic SBFT augmented by these innovations likely demonstrates mucosal abnormalities better than cross-sectional imaging unless transmural manifestations are also present.[16] In a report comparing CT enterography with CTE, the conclusion was made that CT enterography "compared favorably" with CTE in the diagnosis of SB Crohn's disease.[184] An invited commentary on the report concluded that the comparison was flawed. The research actually compared 2 forms of CT enterography, one with enteral contrast orally ingested (enterography) and the other with enteral contrast hand injected through a tube (labeled as CTE). Contrast was not continuously infused during CT acquisition as should be in a technically satisfactory CTE. Distention of the SB was similar as expected. The disease phenotype was not categorized.[184] An evaluation of published reports does not show an illustration of aphthoid lesions as the only manifestation of SB Crohn's disease with cross-sectional imaging as the method of examination. Aphthoid lesions are sometimes labeled but are associated with more advanced manifestations in the same or in adjacent segments. In addition, the labeled abnormality seems to be deeper ulcerations with transmural involvement and not only early mucosal lesions. The demonstration of aphthoid lesions by barium examinations requires fluoroscopic experience; false-positive results should be avoided particularly in patients with slow transit. In our experience, stasis results in admixture defects, which can be mistaken as aphthoid lesions and suboptimal mucosal coating.

Radiologists must understand that when reporting the SB examination of patients with Crohn's disease, the disease phenotype, sites of involvement, and severity are categorized. Phenotype classification of SB Crohn's disease using all imaging modalities has been previously reported.[199] This is central information for referring clinicians in formulating a course of management. It is no longer enough to state that the findings are consistent with SB Crohn's disease.

CTE and MRE have been compared with biphasic barium enteroclysis. CTE has been proved to be significantly superior to enteroclysis in depicting Crohn's disease–associated intramural and extramural abnormalities.[200] The best current evidence-based analysis shows that CTE is a good test for the diagnosis of SB Crohn's disease but barium enteroclysis is required in the group of patients with high clinical suspicion of disease with a negative CTE.[62] In the clinical scenario where there is a high pretest probability (eg, 85%), a positive CTE result confirms the presence of disease (0.99) but a negative test result is equivocal (0.5). Further investigation with barium enteroclysis was recommended.[62,201] A similar conclusion was made in a report comparing MRE with barium enteroclysis and CTE.[202] In another report, it was concluded that MRE does not perform as well as barium enteroclysis but the additional extraluminal details and absence of ionizing radiation enhances its overall performance.[203] MR imaging is able to depict morphologic changes in the assessment of SB Crohn's disease.[204] In another evidence-based comparison between CTE and barium enteroclysis, Minordi and colleagues[62] concluded that CTE is a good test for the diagnosis of SB Crohn's disease but barium enteroclysis is required in patients with high clinical suspicion of disease

with a negative result on CTE. Further investigation with barium enteroclysis was also recommended (**Fig. 13**). Aphthoid lesions are below the spatial resolution of currently used cross-sectional imaging (CT or MR). These abnormalities become perceptible with cross-sectional imaging when submucosal and transmural abnormalities become manifest. They are subtle with DC barium enteroclysis and are easier to diagnose when accompanied by submucosal edema.[205–207] In the symptomatic patient, however, with mucosal hyperenhancement by cross-sectional imaging in an adequately distended segment, particularly when accompanied by submucosal edema, early SB Crohn's disease should be considered, but further confirmation should be recommended. A false-positive diagnosis of SB Crohn's disease has significant ramifications to patients. The Minordi report[62] used the biphasic enteroclysis method with methylcellulose, the latter having been shown to efface surface markings of the SB.[69,122,123]

An insight into the problem of the diagnosis of early SB Crohn's disease was also provided in another evidence-based analysis comparing CT enterography, MR enterography, and the SBFT.[191] Phenotype classification using an endoscopic grading of disease severity[187] was used as the reference standard. All 3 methods of investigation showed similar high sensitivity and specificity, but the SBFT was only 76% effective compared with 87% for both CT and MR enterographies. The SBFT had the worst interobserver agreement (35%). The negative predictive values (CT enterography 67%, MR enterography 63%, and SBFT 35%) allow an understanding of the problems in the diagnosis of early SB Crohn's disease using nonenteral volume-challenged examinations and examinations in which mucosal

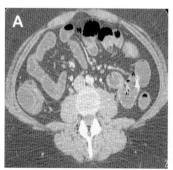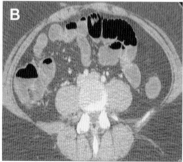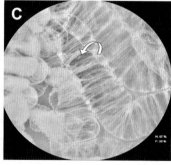

Fig. 13. Limitations of cross-sectional imaging in the diagnosis of aphthoid lesions of early SB Crohn's disease. (*A, B*) Images show no evidence of hyper enhancement, transmural edema, or wall thickening on CTE done to rule out SB Crohn's disease. Upper and lower endoscopies were not informative. (*C*) DC barium enteroclysis shows diffuse aphthous ileitis with tiny ulcers and beginning submucosal edema evidence by mild thickening of plicae circulares (*curved arrow*). Inflammatory disease markers were abnormal. Patient also had unexplained lower GI bleed.

coating is not optimized and abnormalities are smaller than the spatial resolution of the modality. The use of CE early in the investigation may be a rational approach compared with cross-sectional imaging in practices with no expertise in performing DC barium enteroclysis despite its shortcomings.[123] A comparison between CE and the various modifications of enteroclysis[48,69,123,208] has further shown that cross-sectional imaging (CT or MR) does not show the aphthae of early SB Crohn when it is the only manifestation of the disease.

A review of the literature has shown that the DC barium enteroclysis technique as popularized by Japanese practitioners and others[116,205,206,209,210] and later modified to shorten examination time and decrease discomfort[85] can show aphthae when it is the only manifestation of the disease. Cross-sectional imaging (CT or MR) shows mural involvement and extraintestinal complications but does not exclude or demonstrate the aphthoid lesions of early disease when they are the only manifestation. Endoscopic grades 0 (normal) to grade 2 (aphthous enteritis) SB Crohn's disease[187] are not excluded by CT or MR imaging. Cross-sectional imaging performance for endoscopic grade 3 (diffuse aphthous ileitis with inflamed mucosa) is variable. All cross-sectional imaging methods are excellent with endoscopic grades 4 (diffuse inflammation with large ulcers) and 5 (ulcerated stenosis) including sonography.[211] Sonography has limited use in the United States because of operator dependence but should be used for staging where radiologists with special interest in this technique are available.[77,212] Evidence-based use of imaging in the investigation of SB Crohn's disease should therefore depend on the clinical query and should be taken into consideration when advocating diagnostic pathways or algorithms in clinical practice. DC barium enteroclysis is the most sensitive radiological method for the demonstration of mucosal lesions of early SB Crohn's disease. In practices in which expertise in performing this method is not available, peroral pneumocolon has validity, as the terminal ileum is the most frequent site of SB Crohn's disease.[192–196] MR imaging and sonography should be considered local resources and expertise permitting in the follow-up of SB Crohn's disease in children.[211] Radiation dose is a greater concern in children with Crohn's disease because repeated examinations are done during their lifetime.[213]

Several of these evidence-based comparisons predated CE or newer methods of enteroscopy. Most patients had known disease or were highly suspected of having SB Crohn's disease, and the phenotype of SB Crohn's disease was not categorized. In addition, there were heterogeneous tests used as reference standards, including the SBFT, biphasic methylcellulose enteroclysis, or subjective indices. In another meta-analysis, CE was shown to have an incremental yield of 31% more than CT enterography.[214,215] In other reports, DC barium enteroclysis and both modifications of CTE compared favorably with CE in the evaluation of suspected Crohn's disease and obscure GI bleeding.[69,123]

SB Tumors

Changes in the practice of radiology in the past 3 decades and knowledge of the long-term survival of patients with malignant tumors of the SB are reminders to referring physicians and radiologists of the important role of imaging in the evaluation of SB tumors. Although the small intestine represents nearly three-quarters of the total length of the GI tract and almost 90% of its mucosal surface, SB neoplasms remain rare; they account for less than 5% of all GI tumors.[216] Colon cancer is 50 times more common than SB cancer.[217] Adenocarcinoma mostly located in the duodenum and proximal jejunum makes up 30% to 40% of cancers. Carcinoid, mostly in the ileum and uncommon in the proximal SB makes up 35% to 42%; lymphomas mostly in the ileum and jejunum, approximately 15% to 20%; and sarcomas, which is evenly distributed, approximately 10% to 15%.[218] The incidence of SB cancer has increased during the past several decades: fourfold for carcinoid, less dramatic for adenocarcinoma and lymphoma, and stable for lymphoma. The incidence is higher in North America, Western Europe, and Oceania than in Asia.[219]

An increase in the 5-year relative survival (US SEER data 1992–2005) particularly for carcinoid (80.7%) has been noted.[220] This is secondary to novel adjuvant therapies and not to imaging. The relative contribution of imaging to this improvement has not been evaluated. The relative survival is 64.1% for lymphoma, 57.9% for sarcomas, and 28.0% for adenocarcinoma. There is, however, no significant change in the long-term survival for any of the histologic types.[220] This has been attributed to most patients being diagnosed late, with local extension or distant tumor spread at the time of surgery and the long interval between the onset of symptoms and the time of diagnosis. Reports have shown 40% local spread and 30% distant spread (**Fig. 14**).[221,222] A prior analysis of why these delays occur showed that the major delay was after medical help was sought, longest after a false-negative result of radiological examination.[222] In this report, the delay due to the patient failing to

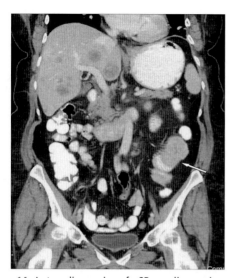

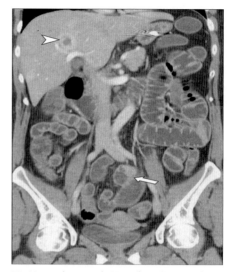

Fig. 14. Late diagnosis of SB malignancies. CT abdomen and pelvis with IV contrast in patient with chronic recurrent nausea and vomiting. Coronal images show a mass in proximal jejunum (*arrow*) consistent with proximal SB malignancy; also note liver metastases. Surgical pathologic findings showed adenocarcinoma.

Fig. 15. Neutral enteral CTE of patient with anemia shows a hyperenhancing mass in the left lower abdomen consistent with carcinoid; also note liver metastases (*arrowheads*). Patient had vague abdominal symptoms and was referred for CTE because of heme-positive stools.

report symptoms was less than 2 months, the physician not ordering an appropriate diagnostic test about 8 months, and the radiologist failing to make the diagnosis approximately 12 months. This is a lag time of approximately 2 years, longest after a false-negative result of radiological examination.[222] The vague clinical presentation of these tumors, usually abdominal pain and less often GI bleeding, is also contributory. These data underlie the need for a reliable method of examination when there is a possibility of SB neoplasm or unexplained abdominal symptom when upper and lower GI evaluations are unrevealing. The role of imaging in these patients is to reliably rule out or confirm early SB tumor. SB tumors are rare and frequently underdiagnosed or diagnosed late (Fig. 15). Curative resection remains the only curative therapy for SB malignancies.[223]

There is no rigorous imaging comparison evaluating multiple peroral SB examinations and intubation-infusion distended SB modifications. A prior comparison of orally ingested SB barium examination with enteral volume-challenged examinations showed the sensitivity of orally ingested SB examination to be 61%, whereas that of enteroclysis was 95%.[224] This result highlights the difference in diagnosing filling defects when the SB is distended. There is no rigorous head-to-head comparison between CTE and MRE or between CT enterography and MR enterography. MR imaging is frequently recommended because

of the lack of ionizing radiation.[202] Both CTE and MRE have been shown to have high accuracies +90%,[30,59,120,225,226] but the discomfort of intubation has been a deterrent and hence the rationale for recommending MR enterography. This deterrent is not an issue when appropriate conscious sedation is administered and may even be preferred by patients who do not want to drink the large amount of oral contrast and who want to have no recall of their experience.[118]

An important factor for radiologists to consider is that there is a lack of knowledge on the part of ordering physicians who want to do what is best for their patients but do not understand which imaging study is the most reliable to answer questions relevant to patient workup and management in the evaluation of SB diseases, particularly when the possibility of SB neoplasm is concerned. Radiologists must function as consultants so that when orally ingested SB examinations are not informative and unexplained abdominal symptoms persist, recommendation to refer these patients to centers where enteral volume-challenged examinations are routinely performed should be made.

An added role of imaging in the workup of SB neoplasm is to guide the enteroscopist on which route to take in the evaluation of patients who may require biopsy or endoscopic removal of SB lesions. The precise location of the largest lesion when multiple defects are present is readily estimated by CTE using currently available software. Although this can be done with neutral enteral CTE, the positive enteral CTE modification is simpler to use with vessel analysis software (**Fig. 16**).

Miscellaneous Indications

When the cause of blood loss from the GI tract is still not clear after upper and lower endoscopies (obscure GI bleed), the literature has recommended several options, each with their own proponents, which may present as a long-term and difficult management problem. Angioectasias are the most common cause of obscure GI bleeding and are only visible on endoscopy or potentially on arterial-phase catheter-based or CT angiography.

Imaging studies are insensitive to these small flat vascular lesions. A 3-phase CT enterography has been described with the goal of detecting angioectasias and other arterial-phase dominant lesions.[227–229] The radiation burden (effective dose 59 mSv per examination) and the relative risks should be considered in young patients. Unless the patient is slowly or actively bleeding at the time of acquisition, CT enterography or CTE will not demonstrate the angioectasias that can be seen on endoscopy or SB enteroscopy. CTE has the advantage of reliably excluding small SB neoplasms because it examines the entire small intestine and mesentery. In centers where expertise

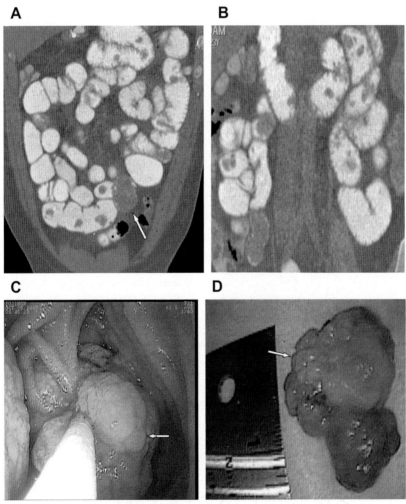

Fig. 16. Use of CTE to guide enteroscopic approach in a patient with multiple SB abnormalities. (*A*) Coronal image of a positive enteral contrast CTE on a patient with Peutz-Jeghers syndrome done because of symptoms of mechanical SBO. Multiple filling defects are seen throughout the mesenteric SB and duodenum. The largest (*arrow*) showed intermittent intussusception on real-time (fluoroscopic) phase of examination. (*B*) Multiple small polyps in the duodenum, proximal jejunum, and midileum. (*C*) Enteroscopic image shows the largest polypoid mass (*arrow*). (*D*) Hamartomatous mass (*arrow*) removed during double-balloon enteroscopy done using the oral approach. The use of "vessel analysis" software allows determination of the distance of an abnormality from either the ligament of Treitz or ileocecal valve. ([*B, C*] *Courtesy of* M. Chiorean, MD.)

in performing DC barium air enteroclysis is available, it should be performed when NSAID enteropathy is a clinical possibility and cross-sectional imaging is not informative. A history of heme-positive stools or hematochezia indicates that mucosal abrasion or ulceration is present, and examinations that depict the mucosa should be considered, such as DC barium enteroclysis in the nonemergent setting. The need to perform a SB examination in the emergent setting on a bleeding patient after endoscopic examinations with negative results make CT enterography a practical approach. DC barium enteroclysis should be recommended in the group of patients with equivocal or noninformative cross-sectional imaging studies or CE with a heme-positive stool examination. This method allows exclusion of SB neoplasm, early Crohn's disease, NSAID enteropathy, and other SB abnormalities (**Fig. 17**).

PITFALLS IN THE IMPLEMENTATION AND PERFORMANCE OF ENTEROCLYSIS IN PRACTICE

The secret of patient care is caring for the patient.
—*Francis Peabody, 1927.*[230]

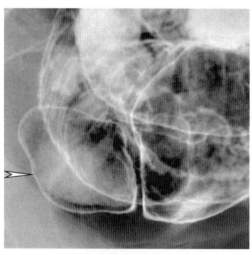

Fig. 17. Role of imaging in occult GI bleeding. Teen-aged patient with heme-positive stools with negative results by upper and lower endoscopies, CT enterography, and Meckel scan and CE. DC barium enteroclysis shows a small Meckel diverticulum (*arrowhead*). Small ulcerations were seen in the surgical specimen. Enteroclysis with careful fluoroscopic evaluation is the most accurate method of diagnosing Meckel diverticulum. (*Data from* Maglinte DD, et al. Meckel diverticulum: radiologic demonstration by enteroclysis. AJR Am J Roentgenol 1980;134(5):925–32.)

The discomfort and pain associated with nasoenteric intubation is the most significant factor that has limited the implementation of enteroclysis and its cross-sectional modifications in clinical practice despite its diagnostic accuracy.[231] The fact that patients have been able to undergo enteroclysis without conscious sedation does not indicate that it is a well-tolerated procedure. A stoic patient can undergo the examination but cannot forget the discomfort and pain endured during the procedure. Several studies have shown that physicians underestimate discomfort during intubation procedures, and like their patient, are unwilling to undergo intubation procedures on themselves without sedation/analgesia.[232–237] This basic pitfall seemingly forgotten by most radiologists is obviated by the use of conscious sedation, which allows patients to tolerate unpleasant procedures while maintaining adequate cardiopulmonary function and the ability to respond purposefully to verbal commands.[238] Many patients tolerate enteroclysis with the use of only a sedative as initially reported[117]; however, their recall of nasal pain, gagging, and occasional vomiting are good. A recent survey of the safety and patient-reported effectiveness comparing a protocol of using only a sedative and intranasal gel with a regimen combining an amnesic and analgesic and a local nasal anesthetic and intranasal gel showed that the latter is better tolerated; when an adequate amnesic dose is administered, patients forget the discomfort.[118] The addition of a local nasal anesthesia to the amnesic/analgesic medication is likely the underpinning of the success of our busy patient-friendly enteroclysis practice.[118] Unless contraindicated, our conscious sedation protocol uses a combination of midazolam (2–7 mg) given at increments of 1 mg and fentanyl (50–150 µg) given at increments of 25 µg intravenously, carefully monitored by a radiology sedation nurse. This regimen is safe and effective. Radiologists who want to start a conscious sedation protocol for enteroclysis should make arrangements with interventional radiology sections who have use dedicated radiology nurses for their procedures.[239]

Performance pitfalls of enteroclysis relate more to experience and familiarity with catheters, balloons, pumps, and various oral contrast agents, which have all been recently described.[19] Nuances related to catheterization, rates of infusion, and the type of modification to be used depending on the clinical indication have also been previously described.[54,85–87,240,241] It would be time well spent if 2 to 3 days are spent observing a practice that performs these procedures daily.

There has been a prevalent misconception that enteroclysis is simply positioning a nasoenteric catheter and infusing contrast. This is the recipe for an "enterocrisis"! Every patient is different, and optimizing the protocol for every modification of enteroclysis depending on the clinical indication and addressing multiple technical variables require understanding of basic principles, which are unfortunately not intuitive. Understanding the various pitfalls and limitations in the evaluation of SB disease and optimizing SB imaging techniques decrease errors in the performance of these procedures.

RADIATION CONSIDERATIONS

A recent report by the National Council on Radiation Protection and Measurements, an advisory body to the US Government that routinely publishes reports on topics related to radiation measurements and protection, has drawn attention to the need for improved radiation dose optimization and radiation dose-reducing strategies in medical imaging procedures and the need to examine the appropriateness of each medical imaging procedure that uses radiation.[242,243]

Cancer is the bioeffect of concern with CT and radiography and is of no concern with MR imaging. The fear of low-level radiation causing an increased incidence of cancer and cancer deaths has resurfaced based on reports of estimated radiation risks, associated with full-body CT screening.[244–251] An estimated risk of 0.08% with a single examination to 1.9% risk for 30 full-body screening CT scans has been shown based on extrapolations from Hiroshima atomic bomb survivors.[252] It was also estimated that radiation-induced cancer was 1.5% to 2% of all current cancers.[244,250,253–256] This fact became relevant because among the different categories of medical procedures, the greatest contribution is from CT examinations (increased use of CT at a rate of 8%–15% during the past 7–10 years [62 million scans in 2006]).[249,252,257–259] This controversy is not new, as older radiologists are familiar with the "linear nonthreshold model," which states that any radiation dose is thought to increase the risk of developing cancer as opposed to the "concept of hormesis" hypothesis, which states that low doses of radiation, including levels of radiation delivered by CT, are harmless or may actually be therapeutic (stimulation of the immune system).[257,260,261] Accumulated evidence does not point to the increase in cancer and death incidence in this direction. In a study involving airline pilots who receive 0.4 mSv/100 h of flight time averaging 2 mSv per year (with some crews receiving 10 mSv), no increase in the incidence of cancer has been seen in longitudinal studies spanning 30 to 50 years.[262] In a more recent large cohort study,[263] no increased cancer risk in children exposed to low x-ray radiation doses was found. Another review[264] concluded that the cancer risks associated with imaging are very low for an individual compared with the lifetime risk of developing cancer from all other causes. In spite of the exponential increase in the use of CT, the Centers for Disease Control and Prevention has reported that there is decreasing incidence in recent years of all common cancers in the United States (including lung, breast, colorectal, and prostate cancers). The cancer risk of low-level radiation made MR imaging an alternative. Many reports were embraced regardless of the science because of the fear of low-level radiation inducing cancer. The low-level radiation from CT and fluoro/radiography are not comparable to the radiation from the atomic bomb. The issue of radiation exposure in CT scanning and risk has been recently updated by Thrall.[265] The use of the linear no-threshold extrapolation model for estimating cancer risk has remained controversial despite its widespread use and endorsement in the BEIR V11 report.[266–268] Hendee and O'Connor[269] have reviewed the issue in the Annual Oration of the 2011 Radiological Society of North America. Highly speculative articles that predict cancer incidence and death in populations receiving small doses of radiation from medical imaging are not without their own health risks. The debate about extrapolation models is unwinnable on either side without more information.[265–268] No prospective epidemiologic study with nonirradiated control subjects has quantitatively demonstrated adverse effects of radiation at doses less than 100 mSv.[269]

The Health Physics Society issued a Position Statement on Radiation Risks from Medical Imaging Procedures,[270] which stated "Risk of medical imaging at effective doses below 50 mSv for single procedure or 100 mSv for multiple procedures over short time periods are too low to be detectable and may be nonexistent. Predictions of hypothetical cancer incidence and deaths in patient populations exposed to such low doses are highly speculative and should be discouraged. These predictions are harmful because they lead to sensationalistic articles in the public media that cause some patients and parents to refuse medical imaging procedures, placing them at substantial risk by not receiving the clinical benefits of the prescribed procedures." Improved radiation dose optimization and radiation dose-reducing strategies are currently available and used in CT technology tools, and future dose-lowering methods are in the pipeline.[271] When ordering SB imaging procedures unlike other abdominal organs, it should be realized that the incidence of SB diseases is low and the clinical presentation not specific so that methods of examinations that have a high negative predictive value and high sensitivity should be performed first where expertise is available.[3,4,7,13,15,16,96,123,147,207,224] In SB imaging, the examination that reliably excludes SB disease or confirms early or small abnormalities and gives clinicians confidence in formulating a treatment should be given primary consideration. Procedures that provide equivocal or inconclusive information and that do not provide referring physicians the confidence to formulate a management plan should not be used repeatedly. Enteroclysis and its modifications when done appropriately with due consideration for patient comfort fulfills this role. Few reports that show the superiority of enteroclysis and its modifications are based on well-controlled trials. Only recently have clinically important advances been based predominantly on evidence generated from well-controlled trials,[135,157,272–281] which may not be possible in SB imaging.[1] The number of well-controlled trials in SB imaging is few and will likely remain this way. Referring physicians and radiologists must rely on the "art" of medicine to fill in the deficiency.[273] In the literature, there is enough clinical evidence to show the superiority of enteroclysis and its modifications over orally ingested enteral SB examinations.

SUMMARY

Evidence- and experience-based analyses show that there are no shortcuts to reliable SB imaging. When properly performed, the added value of enteral volume-challenged examinations to patient care is not difficult to understand. Examinations that distend the SB diagnose smaller/early lesions and allow confident exclusion of SB disease, an important variable to consider when imaging the patient for possible SB disease. As stated by Reed,[135] it may not be necessary to establish the true scientific accuracy of an imaging evaluation to understand its efficacy.

ACKNOWLEDGMENTS

The author thanks K. Sandrasegaran, MD, and Kenneth Buckwalter, MD, for help in the preparation of the illustrations.

REFERENCES

1. Gunderman RB, Chou HY. Effective argumentation. AJR Am J Roentgenol 2011;196(6):1345–9.

2. Maglinte DD. Small bowel imaging – a rapidly changing field and a challenge to radiology. Eur Radiol 2006;16(5):967–71.

3. Antes G. Why not enteroclysis? N Engl J Med 1980; 303(24):1420.

4. Barloon TJ, Lu CC, Honda H, et al. Does a normal small-bowel enteroclysis exclude small-bowel disease? A long-term follow-up of consecutive normal studies. Abdom Imaging 1994;19(2):113–5.

5. Bartram CI. Small bowel enteroclysis: cons. Abdom Imaging 1996;21(3):245–6.

6. Bender GN. Radiographic examination of the small bowel. An application of odds ratio analysis to help attain an appropriate mix of small bowel follow through and enteroclysis in a working-clinical environment. Invest Radiol 1997;32(6):357–62.

7. Bender GN, et al. CT enteroclysis: a superfluous diagnostic procedure or valuable when investigating small-bowel disease? AJR Am J Roentgenol 1999; 172(2):373–8.

8. Bender GN, et al. Computed tomographic enteroclysis: one methodology. Invest Radiol 1996; 31(1):43–9.

9. Chernish SM, Maglinte DD, O'Connor K. Evaluation of the small intestine by enteroclysis for Crohn's disease. Am J Gastroenterol 1992;87(6):696–701.

10. Diner WC, Hoskins EO, Navab F. Radiologic examination of the small intestine: review of 402 cases and discussion of indications and methods. South Med J 1984;77(1):68–74.

11. Dixon PM, Roulston ME, Nolan DJ. The small bowel enema: a ten year review. Clin Radiol 1993;47(1): 46–8.

12. Halpert RD, et al. Enteroclysis for the examination of the small bowel. Henry Ford Hosp Med J 1985; 33(2–3):116–21.

13. Herlinger H. Why not enteroclysis? J Clin Gastroenterol 1982;4(3):277–83.

14. Lappas JC. Small bowel imaging. Curr Opin Radiol 1992;4(3):32–8.

15. Maglinte DD, et al. Current status of small bowel radiography. Abdom Imaging 1996;21(3):247–57.

16. Maglinte DD, et al. Small bowel radiography: how, when, and why? Radiology 1987;163(2):297–305.

17. Nolan DJ. Small bowel enteroclysis: pros. Abdom Imaging 1996;21(3):243–4.

18. Nolan DJ. The true yield of the small-intestinal barium study. Endoscopy 1997;29(6):447–53.

19. Gollub MJ, Maglinte DT. CT enterography and CT enteroclysis. In: Shirkhoda A, editor. Variants and pitfalls in imaging. Philadelphia: Lippincott; 2011. p. 328–62.

20. Maglinte D. Invited commentary. Radiographics 2006;26:657–62.

21. Horsthuis K. Inflammatory bowel disease diagnosed with US, MR, scintigraphy, and CT: meta-analysis of prospective studies. Radiology 2008;247(1):64–79.

22. Gourtsoyiannis N, et al. MR imaging of the small bowel with a true-FISP sequence after enteroclysis with water solution. Invest Radiol 2000;35(12): 707–11.

23. Kloppel VR. The Sellink CT method. Rofo 1992; 156(3):291–2.

24. Maglinte DD, Siegelman ES, Kelvin FM. MR enteroclysis: the future of small-bowel imaging? Radiology 2000;215(3):639–41.

25. Umschaden HW, et al. Small-bowel disease: comparison of MR enteroclysis images with conventional enteroclysis and surgical findings. Radiology 2000;215(3):717–25.

26. Adamek HE, et al. Ultra-high-field magnetic resonance enterography in the diagnosis of ileitis (neo-)terminalis: a prospective study. J Clin Gastroenterol 2012;46(4):311–6.

27. Apostolopoulos P, et al. The role of wireless capsule endoscopy in investigating unexplained iron deficiency anemia after negative endoscopic evaluation of the upper and lower gastrointestinal tract. Endoscopy 2006;38(11):1127–32.

28. Baker ME, Einstein DM, Veniero JC. Computed tomography enterography and magnetic resonance enterography: the future of small bowel imaging. Clin Colon Rectal Surg 2008;21(3):193–212.

29. Biscaldi E, et al. Bowel endometriosis: CT-enteroclysis. Abdom Imaging 2007;32(4):441–50.

30. Boudiaf M, et al. Small-bowel diseases: prospective evaluation of multi-detector row helical CT enteroclysis in 107 consecutive patients. Radiology 2004;233(2):338–44.

31. Broglia L, et al. Magnetic resonance enteroclysis imaging in Crohn's disease. Radiol Med 2003; 106(1–2):28–35.

32. Cappabianca S, et al. The role of nasoenteric intubation in the MR study of patients with Crohn's disease: our experience and literature review. Radiol Med 2011;116(3):389–406.

33. Cohen ME, Barkin JS. Enteroscopy and enteroclysis: the combined procedure. Am J Gastroenterol 1989;84(11):1413–5.

34. Dave-Verma H, et al. Computed tomographic enterography and enteroclysis: pearls and pitfalls. Curr Probl Diagn Radiol 2008;37(6):279–87.

35. Di Mizio R, et al. Multidetector-row helical CT enteroclysis. Radiol Med 2006;111(1):1–10.

36. Doerfler OC, et al. Helical CT of the small bowel with an alternative oral contrast material in patients with Crohn disease. Abdom Imaging 2003;28(3): 313–8.

37. Feuerbach S. MRI enterography: the future of small bowel diagnostics? Dig Dis 2010;28(3):433–8.

38. Fidler J. MR imaging of the small bowel. Radiol Clin North Am 2007;45(2):317–31.

39. Fidler JL, Guimaraes L, Einstein DM. MR imaging of the small bowel. Radiographics 2009;29(6):1811–25.

40. Finke M. Enteroclysis: double contrast examination of the small bowel. Radiol Technol 1987;59(2):143–9.

41. Furukawa A, et al. Helical CT in the diagnosis of small bowel obstruction. Radiographics 2001; 21(2):341–55.

42. Gasparaitis AE, MacEneaney P. Enteroclysis and computed tomography enteroclysis. Gastroenterol Clin North Am 2002;31(3):715–30, v.

43. Gerson LB, Van Dam J. Wireless capsule endoscopy and double-balloon enteroscopy for the diagnosis of obscure gastrointestinal bleeding. Tech Vasc Interv Radiol 2004;7(3):130–5.

44. Gollub MJ. Multidetector computed tomography enteroclysis of patients with small bowel obstruction: a volume-rendered "surgical perspective". J Comput Assist Tomogr 2005;29(3):401–7.

45. Gollub MJ, DeCorato D, Schwartz LH. MR enteroclysis: evaluation of small-bowel obstruction in a patient with pseudomyxoma peritonei. AJR Am J Roentgenol 2000;174(3):688–90.

46. Jain TP, et al. CT enteroclysis in the diagnosis of obscure gastrointestinal bleeding: initial results. Clin Radiol 2007;62(7):660–7.

47. Kerr JM. Small bowel imaging: CT enteroclysis or barium enteroclysis? Critically appraised topic. Abdom Imaging 2008;33(1):31–3.

48. Kohli MD, Maglinte DD. CT enteroclysis in small bowel Crohn's disease. Eur J Radiol 2009;69(3): 398–403.

49. Kohli MD, Maglinte DD. CT enteroclysis in incomplete small bowel obstruction. Abdom Imaging 2009;34(3):321–7.

50. Korman U, Kurugoglu S, Ogut G. Conventional enteroclysis with complementary MR enteroclysis: a combination of small bowel imaging. Abdom Imaging 2005;30(5):564–75.

51. La Seta F, et al. Multidetector-row CT enteroclysis: indications and clinical applications. Radiol Med 2006;111(2):141–58.

52. Lalitha P, et al. Computed tomography enteroclysis: a review. Jpn J Radiol 2011;29(10):673–81.

53. Maglinte DD, et al. Multidetector-row helical CT enteroclysis. Radiol Clin North Am 2003;41(2): 249–62.

54. Maglinte DD, et al. Technical refinements in enteroclysis. Radiol Clin North Am 2003;41(2):213–29.

55. Masselli G, et al. Crohn disease: magnetic resonance enteroclysis. Abdom Imaging 2004;29(3): 326–34.

56. Masselli G, et al. Magnetic resonance enteroclysis imaging of Crohn's. Radiol Med 2005;110(3):221–33.

57. Masselli G, et al. Comparison of MR enteroclysis with MR enterography and conventional enteroclysis in patients with Crohn's disease. Eur Radiol 2008;18(3):438–47.

58. Masselli G, et al. Assessment of Crohn's disease in the small bowel: prospective comparison of

magnetic resonance enteroclysis with conventional enteroclysis. Eur Radiol 2006;16(12):2817–27.

59. Masselli G, Gualdi G. Evaluation of small bowel tumors: MR enteroclysis. Abdom Imaging 2010; 35(1):23–30.

60. Matsumoto T, et al. Double-contrast barium enteroclysis as a patency tool for nonsteroidal anti-inflammatory drug-induced enteropathy. Dig Dis Sci 2011;56(11):3247–53.

61. McGovern R, Barkin JS. Enteroscopy and enteroclysis: an improved method for combined procedure. Gastrointest Radiol 1990;15(4):327–8.

62. Minordi LM, et al. Multidetector CT enteroclysis versus barium enteroclysis with methylcellulose in patients with suspected small bowel disease. Eur Radiol 2006;16(7):1527–36.

63. Minordi LM, et al. CT enteroclysis: multidetector technique (MDCT) versus single-detector technique (SDCT) in patients with suspected small-bowel Crohn's disease. Radiol Med 2007; 112(8):1188–200.

64. Nygaard A, et al. Magnetic resonance enteroclysis in the diagnosis of small-intestinal Crohn's disease: diagnostic accuracy and inter- and intra-observer agreement. Acta Radiol 2006; 47(10):1008–16.

65. Neu B, et al. Capsule endoscopy versus standard tests in influencing management of obscure digestive bleeding: results from a German multicenter trial. Am J Gastroenterol 2005;100(8): 1736–42.

66. Parrish FJ. Small bowel CT-enteroclysis: technique, pitfalls and pictorial review. Australas Radiol 2006; 50(4):289–97.

67. Patak MA, et al. Non-invasive distension of the small bowel for magnetic-resonance imaging. Lancet 2001;358(9286):987–8.

68. Prassopoulos P, et al. MR enteroclysis imaging of Crohn disease. Radiographics 2001;21(Spec No): S161–72.

69. Rajesh A, et al. Comparison of capsule endoscopy with enteroclysis in the investigation of small bowel disease. Abdom Imaging 2009;34(4):459–66.

70. Schmidt S, et al. Multidetector CT enteroclysis: comparison of the reading performance for axial and coronal views. Eur Radiol 2005;15(2):238–46.

71. Schmidt S, et al. CT enteroclysis: technique and clinical applications. Eur Radiol 2006;16(3): 648–60.

72. Schmidt S, et al. Prospective comparison of MR enteroclysis with multidetector spiral-CT enteroclysis: interobserver agreement and sensitivity by means of "sign-by-sign" correlation. Eur Radiol 2003;13(6):1303–11.

73. Suzuki T, et al. Clinical utility of double-balloon enteroscopy for small intestinal bleeding. Dig Dis Sci 2007;52(8):1914–8.

74. Torregrosa A, et al. Magnetic resonance enterography: technique and indications. Findings in Crohn's disease. Radiologia 2012. [Epub ahead of print].

75. Turetschek K, et al. Findings at helical CT-enteroclysis in symptomatic patients with Crohn disease: correlation with endoscopic and surgical findings. J Comput Assist Tomogr 2002;26(4): 488–92.

76. Umschaden HW, Gasser J. MR enteroclysis. Radiol Clin North Am 2003;41(2):231–48.

77. Valek V, Kysela P, Vavrikova M. Crohn's disease at the small bowel imaging by the ultrasound-enteroclysis. Eur J Radiol 2007;62(2):153–9.

78. Van Weyenberg SJ, et al. MR enteroclysis in the diagnosis of small-bowel neoplasms. Radiology 2010;254(3):765–73.

79. Wiarda BM, et al. Jejunum abnormalities at MR enteroclysis. Eur J Radiol 2008;67(1):125–32.

80. Wiarda BM, et al. MR enteroclysis of inflammatory small-bowel diseases. AJR Am J Roentgenol 2006;187(2):522–31.

81. Wiarda BM, et al. MR enteroclysis: imaging technique of choice in diagnosis of small bowel diseases. Dig Dis Sci 2005;50(6):1036–40.

82. Willis JR, et al. Enteroscopy-enteroclysis: experience with a combined endoscopic-radiographic technique. Gastrointest Endosc 1997;45(2):163–7.

83. Wold PB, et al. Assessment of small bowel Crohn disease: noninvasive peroral CT enterography compared with other imaging methods and endoscopy-feasibility study. Radiology 2003; 229(1):275–81.

84. Masselli G, Gualdi G. MR imaging of the small bowel. Radiology 2012;264(2):333–48.

85. Maglinte DD, et al. Air (CO2) double-contrast barium enteroclysis. Radiology 2009;252(3):633–41.

86. Maglinte DD, Sandrasegaran K, Lappas JC. CT enteroclysis: techniques and applications. Radiol Clin North Am 2007;45(2):289–301.

87. Maglinte DD, et al. CT enteroclysis. Radiology 2007;245(3):661–71.

88. Pesquera GS. Method for direct visualization of lesions in the small intestine. AJR Am J Roentgenol 1929;22:254–7.

89. Ghelew B, Mengis O. Mise en evidence de l'intestin grele par une nouvelle technique radiologique. Presse Med 1938;46:444–5.

90. Gershon-Cohen J, Shay H. Barium enteroclysis method for direct immediate examination of the small intestine by single and double contrast. AJR Am J Roentgenol 1939;42:456.

91. Schatzki R. Small bowel enema. AJR Am J Roentgenol 1943;50:743–51.

92. Lura A. Radiology of the small intestine. IV. Enema of the small intestine with special emphasis on the diagnosis of tumors. Br J Radiol 1951;24:264–70.

93. Herlinger H, Maglinte D. Historial aspects. In: Clinical radiology of the small intestine. Philadelphia: W.B. Saunders; 1989. p. 41–4.

94. Sellink JL. Examination of the small intestine by means of duodenal intubation. Acta Radiol 1971; 15:318.

95. Scott-Harden W. Examination of the small bowel. In: McLaren J, editor. Modern trends in diagnostic radiology. London: Butterworth; 1960. p. 84–7.

96. Maglinte DD, Burney BT, Miller RE. Lesions missed on small-bowel follow-through: analysis and recommendations. Radiology 1982;144(4):737–9.

97. Pygott F, Street DF, Shellshear MF, et al. Radiological investigation of the small intestine by small bowel enema technique. Gut 1960;1:366–70.

98. Herlinger H. A modified technique for the double contrast small bowel enema. Gastrointest Radiol 1978;3:201–7.

99. Sellink JL. Proceedings: why enteroclysis of the small intestine? Br J Radiol 1976;49(579):288–9.

100. Bilbao MK, Frische LH, Dotter CT, et al. Hypotonic duodenography. Radiology 1967;89:438–43.

101. Maglinte DD. Balloon enteroclysis catheter. AJR Am J Roentgenol 1984;143(4):761–2.

102. Maglinte DD, et al. Nasointestinal tube for decompression or enteroclysis: experience with 150 patients. Abdom Imaging 1994;19(2):108–12.

103. Maglinte DD, et al. Dual-purpose tube for enteroclysis and nasogastric-nasoenteric decompression. Radiology 1992;185(1):281–2.

104. Maglinte D, Kelvin FM, Rowe M, et al. Small-bowel obstruction: optimizing radiologic investigation and nonsurgical management. Radiology 2001;218(1): 39–46.

105. Nolan DJ. Barium examination of the small intestine. Br J Hosp Med 1994;52(4):136–41.

106. Nolan DJ. Imaging of the small intestine. Schweiz Med Wochenschr 1998;128(4):109–14.

107. Nolan DJ. Enteroclysis of non-neoplastic disorders of the small intestine. Eur Radiol 2000;10(2): 342–53.

108. Nolan DJ, Cadman PJ. The small bowel enema made easy. Clin Radiol 1987;38(3):295–301.

109. Nolan DJ, Cadman PJ, Jeffree MA. Re: detailed per-oral small-bowel examination versus enteroclysis. Radiology 1985;157(3):836–7.

110. Trickey SE, Halls J, Hodson CJ. A further development of the small bowel enema. Proc R Soc Med 1963;56:1070–3.

111. Maglinte D, Herlinger H. Single contrast and biphasic enteroclysis. In: Maglinte D, Herlinger H, editors. Clinical radiology of the small intestine. Philadelphia: W.B. Saunders Co.; 1989. p. 107–18.

112. Kobayashi S, et al. Double contrast study of the small bowel. Jpn J Clin Radiol 1974;19:619–25.

113. Nakamura Y, et al. X-ray examination of the small intestine by means of duodenal intubation-double contrast study of the small bowel. Stom Intest 1974;9:1461–9.

114. Kobayashi S, Nishizawa M. X-ray examination of small intestine-double contrast method by duodenal intuation. Stom Intest 1976;11:157–65.

115. Ushio K, et al. The double contrast method of the small bowel compared with the peroral and compression methods hitherto employed. Stom Intest 1982;17:857–69.

116. Shirakabe H, Kobayashi S. Air double contrast barium study of the small bowel. In: Maglinte D, Herlinger H, editors. Clinical radiology of the small intestine. Philadelphia: W.B. Saunders Co.; 1989. p. 139–50.

117. Maglinte DD, et al. Improved tolerance of enteroclysis by use of sedation. AJR Am J Roentgenol 1988;151(5):951–2.

118. Maglinte DD, et al. Conscious sedation for patients undergoing enteroclysis: comparing the safety and patient-reported effectiveness of two protocols. Eur J Radiol 2009;70(3):512–6.

119. Rajesh A, Maglinte DD. Multislice CT enteroclysis: technique and clinical applications. Clin Radiol 2006;61(1):31–9.

120. Romano S, et al. Multidetector computed tomography enteroclysis (MDCT-E) with neutral enteral and IV contrast enhancement in tumor detection. Eur Radiol 2005;15(6):1178–83.

121. Maglinte D, et al. Multidetector-row helical CT enteroclysis. In: Maglinte D, Rubesin S, editors. Radiologic clinics of North America. Philadelphia: W.B. Saunders Co.; 2003. p. 249–62.

122. Liangpunsakul S, et al. Wireless capsule endoscopy detects small bowel ulcers in patients with normal results from state of the art enteroclysis. Am J Gastroenterol 2003;98(6):1295–8.

123. Maglinte DD, et al. Radiologic investigations complement and add diagnostic information to capsule endoscopy of small-bowel diseases. AJR Am J Roentgenol 2007;189(2):306–12.

124. Biscaldi E, et al. Multislice CT enteroclysis in the diagnosis of bowel endometriosis. Eur Radiol 2007;17(1):211–9.

125. Biscaldi E, et al. MDCT enteroclysis urography with split-bolus technique provides information on ureteral involvement in patients with suspected bowel endometriosis. AJR Am J Roentgenol 2011; 196(5):W635–40.

126. Rollandi G, Curone PF, Biscaldi E, et al. Spiral CT of the abdomen after distention of small bowel loops with transparent enema in patients with Crohn's disease. Abdom Imaging 1999;24(6):544–9.

127. Holzknecht N, Helmberger T, von Ritter C, et al. MRI of the small intestine with rapid MRI sequences in Crohn disease after enteroclysis with oral iron particles [in German]. Radiologe 1998;38(1):29–36.

128. Gourtsoyiannis N, et al. MR enteroclysis protocol optimization: comparison between 3D FLASH with fat saturation after intravenous gadolinium injection and true FISP sequences. Eur Radiol 2001;11(6):908–13.

129. Gourtsoyiannis N, et al. MR enteroclysis: technical considerations and clinical applications. Eur Radiol 2002;12(11):2651–8.

130. Gourtsoyiannis NC, Papanikolaou N. Magnetic resonance enteroclysis. Semin Ultrasound CT MR 2005;26(4):237–46.

131. Papanikolaou N, et al. Technical challenges and clinical applications of magnetic resonance enteroclysis. Top Magn Reson Imaging 2002;13(6):397–408.

132. Papanikolaou N, et al. Optimization of a contrast medium suitable for conventional enteroclysis, MR enteroclysis, and virtual MR enteroscopy. Abdom Imaging 2002;27(5):517–22.

133. Gourtsoyiannis NC, Papanikolaou N, Karantanas A. Magnetic resonance imaging evaluation of small intestinal Crohn's disease. Best Pract Res Clin Gastroenterol 2006;20(1):137–56.

134. Hillman BJ. The irresistible march of technology. J Am Coll Radiol 2009;6(12):823.

135. Reed MH. Evidence in diagnostic imaging: going beyond accuracy. J Am Coll Radiol 2012;9(2):90–2.

136. Herlinger H, Maglinte D. Small bowel obstruction clinical radiology of the small intestine. Philadelphia: W.B. Saunders Co.; 1989.

137. Maglinte D, et al. The role of radiology in the diagnosis of small-bowel obstruction. AJR Am J Roentgenol 1997;168(5):1171–80.

138. Maglinte D, Howard TJ, Lillemoe K, et al. Small-bowel obstruction: state-of-the-art imaging and its role in clinical management. Clin Gastroenterol Hepatol 2008;6:130–9.

139. Maglinte D, Kelvin FM, Sandrasegaran K, et al. Radiology of small-bowel obstruction: contemporary approach and controversies. Abdom Imaging 2005;30(2):160–78.

140. Fukuya T, Hawes DR, Lu C, et al. CT diagnosis of small-bowel obstruction: efficacy in 60 patients. AJR Am J Roentgenol 1992;158:765–9.

141. Megibow A, Balthazar EJ, Cho K. Bowel obstruction: evaluation with CT. Radiology 1991;180:313–8.

142. Maglinte DD, et al. Obstruction of the small intestine: accuracy and role of CT in diagnosis. Radiology 1993;188(1):61–4.

143. Maglinte DD, et al. Enteroclysis in partial small bowel obstruction. Am J Surg 1984;147(3):325–9.

144. Maglinte DD, et al. Reliability and role of plain film radiography and CT in the diagnosis of small-bowel obstruction. AJR Am J Roentgenol 1996;167(6):1451–5.

145. Shrake PD, et al. Radiographic evaluation of suspected small bowel obstruction. Am J Gastroenterol 1991;86(2):175–8.

146. Maglinte D, Reyes B. Computed tomographic diagnosis of partial small-bowel obstruction secondary to anterior peritoneal adhesions: relevance to laparoscopic cholecystectomy. Emerg Radiol 1996;3:84–6.

147. Maglinte DD, et al. Detection of surgical lesions of the small bowel by enteroclysis. Am J Surg 1984;147(2):225–9.

148. Antes G. Radiolology of small-bowel motility disorders. In: Gourtsoyiannis NC, editor. Radiological imaging of the small intestine. Berlin: Springer-Verlag; 2002. p. 235–46.

149. O'Connor OJ, et al. Role of radiologic imaging in irritable bowel syndrome: evidence-based review. Radiology 2012;262(2):485–94.

150. Walsh D, Bender G, Timmons J. Comparison of computed tomography-enteroclysis and traditional computed tomography in the setting of suspected partial small-bowel obstruction. Emerg Radiol 1998;5:29–37.

151. Caroline D, Herlinger H, Laufer I, et al. Small-bowel enema in the diagnosis of adhesive obstruction. AJR Am J Roentgenol 1984;143:1133–9.

152. Bender GN, et al. Malignant melanoma: patterns of metastasis to the small bowel, reliability of imaging studies, and clinical relevance. Am J Gastroenterol 2001;96(8):2392–400.

153. Bass KN, Jones B, Bulkley GB. Current management of small-bowel obstruction. Adv Surg 1997;31:1–34.

154. Hayanga AJ, Bass-Wilkins K, Bulkley GB. Current management of small-bowel obstruction. Adv Surg 2005;39:1–33.

155. Bender G, Maglinte D. Small bowel obstruction: the need for greater radiologist involvement. Appl Radiol 1999;28:7–9.

156. Staunton M, Malone DE. Can diagnostic imaging reliably predict the need for surgery in small bowel obstruction? Critically appraised topic. Can Assoc Radiol J 2005;56(2):79–81.

157. Glazer GM, Ruiz-Wibbelsmann JA. Decades of perceived mediocrity: prestige and radiology. Radiology 2011;260(2):311–6.

158. Bender GN, Maglinte D. Small-bowel obstruction: the need for greater radiologists involvement [editorial]. Emerg Radiol 1997;4:337–9.

159. Yamauchi FI, et al. Multidetector CT evaluation of the postoperative pancreas. Radiographics 2012;32(3):743–64.

160. Scialpi M, et al. Imaging evaluation of post pancreatic surgery. Eur J Radiol 2005;53(3):417–24.

161. Agarwal A, et al. Internal hernia after pancreas transplantation with enteric drainage: an unusual cause of small bowel obstruction. Transplantation 2005;80(1):149–52.

162. Sandrasegaran K, Maglinte DD. Imaging of small bowel-related complications following major abdominal surgery. Eur J Radiol 2005;53(3):374–86.

163. Sandrasegaran K, et al. Surgery for chronic pancreatitis: cross-sectional imaging of postoperative anatomy and complications. AJR Am J Roentgenol 2005;184(4):1118–27.

164. Sandrasegaran K, et al. Small-bowel complications of major gastrointestinal tract surgery. AJR Am J Roentgenol 2005;185(3):671–81.

165. Sandrasegaran K, et al. CT of acute biliopancreatic limb obstruction. AJR Am J Roentgenol 2006; 186(1):104–9.

166. Lall CG, et al. Bowel complications seen on CT after pancreas transplantation with enteric drainage. AJR Am J Roentgenol 2006;187(5):1288–95.

167. Sandrasegaran K, et al. Enteric drainage pancreatic transplantation. Abdom Imaging 2006;31(5): 588–95.

168. Maglinte DD, et al. Current concepts in imaging of small bowel obstruction. Radiol Clin North Am 2003;41(2):263–83, vi.

169. Frager D, et al. CT of small-bowel obstruction: value in establishing the diagnosis and determining the degree and cause. AJR Am J Roentgenol 1994;162(1):37–41.

170. Frager DH, et al. Distinction between postoperative ileus and mechanical small-bowel obstruction: value of CT compared with clinical and other radiographic findings. AJR Am J Roentgenol 1995; 164(4):891–4.

171. Romano S, Bartone G, Romano L. Ischemia and infarction of the intestine related to obstruction. Radiol Clin North Am 2008;46(5):925.

172. Romano S, et al. Ischemia and infarction of the small bowel and colon: spectrum of imaging findings. Abdom Imaging 2006;31(3):277–92.

173. Staunton M, Malone DE. Can acute mesenteric ischemia be ruled out using computed tomography? Critically appraised topic. Can Assoc Radiol J 2005;56(1):9–12.

174. Seror D, Feigin E, Szold A, et al. How conservatively can postoperative small-bowel obstruction be treated? Am J Surg 1993;165:121–6.

175. Ha H, Rha S, Kim J, et al. CT diagnosis of strangulation in patients with small-bowel obstruction: current status and future direction. Emerg Radiol 2000;7:47–55.

176. Gazelle G, Goldberg MA, Wittenberg J, et al. Efficacy of CT in distinguishing small-bowel obstruction from other causes of small-bowel dilatation. AJR Am J Roentgenol 1994;162:43–7.

177. Frager D, Baer JW, Medwid S. Detection of intestinal ischemia in patients with acute small-bowel obstruction due to adhesions or hernia: efficacy of CT. AJR Am J Roentgenol 1996;166: 67–71.

178. Balthazar E, Bauman JS, Megibow A. CT diagnosis of closed-loop obstruction. J Comput Assist Tomogr 1985;9:953–5.

179. Balthazar E, Birnbaum BA, Megibow A, et al. Closed-loop and strangulating intestinal obstruction: CT signs. Radiology 1992;185:769–75.

180. Barnett WO, Petro AB, Williamson JW. A current appraisal of problems with gangrenous bowel. Ann Surg 1976;183(6):653–9.

181. Otamiri T, Sjodahl R, Ihse I. Intestinal obstruction with strangulation of the small bowel. Acta Chir Scand 1987;153(4):307–10.

182. Goldberg HI, et al. Radiographic findings of the National Cooperative Crohn's Disease Study. Gastroenterology 1979;77(4 Pt 2):925–37.

183. Zamboni GA, Raptopoulos V. CT enterography. Gastrointest Endosc Clin N Am 2010;20(2): 347–66.

184. Paulsen SR, et al. CT enterography as a diagnostic tool in evaluating small bowel disorders: review of clinical experience with over 700 cases. Radiographics 2006;26(3):641–57 [discussion: 657–62].

185. Rosen MP, et al. Value of abdominal CT in the emergency department for patients with abdominal pain. Eur Radiol 2003;13(2):418–24.

186. Thompson SE, et al. Abdominal helical CT: milk as a low-attenuation oral contrast agent. Radiology 1999;211(3):870–5.

187. Colombel JF, et al. Quantitative measurement and visual assessment of ileal Crohn's disease activity by computed tomography enterography: correlation with endoscopic severity and C reactive protein. Gut 2006;55(11):1561–7.

188. Hara AK, et al. Small bowel: preliminary comparison of capsule endoscopy with barium study and CT. Radiology 2004;230(1):260–5.

189. Bodily KD, et al. Crohn disease: mural attenuation and thickness at contrast-enhanced CT enterography–correlation with endoscopic and histologic findings of inflammation. Radiology 2006;238(2): 505–16.

190. Paulsen SR, Huprich JE, Hara AK. CT enterography: noninvasive evaluation of Crohn's disease and obscure gastrointestinal bleed. Radiol Clin North Am 2007;45(2):303–15.

191. Lee SS, et al. Crohn disease of the small bowel: comparison of CT enterography, MR enterography, and small-bowel follow-through as diagnostic techniques. Radiology 2009;251(3):751–61.

192. Pickhardt PJ. The peroral pneumocolon revisited: a technique for ileocecal evaluation. Abdom Imaging 2012;37(3):313–25.

193. Kressel H, Evers K, et al. The peroral pneumocolon examination: technique and indications. Radiology 1982;144:41–416.

194. Kelvin F, Gedgaudas RK, Thompson W, et al. The peroral pneumocolon: it's role in evaluating the terminal ileum. AJR Am J Roentgenol 1982;139: 115–21.

195. Fitzgerald E, Thompson GT, Somers S, et al. Pneumocolon as an aid to small bowel studies. Clin Radiol 1985;36:633–7.

196. Kellet M, Zboralske FF, Margulis A. Peroral pneumocolon examination of the ileocecal region. Gastrointest Radiol 1977;1:361–5.

197. Fraser GM, Preston PG. The small bowel follow-through enhanced with an oral effervescent agent. Clin Radiol 1983;34:673–9.

198. Herlinger H, Maglinte D. Nonintubation barium methods. In: Maglinte D, Herlinger H, editors. Clinical radiology of the small intestine. Philadelphia: W.B. Saunders Co.; 1989. p. 71–83.

199. Maglinte DD, et al. Classification of small bowel Crohn's subtypes based on multimodality imaging. Radiol Clin North Am 2003;41(2):285–303.

200. Sailer J, et al. Diagnostic value of CT enteroclysis compared with conventional enteroclysis in patients with Crohn's disease. AJR Am J Roentgenol 2005; 185(6):1575–81.

201. Minordi LM, et al. CT findings and clinical activity in Crohn's disease. Clin Imaging 2009;33(2):123–9.

202. Ryan ER, Heaslip IS. Magnetic resonance enteroclysis compared with conventional enteroclysis and computed tomography enteroclysis: a critically appraised topic. Abdom Imaging 2008; 33(1):34–7.

203. Gourtsoyiannis N, et al. Imaging of small intestinal Crohn's disease: a comparison of MR enteroclysis and conventional examination. Eur Radiol 2006; 16(9):1915–25.

204. Malago R, et al. Assessment of Crohn's disease activity in the small bowel with MR-enteroclysis: clinico-radiological correlations. Abdom Imaging 2008;33(6):669–75.

205. Ekberg O. Crohn's disease of the small bowel examined by double contrast technique: a comparison with oral technique. Gastrointest Radiol 1977; 1(4):355–9.

206. Ekberg O. Double contrast examination of the small bowel. Gastrointest Radiol 1977;1(4):349–53.

207. Ekberg O, Fork FT, Hildell J. Predictive value of small bowel radiography for recurrent Crohn disease. AJR Am J Roentgenol 1980;135(5):1051–5.

208. Sandrasegaran K, et al. Capsule endoscopy and imaging tests in the elective investigation of small bowel disease. Clin Radiol 2008;63(6):712–23.

209. Tanaka K, et al. Double contrast study of the minute lesions of Crohn's disease of the small intestine. Stomach Intest 1982;871–82.

210. Yao T. Double contrast enteroclysis with air. In: Stevenson G, Freeny PC, editors. Alimentary tract radiology. St Louis (MO): Mosby; 1995. p. 548–55.

211. Martinez MJ, et al. Assessment of the extension and the inflammatory activity in Crohn's disease: comparison of ultrasound and MRI. Abdom Imaging 2009;34(2):141–8.

212. Wilson S. Evaluation of small intestine by ultrasonography. In: Gourtsoyiannis N, editor. Radiological imaging of the small intestine. Berlin: Springer-Verlag; 2002. p. 73–86.

213. Desmond AN, et al. Crohn's disease: factors associated with exposure to high levels of diagnostic radiation. Gut 2008;57(11):1524–9.

214. Triester SL, et al. A meta-analysis of the yield of capsule endoscopy compared to other diagnostic modalities in patients with obscure gastrointestinal bleeding. Am J Gastroenterol 2005;100(11):2407–18.

215. Triester SL, et al. A meta-analysis of the yield of capsule endoscopy compared to other diagnostic modalities in patients with non-stricturing small bowel Crohn's disease. Am J Gastroenterol 2006; 101(5):954–64.

216. Schottenfield J, et al. Histological subtypes of small intestinal cancers. Ann Epidemiol 2009;19:439–522.

217. Wheeler JM, et al. An insight into the genetic pathway of adenocarcinoma of the small intestine. Gut 2002;50(2):218–23.

218. Schottenfield J, et al. 40 Histological subtypes of small intestinal cancers. Ann Epidemiol 2009;19.

219. Haselkorn T, Whittemore AS, Lilienfeld DE. Incidence of small bowel cancer in the United States and worldwide: geographic, temporal, and racial differences. Cancer Causes Control 2005;16(7): 781–7.

220. Pan SY, Morrison H. Epidemiology of cancer of the small intestine. World J Gastrointest Oncol 2011; 3(3):33–42.

221. Bilimoria KY, Bentrem DJ, Wayne JD. Small bowel cancer in the United States: changes in survival over the last 20 years. Ann Surg 2009;249(1):63–71.

222. Maglinte DD, et al. The role of the physician in the late diagnosis of primary malignant tumors of the small intestine. Am J Gastroenterol 1991;86(3):304–8.

223. Talamonti S, et al. Primary cancers of the SB: analysis of prognostic factors. Arch Surg 2002;137.

224. Bessette JR, et al. Primary malignant tumors in the small bowel: a comparison of the small-bowel enema and conventional follow-through examination. AJR Am J Roentgenol 1989;153(4):741–4.

225. Gourtsoyiannis NC, et al. Benign tumors of the small intestine: preoperative evaluation with a barium infusion technique. Eur J Radiol 1993; 16(2):115–25.

226. Masselli G, et al. Small-bowel neoplasms: prospective evaluation of MR enteroclysis. Radiology 2009; 251(3):743–50.

227. Huprich JE, et al. Prospective blinded comparison of wireless capsule endoscopy and multiphase CT enterography in obscure gastrointestinal bleeding. Radiology 2011;260(3):744–51.

228. Huprich JE. Multi-phase CT enterography in obscure GI bleeding. Abdom Imaging 2009;34(3):303–9.

229. Huprich JE, et al. Obscure gastrointestinal bleeding: evaluation with 64-section multiphase CT enterography–initial experience. Radiology 2008;246(2):562–71.

230. Peabody FW. The care of the patient. JAMA 1927; 88:877–82.

231. Barloon TJ, et al. Small bowel enteroclysis survey. Gastrointest Radiol 1988;13(3):203–6.

232. Redmond PL, Kumpe DA. Fentanyl and diazepam for analgesia and sedation during radiologic special procedures. Radiology 1987;164(1):284.

233. Trevisani L, et al. Upper gastrointestinal endoscopy: are preparatory interventions or conscious sedation effective? A randomized trial. World J Gastroenterol 2004;10(22):564–70.

234. Zaman A, et al. A randomized trial of peroral versus transnasal unsedated endoscopy using an ultrathin videoendoscope. Gastrointest Endosc 1999; 49(3 Pt 1):279–84.

235. Madan A, Minocha A. Who is willing to undergo endoscopy without sedation: patients, nurses or the physicians? South Med J 2004;97(9):800–5.

236. Singer AJ, et al. Comparison of patient and practitioner assessments of pain from commonly performed emergency department procedures. Ann Emerg Med 1999;33(6):652–8.

237. Maglinte DD, Cordell WH. Strategies for reducing the pain and discomfort of nasogastric intubation. Acad Emerg Med 1999;6(3):166–9.

238. American Society of Anesthesiologists Task Force on Sedation and Analgesia by Non-Anesthesiologists. Practice guidelines for sedation and analgesia by non-anesthesiologists. Anesthesiology 2002;96:1004–17.

239. Muller P, Wittenberg KH, Kaufman J. Patterns of analgesia and nursing care for interventional radiology procedures: a national survey of physician practices and preferences. Radiology 1997;202:339–43.

240. Maglinte DD, et al. Intubation routes for enteroclysis. Radiology 1986;158(2):553–4.

241. Maglinte DD, Miller RE. A comparison of pumps used for enteroclysis. Radiology 1984;152(3):815.

242. Mahesh M. NCRP Report Number 160: its significance to medical imaging. J Am Coll Radiol 2009;6(12):890–2.

243. National Council on Radiation Protection and Measurements. Our mission. Available at: http://www.ncrponline.org/AboutNCRP/Our_Mission.html. Accessed October 2, 2009.

244. Brenner D, et al. Estimated risks of radiation-induced fatal cancer from pediatric CT. AJR Am J Roentgenol 2001;176(2):289–96.

245. Hall EJ, Brenner DJ. Cancer risks from diagnostic radiology. Br J Radiol 2008;81(965):362–78.

246. Brenner D, Hricak H. Radiation exposure from medical imaging: time to regulate? JAMA 2010; 304(2):208–9.

247. Brenner DJ. Radiation risks potentially associated with low-dose CT screening of adult smokers for lung cancer. Radiology 2004;231(2):440–5.

248. Brenner DJ. Estimating cancer risks from pediatric CT: going from the qualitative to the quantitative. Pediatr Radiol 2002;32(4):228–33 [discussion: 242–4].

249. Brenner DJ. Should we be concerned about the rapid increase in CT usage? Rev Environ Health 2010;25(1):63–8.

250. Brenner DJ, Elliston CD. Estimated radiation risks potentially associated with full-body CT screening. Radiology 2004;232(3):735–8.

251. Brenner DJ, Sachs RK. Estimating radiation-induced cancer risks at very low doses: rationale for using a linear no-threshold approach. Radiat Environ Biophys 2006;44(4):253–6.

252. Mahesh M, Hevezi JM. Multislice scanners and radiation dose. J Am Coll Radiol 2009;6(2):127–8.

253. Brenner DJ. It is time to retire the computed tomography dose index (CTDI) for CT quality assurance and dose optimization. For the proposition. Med Phys 2006;33(5):1189–90.

254. Brenner DJ, Hall EJ. Computed tomography–an increasing source of radiation exposure. N Engl J Med 2007;357(22):2277–84.

255. Brenner DJ. Slowing the increase in the population dose resulting from CT scans. Radiat Res 2010; 174(6):809–15.

256. Brenner DJ, Shuryak I, Einstein AJ. Impact of reduced patient life expectancy on potential cancer risks from radiologic imaging. Radiology 2011;261(1):193–8.

257. Cohen MD. More on the risks associated with radiation. J Am Coll Radiol 2009;6(6):463.

258. Thrall JH. Radiation exposure: politics and opinion vs science and pragmatism. J Am Coll Radiol 2009;6(3):133–4.

259. Brenner DJ. The linear-quadratic model is an appropriate methodology for determining isoeffective doses at large doses per fraction. Semin Radiat Oncol 2008;18(4):234–9.

260. Cohen BL. Cancer risk from low-level radiation. AJR Am J Roentgenol 2002;179(5):1137–43.

261. Pierce DA, Vaeth M. Age-time distribution of cancer risks to be expected from acute or chronic exposures to general mutagens. Radiat Res 2000; 154(6):727–8 [discussion: 730–1].

262. Pukkala E, et al. Incidence of cancer among Nordic airline pilots over five decades: occupational cohort study. BMJ 2002;325(7364):567.

263. Hammer GP, et al. Childhood cancer risk from conventional radiographic examinations for selected referral criteria: results from a large cohort study. AJR Am J Roentgenol 2011;197(1):217–23.

264. Amis ES Jr. CT radiation dose: trending in the right direction. Radiology 2011;261(1):5–8.

265. Thrall JH. Radiation exposure in CT scanning and risk: where are we? Radiology 2012;264(2): 325–8.

266. Committee to Assess Health Risks from Exposure to Low Levels of Ionizing Radiation, N.R.C. Health risks from exposure to low levels of ionizing radiation: BEIR V11 phase 2. Washington, DC: National Academic Press; 2006.

267. Little MP, et al. Risks associated with low doses and low dose rates of ionizing radiation: why linearity may be (almost) the best we can do. Radiology 2009;251(1):6–12.

268. Tubiana M, et al. The linear no-threshold relationship is inconsistent with radiation biologic and experimental data. Radiology 2009;251(1): 13–22.

269. Hendee WR, O'Connor MK. Radiation risks of medical imaging: separating fact from fantasy. Radiology 2012;264(2):312–21.

270. Health Physics Society. McLean, V. Radiation risk in perspective. 1996. Available at: www.hps.org/document/risk_ps010-1.pdf. Accessed July 18, 2011.

271. McCollough CH, et al. Achieving routine submillisievert CT scanning: report from the summit on management of radiation dose in CT. Radiology 2012;264(2):567–80.

272. Brink JA, Amis ES Jr. Image wisely: a campaign to increase awareness about adult radiation protection. Radiology 2010;257(3):601–2.

273. Brink JA. The art and science of medical guidelines: what we know and what we believe. Radiology 2010;254(1):20–1.

274. Huprich JE, Fletcher JG. CT enterography: principles, technique and utility in Crohn's disease. Eur J Radiol 2009;69(3):393–7.

275. Elsayes KM, et al. CT enterography: principles, trends, and interpretation of findings. Radiographics 2010;30(7):1955–70.

276. Megibow AJ, et al. Evaluation of bowel distention and bowel wall appearance by using neutral oral contrast agent for multi-detector row CT. Radiology 2006;238(1):87–95.

277. Oliva M, Erturk S, Ichikawa T, et al. Abdominal MDCT with neutral oral contrast media (Volumen): comparison with positive oral contrast media and water (abstract no. SSJ06-03). Chicago: Radiological Society of North America; 2005.

278. Arslan H, et al. Peroral CT enterography with lactulose solution: preliminary observations. AJR Am J Roentgenol 2005;185(5):1173–9.

279. Bilimoria KY, et al. Small bowel cancer in the United States: changes in epidemiology, treatment, and survival over the last 20 years. Ann Surg 2009; 249(1):63–71.

280. Krishnaraj A. Standing our ground. J Am Coll Radiol 2010;7:8–9.

281. Lee CI, Forman HP. Radiology health services research: from imperative to legislative mandate. Am J Roentgenol 2011;196(5):1111–4.

Endoscopic Techniques for Small Bowel Imaging

Shabana F. Pasha, MD*, Jonathan A. Leighton, MD

KEYWORDS

- Capsule endoscopy • Double-balloon enteroscopy • Single-balloon enteroscopy
- Spiral enteroscopy • Obscure gastrointestinal bleeding • Crohn's disease • Small bowel tumors
- Polyposis syndromes

KEY POINTS

- Capsule endoscopy is a noninvasive test that allows diagnostic evaluation of the entire small bowel.
- Deep enteroscopy techniques (balloon-assisted and spiral enteroscopy) allow endoscopic management of small bowel disorders, including biopsies, polypectomy, dilation of strictures, tattooing, and retrieval of retained capsules.
- The deep enteroscopy techniques have a comparable diagnostic and therapeutic yield in the management of small bowel disorders.
- Capsule endoscopy and deep enteroscopy are considered complementary tests, and capsule endoscopy is often used as a screening tool before deep enteroscopy.
- Double-balloon enteroscopy appears to have the highest success rate for total enteroscopy among all deep enteroscopy techniques, and should therefore be the procedure of choice when total enteroscopy is a desired goal.

INTRODUCTION

Significant advances in small bowel enteroscopy over the last decade have facilitated both the diagnostic evaluation and therapeutic management of small bowel disorders. The small bowel, therefore, is no longer considered the "black box" of the gastrointestinal tract. Multiple enteroscopic tools are now available that differ in their technique and capabilities. Capsule endoscopy enables visualization of the entire small bowel in a noninvasive manner, but is a purely diagnostic test. The deep enteroscopy techniques, which include balloon-assisted and spiral enteroscopy, allow therapeutic interventions in the deeper portions of the small bowel, but are relatively invasive and often protracted procedures. The selection of the appropriate enteroscopy tool is determined by several factors, including clinical presentation of the patient, index of suspicion for a small bowel lesion, and the suspected location of the lesion. This article reviews the use of the enteroscopy techniques, and their advantages and limitations in the evaluation of the small bowel.

ANATOMY OF THE SMALL BOWEL

The small bowel is a tubular organ that is 600 to 800 cm in length, and extends between the pylorus and the ileocecal (IC) valve. It is divided into 3 segments: duodenum, jejunum, and ileum. The duodenum is the most proximal and shortest segment of the small bowel, with a mean length of 25 cm. It is shaped like a C loop. This segment

The authors have no conflict of interest or financial involvement with this article.
Division of Gastroenterology, Department of Internal Medicine, Mayo Clinic College of Medicine, Scottsdale, 13400 East Shea Boulevard, AZ 85259, USA
* Corresponding author.
E-mail address: pasha.shabana@mayo.edu

is the only one located in the retroperitoneal space, and is therefore relatively fixed. It includes the bulb, second, third, and fourth portions, and extends up to the ligament of Treitz. The ampulla of Vater lies in the second portion of the duodenum. The remainder of the small bowel is suspended in the peritoneal cavity by a broad-based mesentery, and is freely mobile. The proximal 40% of this portion is the jejunum and the distal 60% the ileum. The luminal surface of the small bowel has numerous folds called the plicae circularis. The plicae are most prominent in the proximal small bowel, and decrease in number distally.[1]

Historically, gastrointestinal sources of bleeding were classified as proximal and distal to the ligament of Treitz. Since the introduction of the deep enteroscopy techniques, the gastrointestinal tract is now divided into 3 segments: proximal to the ligament of Treitz, distal to IC valve, and midgut, which refers to the portion of the small bowel that is located between the ampulla and IC valve.[2]

VIDEO CAPSULE ENDOSCOPY

Capsule endoscopy (CE) was introduced in the year 2000, and was the first endoscopic test that enabled visualization of the entire small bowel. There are 4 CE systems currently available. The CE systems used in the United States are Pillcam SB2 (Given Imaging, Yoqneam, Israel) and Endo Capsule (Olympus America Inc, Center Valley, PA). The systems include a capsule endoscope, 8-point sensory array, and a portable data recorder. Both the Pillcam SB2 and Endo Capsule measure 11 × 26 mm, and contain light-emitting diodes, silver oxide batteries, lens, radiofrequency transmitter, and antenna. The Pillcam SB2 contains a metal oxide semiconductor whereas the Endo Capsule has a charged coupled device.

CE is a noninvasive procedure that can be performed in the outpatient ambulatory setting. Patients are required to fast for an 8-hour period, and most centers recommend a bowel preparation (2 L oral polyethylene glycol) on the night before capsule ingestion. The capsule is usually swallowed by the patient, but can also be delivered directly into the small bowel by endoscopic assistance in patients with dysphagia or risk factors for an incomplete study.[3,4] It is propelled through the small bowel by peristalsis over an 8- to 12-hour period. Images are captured by the camera at the rate of 2 frames per second and transferred by wireless technology to a data recorder that is strapped to the patient's waist. The images can then be downloaded and viewed on a computer that contains the appropriate software. The average physician time for viewing the images ranges from 45 to 120 minutes.[5] The software has features that include multiviewing by simultaneous display of 2 to 4 consecutive images, and a suspected blood indicator.

CE allows visualization of the entire small bowel in 79% to 90% of patients.[6] The test is approved by the Food and Drug Administration for use in patients older than 10 years for the evaluation of obscure gastrointestinal bleeding (OGIB), Crohn's disease, celiac sprue, polyposis syndromes, small bowel abnormalities on imaging studies, and clinical symptoms.

The main disadvantage of CE is its purely diagnostic capability and, therefore, necessity for additional therapeutic procedures in patients with positive CE findings. There also is a high rate of incidental findings in up to 23% of healthy controls,[7] which may result in unnecessary invasive procedures. CE may be limited by incomplete visualization of the small bowel in 15% to 20% of patients.[8] The most important complication is small bowel retention in patients with an underlying stricture or obstruction. This risk ranges from less than 1% in patients with OGIB, up to 13% in patients with Crohn's disease, and 17% in patients with small bowel tumors.[9,10]

Patency Capsule

The patency capsule (PC) is useful for minimizing the risk of retention in patients with a suspected small bowel stricture or obstruction, by selection of those patients who can safely undergo CE. The system includes a PC, scanner, and TesTag. The capsule is 26 × 11 mm in size, and contains a body with a radiofrequency identification tag (RFID) covered with lactose and barium, and a timer plug on either side of the capsule. The PC is designed to dissolve in gastrointestinal secretions 30 hours after ingestion. Patency of the gastrointestinal tract can be confirmed if the patient witnesses passage of the patency capsule or if the RFID tag is not detected with the scanner at or before 30 hours after ingestion. Fluoroscopy is used in place of the scanner for accurate localization of the RFID tag and in patients with pacemakers.

In a study of 27 patients with suspected obstruction, the PC was excreted intact in 63% of patients over a mean transit time of 25.6 hours. CE was performed in all these patients without any complications of retention.[11] Another large study evaluated 106 patients using PC. Fifty-six percent of patients excreted the capsule intact, and subsequently underwent CE without retention.[12] A study that compared patency capsule with radiologic tests showed similar sensitivity (57% vs 71%; P = 1.00) and specificity (86% vs 97%; P = .22) for the detection of clinically significant strictures. Pooled results using both the PC and radiologic tests had the highest sensitivity (100%) and negative predictive value (NPV) (100%).[13]

DOUBLE-BALLOON ENTEROSCOPY

The double-balloon enteroscope (Fujinon Inc, Tokyo, Japan) was the first therapeutic deep enteroscopy tool that was introduced in 2004. The double-balloon enteroscopy (DBE) system comprises an enteroscope, an overtube, and a balloon-pump system. Two double-balloon enteroscopes are currently available, diagnostic (EN-450P5) and therapeutic EN-450T5. The enteroscope has a working length of 200 cm and an overtube made of polyurethane, which is 140 cm in length. Both the enteroscope and overtube have latex balloons at their distal ends. The balloons can be inflated to a pressure of 45 mm Hg. The EN-450T5 has an external diameter of 9.4 mm and an accessory channel of 2.8 mm, compared with 8.5 mm and 2.2 mm, respectively, with the EN-450P5.

DBE may be performed by the oral (antegrade) or aboral (retrograde) route. Advancement through the small bowel is achieved with a series of cycles using a push-and-pull technique. In this technique, the enteroscope and overtube are advanced into the small bowel to the maximal extent without looping. Once looping is encountered, the balloon on the overtube is inflated and the enteroscope is advanced further into the small bowel. The balloon on the enteroscope is inflated after full advancement. After deflation of its balloon, the overtube is advanced over the enteroscope. With both balloons inflated, the enteroscope and overtube are slowly pulled back, which allows the small bowel to pleat over the enteroscope. By repeating this series of steps, a greater depth of small bowel can be intubated than with push enteroscopy (PE) or ileoscopy.[14] General anesthesia is often used for antegrade procedures, whereas retrograde procedures are more often performed under conscious sedation at many centers. The procedure requires additional personnel for handling of the overtube.

The depth of intubation with DBE ranges from 240 to 360 cm with the antegrade approach, and from 102 to 140 cm with the retrograde approach.[15–18] A "targeted enteroscopy" is performed when there is a preidentified lesion on prior CE or small bowel imaging, and the route of DBE is based on suspected location of the lesion. The antegrade route is used for lesions suspected to lie within the proximal 75%, whereas the retrograde route is used for lesions in the distal 25% of the small bowel, based on capsule transit times.[19] Total enteroscopy is defined as intubation of the entire small bowel by one or both routes. This approach is useful in patients with multiple small bowel lesions, negative initial DBE, or high clinical suspicion for a small bowel lesion after a negative CE. The success rate for total enteroscopy ranges from 0% to 86%, and is highest in the Asian population.[14,16,17,20]

The diagnostic yield of DBE ranges from 43% to 80%. The test enables the performance of therapeutic interventions, including biopsies, injection, polypectomy, stricture dilation, hemostatic techniques (argon-plasma coagulation, electrocoagulation, and hemoclips), and retrieval of foreign bodies, including retained capsules.[15,21,22]

One of the main limitations of DBE and other deep enteroscopy techniques is the lack of a validated method for estimating the depth of small bowel intubation. The method currently used is based on subjective perception by the endoscopist of depth of insertion with each advancement cycle.[23] The overall complication rate of DBE is 0.8% for diagnostic and upto 4% for therapeutic procedures, and the most common complications include bleeding and perforation. Pancreatitis has also been reported, but its incidence appears to have decreased over time.[24,25]

SINGLE-BALLOON ENTEROSCOPY

The single-balloon enteroscope (Olympus Optical, Tokyo, Japan) was introduced in 2007. In contrast to the double-balloon enteroscope, this device has only one balloon at the distal end of the overtube. The enteroscope (SIF-Q180) has a length of 200 cm, and the overtube is 140 cm. The outer diameter of the enteroscope is 9.2 mm and the accessory channel is 2.8 mm. The overtube and balloon are made from silicon.

Single-balloon enteroscopy (SBE) is also performed by the push-and-pull technique, but the advancement cycles differ slightly from DBE. In the technique of SBE, the enteroscope is advanced to the maximal depth without looping. The overtube is advanced over the enteroscope and its balloon is inflated. The distal end of the enteroscope is then anchored behind a fold for stabilization, and the enteroscope and overtube are pulled back to allow pleating of the small bowel.[26]

The depth of intubation with SBE ranges from 133 to 256 cm with the antegrade approach and from 73 to 163 cm with the retrograde approach,[27,28] and the success rate of total enteroscopy has been reported as 15% to 25%.[28,29] The diagnostic yield of SBE ranges from 47% to 60%,[27,28,30] and endoscopic therapeutics can be performed, similar to DBE. SBE has a complication rate of 1%, which includes perforation and pancreatitis.[31]

SPIRAL ENTEROSCOPY

The Endo-Ease Discovery SB (Spirus Medical, Stoughtom, MA) is a spiral overtube made of polyvinyl chloride. It measures 118 cm and has a 21-cm raised helix at the distal end. In the technique of spiral enteroscopy, the overtube is placed over a pediatric colonoscope or push enteroscope and locked into place. It is then advanced into the small bowel until the ligament of Treitz is reached. The device is rotated using clockwise movements until the furthest extent possible is reached. The enteroscope is then unlocked and advanced beyond the overtube as far as possible. This series of steps is repeated until the maximal extent has been intubated. The device is withdrawn using counterclockwise rotations.[32]

With the exception of one pilot study of 6 patients using retrograde SE,[33] all studies have described SE using the antegrade approach. The mean depth of intubation with SE ranges from 176 to 250 cm.[34,35] Complications with SE include minor mucosal tears, and perforation has been reported in 0.3% of patients.[36]

OBSCURE GASTROINTESTINAL BLEEDING

OGIB is defined as bleeding from the gastrointestinal tract that persists or recurs after a negative initial evaluation with bidirectional endoscopy and small bowel radiography.[2,37] The majority of patients with OGIB have midgut bleeding, and the small bowel enteroscopy techniques have led to a trend toward endoscopic evaluation and management of these patients.

Capsule Endoscopy

CE has a diagnostic yield ranging from 38% to 83%,[6] and a pooled analysis of 24 trials reported an overall yield of 87% in patients with OGIB.[38] When compared with intraoperative enteroscopy, CE was found to have a sensitivity of 95%, specificity 75%, positive predictive value (PPV) of 95%, and NPV of 86%.[39] Other studies have also reported a high PPV of 94% to 97% and NPV of 83% to 100% with CE in these patients.[40,41]

The yield of CE is dependent on several factors, including clinical presentation and timing. A study of 250 patients with OGIB reported a significantly higher diagnostic yield of 60% in patients with overt bleed, compared with 46% in those with occult bleed. There was a significant difference between patients with overt ongoing bleed (87%) and prior overt bleed (56%).[42] CE was also shown to have a high yield of 91% in patients who undergo the procedure within 2 weeks of the bleeding episode but only 34% if performed after this time frame.[43] Other factors that favorably affect the yield of CE are recurrent bleeding, longer duration of bleeding, and a hemoglobin count of less than 10 g/dL.[44]

CE is superior to PE in the evaluation of OGIB. A meta-analysis of 14 studies found that CE had an incremental yield of 30% over PE for clinically significant findings in the small bowel. Another meta-analysis of 9 studies also showed that CE is superior to other tests, with a rate difference of 37% over PE, small bowel radiography, and enteroclysis. The guidelines of the American Gastroenterological Association and the American Society for Gastrointestinal Endoscopy recommend that CE be performed as the third test in patients with OGIB after negative bidirectional endoscopy.[2,37]

A negative capsule study predicts a low rebleeding rate in patients with OGIB. Two studies reported bleeding rates of 5.6% and 11% at a mean follow-up of 19 and 17 months, respectively.[45,46] Additional invasive testing may therefore be avoided in these patients unless the initial examination has been compromised by suboptimal preparation or incomplete small bowel examination.[47] A repeat CE may be useful in patients who present with recurrent bleeding. Studies have reported a diagnostic yield of 35% and 75% in these patients and a change in management based on repeat CE findings in 63% of patients. Factors that may predict positive findings on repeat CE include a change in clinical presentation from occult to overt bleed, and a drop in hemoglobin of more than 4 g/dL.[48–50]

Double-Balloon Enteroscopy

DBE is superior to PE in the evaluation of OGIB. A study that compared the two tests in 52 patients with OGIB found that DBE allowed a greater depth of intubation (230 cm vs 80 cm) and also had a significantly higher yield (73% vs 44%) compared with push enteroscopy.[51] The diagnostic yield of DBE ranges from 50% to 80%, and endoscopic therapeutics can be successfully performed in up to 75% of patients.[15,16,18,52,53] Based on a systematic review of 13 studies with 906 patients with OGIB, the diagnostic yield with DBE was 66%, and included predominantly angioectasias.[54] The yield is significantly higher in patients with overt ongoing bleed compared with those with a prior overt bleed or occult bleed, and also in patients with multiple episodes or prolonged duration of bleeding.[55,56] The test has a high sensitivity of 92.7%, specificity 96.4%, PPV 98.1%, and NPV 87.1% in the evaluation of these patients.[55]

Favorable outcomes have been reported in patients after DBE. A study that followed 85 patients at 30-month follow-up after DBE reported no rebleeding in 59% of patients.[57] Two other studies that followed patients with small bowel vascular lesions after DBE showed that 54% and 58% remained without rebleeding at a mean follow-up of 36 months and 55 months, respectively. In patients with rebleeding, there was a decrease in transfusion requirements from 60% to 16% after DBE.[58,59]

Single-Balloon Enteroscopy

A large single-center study from the United States evaluated 161 patients with suspected small bowel disorders, 59% with OGIB, using SBE. The yield of SBE was 58% and the most common findings were angioectasias. The concordance between CE and SBE findings was 40%, and SBE detected new findings in 17% of patients.[27] Two smaller studies also reported a diagnostic yield of 47% and 60% in patients with OGIB.[28,30]

Spiral Enteroscopy

A multicenter study using SE that evaluated 148 patients, the majority with OGIB, reported a diagnostic yield of 65%, and the predominant findings were angioectasias.[35] In a study of 56 patients (89% with OGIB), all of whom had abnormal findings on prior CE, the diagnostic yield on SE was 57%, and abnormal findings on CE were detected in 54% of patients. Although SE detected vascular lesions seen on CE, it failed to detect most of the ulcerations and mass lesions.[60]

Comparison of Deep Enteroscopy Techniques in OGIB

Studies comparing DBE and SBE in patients with small bowel disorders (predominantly OGIB) have reported conflicting results. In a study that compared the two techniques using the Fujinon DB enteroscope (using 1 and 2 balloons), there was a significantly higher yield (72% vs 48%) and total enteroscopy rate (66% vs 22%) with DBE.[61] In comparison, another study that compared the Fujinon DB enteroscope with the Olympus SB enteroscope reported a significantly higher yield with the latter technique (70% vs 51%).[62] A third study that was terminated after interim analysis found a significantly higher success rate for total enteroscopy with DBE, but no difference in diagnostic yield (61% vs 50%) or therapeutic outcomes (35% vs 28%) between the tests.[63] A recent randomized multicenter trial in 130 patients showed a comparable depth of intubation, total enteroscopy rate, and diagnostic yield with the two techniques.[64]

Studies have also shown that SE is comparable to DBE. A prospective randomized trial found no significant difference in diagnostic yield (47% vs 33%) or mean depth of intubation with these tests.[65] Similarly, a retrospective study that compared SBE and SE showed no difference in diagnostic yield (43 vs 57%), although mean depth of intubation was significantly greater with SE (301 vs 222 cm).[66]

CE and DBE have a comparable yield in patients with OGIB. Two meta-analyses that compared the tests in patients with suspected small bowel disorders, predominantly OGIB, found no difference in their yield.[67,68] There was also no difference in the detection of vascular lesions (**Fig. 1**), ulcerations, (**Fig. 2**) or neoplasms (**Fig. 3**).[67] CE did have a significantly higher yield when compared

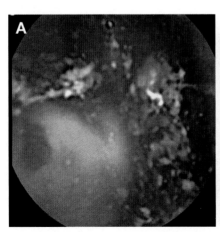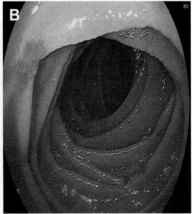

Fig. 1. (*A, B*) Angioectasia seen on capsule endoscopy and double-balloon enteroscopy.

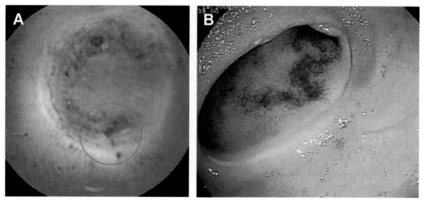

Fig. 2. (*A, B*) NSAID-related ulcerated stenosis seen on capsule endoscopy and double-balloon enteroscopy.

with DBE by a single approach, but there was no difference between the tests when DBE was performed using a combined antegrade and retrograde approach.[68] A recent updated meta-analysis that compared the tests in patients with OGIB also showed no difference in their diagnostic yield (62% with CE and 56% with DBE). However, the yield of DBE was increased significantly after a positive CE (75%) in comparison with a negative CE (27.5%).[69]

These results support the role of using CE as a screening tool before proceeding with therapeutic deep enteroscopy. CE is the preferred initial test of choice, as it allows evaluation of the entire small bowel in a noninvasive manner, and also provides information on location of the small bowel lesion. Additional evaluation and therapeutics may then be pursued with any one of the deep enteroscopy techniques, based on their availability and the endoscopist's experience. However, when total enteroscopy is a desired goal, the best choice of test may be DBE.

CROHN'S DISEASE
Capsule Endoscopy

CE is superior to other tests in the evaluation of patients with Crohn's disease. A meta-analysis showed that CE had an incremental yield of 42% over PE, 37% over small bowel radiography, 39% over computed tomography (CT) enterography, and 15% over ileoscopy for the diagnosis of nonstricturing Crohn's disease. CE was superior to these tests for the diagnosis of patients with suspected as well as established Crohn's disease.[70] The overall yield of CE has been reported to range from 43% to 71%.[71–74]

A prospective study that compared CE with CT enterography, small bowel radiography, and ileocolonoscopy for evaluation of Crohn's disease showed that the sensitivity of CE (83%) was comparable with that of CT enterography (83%), ileocolonoscopy (74%) and small bowel radiography (65%). However, CE had a significantly lower specificity of 53% compared with 100% with the other tests.[75] CE cannot accurately differentiate

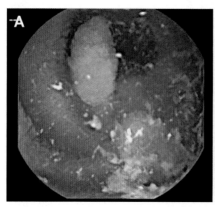
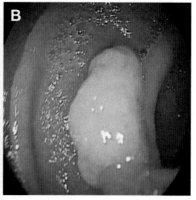

Fig. 3. (*A, B*) Adenomatous polyp seen on capsule endoscopy and double-balloon enteroscopy.

between Crohn's disease and other small bowel inflammatory disorders, and should not be used as a first-line diagnostic test in these patients. It may be useful after a negative evaluation with ileocolonoscopy and CT enterography in patients in whom there is a high clinical suspicion for Crohn's disease. CE is also useful in excluding a diagnosis of Crohn's disease in patients with a low pretest probability, as it has a low miss rate of only 0.5% for small bowel inflammation.[38]

Medical management of patients with Crohn's disease is influenced by findings on CE. A study reported improvement in 70% of patients after CE-guided modifications in treatment.[73,76] Another important role of CE lies in evaluation of patients with indeterminate colitis. Studies have shown that a diagnosis of Crohn's disease can be established on CE in 17% to 38% of patients.[73,77,78] CE is also useful in detecting postoperative recurrence of Crohn's disease. A study that compared CE and ileocolonoscopy found that the latter test had a higher sensitivity than CE (90% vs 62%) for detection of postoperative recurrence, but CE allowed detection of inflammation in locations inaccessible to ileoscopy in 67% of patients.[79]

Double-Balloon Enteroscopy

DBE and other deep enteroscopy techniques are not considered a first-line tool in patients with Crohn's disease, but may be useful for histologic confirmation of small bowel findings on CE or imaging studies, and the performance of therapeutic interventions. The overall yield for small bowel Crohn's disease ranges from 5% to 13% in all patients undergoing DBE, but increases to 74% to 96% in patients with known Crohn's disease.[80,81] Studies have shown that DBE is useful for dilation of Crohn-related small bowel strictures and retrieval of retained capsules.[82,83]

SMALL BOWEL TUMORS

Although small bowel tumors are rare, they are important to recognize because they are often malignant and carry a poor prognosis resulting from a delay in their diagnosis. Deep enteroscopy techniques may allow earlier diagnosis (**Fig. 3**) and, therefore, improved outcomes in these patients. Most small bowel polyps can now be removed endoscopically at deep enteroscopy, but surgery continues to remain the definitive management for tumors.

Capsule Endoscopy

The incidence of small bowel tumors detected on CE ranges from 2% to 10%; these are mostly malignant and include gastrointestinal stromal tumors, adenocarcinomas, and carcinoid tumors.[84–87] A multicenter study showed improved outcomes in patients with small bowel tumors detected on CE. The prevalence of small bowel tumors in this study was 6.3%, most of which were malignant tumors. After detection on CE, curative resection of the tumors was performed in 52% of patients, all of whom remained recurrence free at a mean follow-up period of 38 months.[84]

CE may be useful for surveillance of the small bowel in patients with hereditary polyposis syndromes, including familial adenomatous polyposis and Peutz-Jeghers syndrome. The test is superior to small bowel radiography for the detection of clinically significant small bowel polyps (>1 cm), and is also better tolerated by patients.[88,89] The main limitation of CE is that the location and size of the polyps cannot be determined accurately on the test.[90] A study that compared CE with magnetic resonance (MR) enterography showed a comparable yield for polyps larger than 15 mm, but CE detected a greater number of smaller polyps. However, assessment of size and location was more accurate with MR enterography.[91] Periampullary polyps cannot be accurately diagnosed on CE, as the ampulla may not be visualized consistently in all patients.[92]

The role of CE in detection of small bowel tumors is also limited by a high miss rate of 19%.[38] Studies have reported on small bowel tumors that have been missed on CE and have been detected with other modalities, including PE, CT enterography, and DBE.[93–95] CE also has a high risk of retention (9.8%–17%) in patients with small bowel tumors, but this is considered a "therapeutic complication" because it enables both the detection and localization of the tumor at subsequent surgery.[86,96]

Double-Balloon Enteroscopy

DBE may be useful for the detection of small bowel tumors missed on prior CE.[95] However, its main role in patients with small bowel tumors and polyposis syndromes is the performance of therapeutic interventions including biopsies, polypectomy, tattooing of tumors to enable their detection at surgery, palliative dilation and stent placement, and retrieval of retained capsule endoscopes.[97–100]

SUMMARY

There have been significant advances in small bowel enteroscopy over the last decade. The development of CE as well as other deep enteroscopy techniques has enabled both diagnostic evaluation and therapeutic management of almost all small bowel disorders. The enteroscopic tools have a complementary role in the evaluation of the small bowel, and their selection should be based on clinical presentation and suspected location of the lesion, as well as the necessity for therapeutics.

REFERENCES

1. Kahn E, Daum F. Anatomy, histology, embryology, and developmental anomalies of the small and large intestine. In: Feldman M, Friedman LS, Brandt LJ, editors. Sleisinger and Fordtran's gastrointestinal and liver disease, vol. 96. Philadelphia: Saunders Elsevier; 2010. p. 1615–7.

2. Raju GS, Gerson L, Das A, et al. American Gastroenterological Association (AGA) Institute medical position statement on obscure gastrointestinal bleeding. Gastroenterology 2007;133:1694–6.

3. Lee MM, Jacque A, Lam E, et al. Factors associated with incomplete small bowel examinations. World J Gastroenterol 2010;16:5329–33.

4. Gao YJ, Ge ZZ, Chen HY, et al. Endoscopic capsule placement improves the completion rate of small bowel capsule endoscopy and increases diagnostic yield. Gastrointest Endosc 2010;72:103–8.

5. Levinthal GN, Burke CA, Santisi JM. The accuracy of an endoscopy nurse in interpreting capsule endoscopy. Am J Gastroenterol 2003;98:2669–71.

6. Rondonotti E, Villa F, Mulder CJ, et al. Small bowel capsule endoscopy in 2007; indications, risks and limitations. World J Gastroenterol 2007;13:6140–9.

7. Goldstein JL, Eisen GM, Lewis B, et al. Video capsule endoscopy to prospectively assess small bowel injury with celecoxib, naproxen plus omeprazole, and placebo. Clin Gastroenterol Hepatol 2005;3:133–41.

8. Rondonotti E, Herrerias JM, Pennazio M, et al. Complications, limitations and failures of capsule endoscopy: a review of 733 cases. Gastrointest Endosc 2005;62:712–6.

9. Barkin JS, Freidman S. Surgical indication for capsule retention. Am J Gastroenterol 2002;97:S298.

10. Cave D, Legnani P, de Franchis R, et al. ICCE Consensus for capsule retention. Endoscopy 2005;37:1065–7.

11. Spada C, Shah RK, Riccioni ME, et al. Video capsule endoscopy in patients with known or suspected small bowel stricture previously tested with the dissolving patency capsule. J Clin Gastroenterol 2007;41:576–82.

12. Herrerias JM, Leighton JA, Costamagna G, et al. Agile patency system eliminates risk of capsule retention in patients with known intestinal strictures who undergo capsule endoscopy. Gastrointest Endosc 2008;67:902–9.

13. Yadav A, Heigh RI, Hara AK, et al. Performance of the patency capsule compared with nonenteroclysis radiologic examinations in patients with known or suspected intestinal strictures. Gastrointest Endosc 2011;74:834–9.

14. Yamamoto H, Sekine Y, Sato Y, et al. Total enteroscope with a nonsurgical steerable double-balloon method. Gastrointest Endosc 2001;53:216–20.

15. May A, Nachbar L, Ell C. Double-balloon enteroscopy (push-and-pull enteroscopy) of the small bowel: feasibility and diagnostic and therapeutic yield in patients with suspected small bowel disease. Gastrointest Endosc 2005;62:62–70.

16. Mehdizadeh S, Ross A, Gerson L, et al. What is the learning curve associated with double-balloon enteroscopy? Technical details and early experience in 6 US tertiary care centers. Gastrointest Endosc 2006;64:740–50.

17. Gross SA, Stark ME. Initial experience with double-balloon enteroscopy at a US center. Gastrointest Endosc 2008;67:890–7.

18. Heine GD, Hadithi M, Groenen MJ, et al. Double-balloon enteroscopy: indications, diagnostic yield and complications in a series of 275 patients with suspected small-bowel disease. Endoscopy 2006;38:42–8.

19. Gay G, Delvaux M, Fassler I. Outcome of capsule endoscopy in determining indication and route for push and pull enteroscopy. Endoscopy 2006;38:49–58.

20. Ell C, May A. Mid-gastrointestinal bleeding: capsule endoscopy and push-and-pull enteroscopy give rise to a new medical term. Endoscopy 2006;38:73–5.

21. Yamamoto H, Kita H, Sunada K, et al. Clinical outcomes of double-balloon endoscopy for the diagnosis and treatment of small intestinal diseases. Clin Gastroenterol Hepatol 2004;2:1010–6.

22. Di Caro S, May A, Heine DG, et al. The European experience with double-balloon enteroscopy: indicatios, methodology, safety and clinical impact. Gastrointest Endosc 2005;62:545–50.

23. May A, Nachbar L, Schneider M, et al. Push and pull enteroscopy using the double-balloon technique: methods of assessing depth of insertion and training of the enteroscopy technique using the Erlanger endo-trainer. Endoscopy 2005;37:66–70.

24. Mensink P, Haringsma J, Kucharzik TF, et al. Complications of double-balloon enteroscopy (DBE): a multicenter study. Endoscopy 2007;39:613–5.

25. Groenen MJ, Moreels TG, Orlent H, et al. Acute pancreatitis after double-balloon enteroscopy: an

old pathologic theory revisited as a result of a new endoscopic tool. Endoscopy 2006;38:82–5.

26. Manno M, Barbera C, Bertani H, et al. Single balloon enteroscopy: technical aspects and clinical applications. World J Gastroenterol 2012;4:28–32.

27. Upchurch BR, Sanaka MR, Lopez AR, et al. The clinical utility of single-balloon enteroscopy: a single center experience of 72 procedures. Gastrointest Endosc 2010;71:1218–23.

28. Ramchandani M, Reddy ND, Gupta R, et al. Diagnostic yield and therapeutic impact of single-balloon enteroscopy: a series of 106 cases. J Gastroenterol Hepatol 2009;24:1631–8.

29. Tsujikawa T, Saitoh Y, Andoh A, et al. Novel single-balloon enteroscopy for diagnosis and treatment of the small bowel: preliminary experiences. Endoscopy 2008;40:11–5.

30. Franz DJ, Dellon ES, Grimm IS, et al. Single-balloon enteroscopy: results from an initial experience in a US tertiary care center. Gastrointest Endosc 2010;72:422–6.

31. Aktas H, de Ridder L, Haringsma J, et al. Complications of single-balloon enteroscopy: a prospective evaluation of 166 patients. Endoscopy 2010; 42:365–8.

32. Ackerman PA, Agrawal D, Cantero D, et al. Spiral enteroscopy with the new DSB overtube: a novel technique for deep peroral small-bowel intubation. Endoscopy 2008;40:974–8.

33. Lara LF, Singh S, Sreenarasinhaiah J. Initial experience with retrograde Overture-assisted enteroscopy using a spiral tip Overture. Proc (Bayl Univ Med Cent) 2010;23:130–3.

34. Ackerman PA, Agrawal D, Chen W, et al. Spiral enteroscopy: a novel method of enteroscopy by using the Endo-Ease Discovery SB overtube and a pediatric colonoscope. Gastrointest Endosc 2009;69: 327–32.

35. Morgan D, Upchurch B, Draganov P, et al. Spiral enteroscopy: a prospective US multicenter study in patients with small bowel disorders. Gastrointest Endosc 2010;72:992–8.

36. Ackerman P, Cantero D. Complications of spiral enteroscopy in the first 2950 patients. Gastro 2009. London, November 21–25, 2009.

37. Fisher L, Krinsky L, Anderson MA, et al, ASGE Standards of Practice Committee. The role of endoscopy in the management of obscure GI bleeding. Gastrointest Endosc 2010;72:471–9.

38. Lewis BS, Eisen GM, Friedman S. A pooled analysis to evaluate the results of capsule endoscopy trials. Endoscopy 2005;37:960–5.

39. Hartmann D, Schmidt H, Bolz G, et al. A prospective two center study comparing wireless capsule endoscopy with intraoperative enteroscopy in patients with obscure GI bleeding. Gastrointest Endosc 2005;61:826–32.

40. Pennazio M, Santucci R, Rondonotti E, et al. Outcome of patients with obscure gastrointestinal bleeding after capsule endoscopy: a report of 100 consecutive cases. Gastroenterology 2004; 126:643–53.

41. Delvaux M, Fassler I, Gay G. Clinical usefulness of the endoscopic video capsule as the initial intestinal investigation in patients with obscure digestive bleeding: validation of a diagnostic strategy based on patient outcomes after 12 months. Endoscopy 2004;36:1067–73.

42. Carey EJ, Leighton JA, Heigh R, et al. A single-center experience of 260 consecutive patients undergoing capsule endoscopy for obscure gastrointestinal bleeding. Am J Gastroenterol 2007;102:89–95.

43. Bresci G, Parisi G, Bertoni M, et al. The role of video capsule endoscopy for evaluating obscure gastrointestinal bleeding: usefulness of early use. J Gastroenterol 2005;40:256–9.

44. May A, Wardack A, Nachbar L, et al. Influence of patient selection on the outcome of capsule endoscopy in patients with chronic gastrointestinal bleeding. J Clin Gastroenterol 2005;39:684–8.

45. Lai LH, Wong GL, Chow DK, et al. Long-term follow up of patients with obscure gastrointestinal endoscopy after negative capsule endoscopy. Am J Gastroenterol 2006;101:1224–8.

46. MacDonald J, Porter V, McNamara D. Negative capsule endoscopy in patients with obscure GI bleeding predicts low rebleeding rates. Gastrointest Endosc 2008;68:1122–7.

47. Mergener K, Ponchon T, Gralnek I, et al. Literature review and recommendations for clinical application of small bowel capsule endoscopy, based on a panel discussion by international experts. Consensus statements for small bowel capsule endoscopy 2006/2007. Endoscopy 2007;39: 895–909.

48. Jones BH, Fleischer DE, Sharma VK, et al. Yield of repeat wireless video capsule endoscopy in patients with obscure gastrointestinal bleeding. Am J Gastroenterol 2005;100:1058–64.

49. Barr-Meir S, Eliakim R, Nadler M, et al. Second capsule endoscopy for patients with severe iron deficiency anemia. Gastrointest Endosc 2004;60: 711–3.

50. Viazis N, Papaxoinis K, Vlachogiannakos J, et al. Is there a role of second look capsule endoscopy in patients with obscure GI bleeding after a nondiagnostic first test? Gastrointest Endosc 2009;69: 850–6.

51. May A, Nachbar L, Schneider M, et al. Prospective comparison of push enteroscopy and push-and-pull enteroscopy in patients with suspected small-bowel bleeding. Am J Gastroenterol 2006;101: 2016–24.

52. Kaffes AJ, Siah C, Kii JH. Clinical outcomes after double-balloon enteroscopy in patients with obscure GI bleeding and a positive capsule endoscopy. Gastrointest Endosc 2007;66:304–9.

53. Sun B, Rajan E, Cheng S, et al. Diagnostic yield and therapeutic impact of double-balloon enteroscopy in a large cohort of patients with obscure gastrointestinal bleeding. Am J Gastroenterol 2006;101:2011–5.

54. Pasha SF, Leighton JA, Das A, et al. Diagnostic yield and therapeutic utility of double-balloon enteroscopy (DBE) in patients with obscure gastrointestinal bleeding (OGIB): a systematic review. Gastrointest Endosc 2007;65:AB306.

55. Tanaka S, Mitsui K, Yamada Y, et al. Diagnostic yield of double-balloon enteroscopy in patients with obscure GI bleeding. Gastrointest Endosc 2008;68:683–91.

56. Byeon JS, Ching JW, Choi KD, et al. Clinical features predicting the detection of abnormalities by double-balloon enteroscopy in patients with suspected small bowel bleeding. J Gastroenterol Hepatol 2008;23:1051–5.

57. Gerson LB, Batenic MA, Newsom SL, et al. Long-term outcomes after double balloon enteroscopy for obscure gastrointestinal bleeding. Clin Gastroenterol Hepatol 2009;7:664–9.

58. May A, Friesing-Sosnik T, Manner H, et al. Long-term outcomes after argon-plasma coagulation of small-bowel lesions using double-balloon enteroscopy in patients with mid-gastrointestinal bleeding. Endoscopy 2011;43:759–65.

59. Samaha E, Rahmi G, Landi B, et al. Long term outcome of patients treated with double-balloon enteroscopy for small bowel vascular lesions. Am J Gastroenterol 2012;107:240–6.

60. Buscaglia JM, Richards R, Wilkinson MN, et al. Diagnostic yield of spiral enteroscopy when performed for the evaluation of abnormal capsule endoscopy findings. J Gastroenterol 2011;45:342–6.

61. May A, Farber M, Aschmoneit I, et al. Prospective multicenter trial comparing push-and-pull enteroscopy with the single and double balloon techniques in patients with suspected small-bowel disorders. Am J Gastroenterol 2010;105:575–81.

62. Landaeta JL, Dias C, Rodriguez MJ. Double balloon enteroscopy vs single balloon enteroscopy in obscure gastrointestinal bleeding. Gastrointest Endosc 2009;69:AB187.

63. Takano N, Yamada A, Watabe H, et al. Single-balloon versus double-balloon endoscopy for achieving total enteroscopy: a randomized controlled trial. Gastrointest Endosc 2011;73:734–9.

64. Dogmagk D, Mensink P, Aktas H, et al. Single vs double balloon enteroscopy in small bowel diagnostics: a randomized multicenter trial. Endoscopy 2011;43:472–6.

65. Frieling T, Heise J, Sassenrath W, et al. Prospective comparison between double-balloon and spiral enteroscopy. Endoscopy 2010;42:885–8.

66. Khashab MA, Lennon AM, Dunbar KB, et al. A comparative evaluation of single-balloon enteroscopy and spiral enteroscopy for patients with mid-gut disorders. Gastrointest Endosc 2010;72:766–72.

67. Pasha SF, Leighton JA, Das A, et al. Double-balloon enteroscopy and capsule endoscopy have a comparable diagnostic yield in small bowel disease: a meta-analysis. Clin Gastroenterol Hepatol 2008;6:671–6.

68. Chen X, Ran Z, Tong J. A meta-analysis of the yield of capsule endoscopy compared to double-balloon enteroscopy in patients with small bowel diseases. World J Gastroenterol 2007;13:4372–8.

69. Teshima CW, Kuipers EJ, van Zanten SV, et al. Double-balloon enteroscopy and capsule endoscopy for obscure gastrointestinal bleeding: an updated meta-analysis. J Gastroenterol Hepatol 2011;26:796–801.

70. Dionisio PM, Gurudu SR, Leighton JA. Capsule endoscopy has a significantly higher diagnostic yield in patients with suspected and established Crohn's disease: a meta-analysis. American Journal of Gastroenterology 2009;105:1240–8.

71. Herrerias JM, Caundeo A, Rodriguez-Tellez M, et al. Capsule endoscopy in patients with suspected Crohn's disease and negative endoscopy. Endoscopy 2003;35:564–8.

72. Fireman Z, Mahajna E, Broide E, et al. Diagnosing small bowel Crohn's disease with wireless capsule endoscopy. Gut 2003;52:390–2.

73. Mow WS, Lo SK, Targan SR, et al. Initial experience with wireless capsule endoscopy in the diagnosis and management of inflammatory bowel disease. Clin Gastroenterol Hepatol 2004;2:31–40.

74. Marmo R, Rotondano G, Piscopo R, et al. Capsule endoscopy versus enteroclysis in the detection of small-bowel involvement in Crohn's's disease: a prospective trial. Clin Gastroenterol Hepatol 2005;3:772–6.

75. Solem CA, Loftus EV Jr, Fletcher JG, et al. Small-bowel imaging in Crohn's's disease: a prospective blinded 4 way comparison trial. Gastrointest Endosc 2008;68:255–66.

76. Voderholzer WA, Beinhoelzl J, Rogalla P, et al. Small bowel involvement in Crohn's's disease: a prospective comparison of wireless capsule endoscopy and computed tomography enteroclysis. Gut 2005;54:369–73.

77. Manoury V, Savoye G, Boureille A, et al. Value of wireless capsule endoscopy in patients with indeterminate colitis (inflammatory bowel disease unclassified). Inflamm Bowel Dis 2007;13:152–5.

78. Viazis N, Karamanolis DG. Indeterminate colitis: the role of wireless capsule endoscopy. Aliment Pharmacol Ther 2007;25:859.

79. Boureille A, Jarry M, D'Halluin PN, et al. Wireless capsule endoscopy versus ileocolonoscopy for the diagnosis of post-operative recurrence of Crohn's's disease: a prospective study. Gut 2006;55:978–83.

80. Numata M, Kodama M, Sasaki F, et al. Usefulness of double-balloon enteroscopy as a diagnostic and therapeutic method for small intestinal involvement in patients with inflammatory bowel disease. Gastrointest Endosc 2007;65:AB188.

81. Ross AS, Leighton JA, Schembre D, et al. Double-balloon enteroscopy in Crohn's's disease: findings and impact. Gastroenterology 2007;132:AB654.

82. Pohl J, May A, Nachbar L, et al. Diagnostic and therapeutic yield of push-and-pull enteroscopy for symptomatic small bowel Crohn's disease strictures. Eur J Gastroenterol Hepatol 2007;19:529–34.

83. Tanaka S, Mitsui K, Shirakawa K, et al. Successful retrieval of video capsule endoscopy retained at ileal stenosis of Crohn's's disease using double-balloon endoscopy. J Gastroenterol Hepatol 2006; 21:922–3.

84. Bailey AA, Debinski HS, Appleyard MN, et al. Diagnosis and outcome of small bowel tumors found by capsule endoscopy: a three center Australian experience. Am J Gastroenterol 2006;101:2237–43.

85. Cobrin GM, Pittman RH, Lewis BS. Increased diagnostic yield of small bowel tumors with capsule endoscopy. Cancer 2006;107:22–7.

86. Pasha SF, Fujii L, Sharma VK, et al. Incidence, management and outcomes of small bowel neoplasms in a cohort of 2000 patients undergoing video capsule endoscopy: a single center experience. Gastrointest Endosc 2010;71:AB373.

87. Rondonotti E, Pennazio M, Toth E, et al. Small-bowel neoplasma in patients undergoing video capsule endoscopy: a multicenter European study. Endoscopy 2008;40:488–95.

88. Mata A, Llach J, Castells S, et al. A prospective trial comparing wireless capsule endoscopy and barium contrast series for small bowel surveillance in hereditary GI polyposis syndromes. Gastrointest Endosc 2005;61:721–5.

89. Brown G, Fraser C, Schofield G, et al. Video capsule endoscopy in Peutz-Jegher's syndrome: a blinded comparison with barium follow-through for detection of small-bowel polyps. Endoscopy 2006;38:385–90.

90. Burke CA, Santisi J, Church J, et al. The utility of capsule endoscopy small bowel surveillance in patients with polyposis. Am J Gastroenterol 2005; 100:1498–502.

91. Caspari R, von Falkenhausen M, Krautmacher C, et al. Comparison of capsule endoscopy and magnetic resonance imaging for the detection of polyps of the small intestine in patients with familial adenomatous polyposis or with Peutz Jeghers' syndrome. Endoscopy 2004;36:1054–9.

92. Iaquinto G, Fornasarig M, Quaia M, et al. Capsule endoscopy is useful and safe for small bowel surveillance in familial adenomatous polyposis. Gastrointest Endosc 2008;67:61.

93. Madisch A, Schimming W, Kinzel F, et al. Locally advanced small bowel adenocarcinoma missed primarily by capsule endoscopy but diagnosed by push enteroscopy. Endoscopy 2003;35(10):861–4.

94. Huprich JE, Fletcher JG, Fidler JL, et al. Prospective blinded comparison of wireless capsule endoscopy and multiphase CT enterography in obscure gastrointestinal bleeding. Radiology 2011;260(3):744–51.

95. Ross A, Mehdizadeh S, Tokar J, et al. Double balloon enteroscopy detects small bowel mass lesions missed by capsule endoscopy. Dig Dis Sci 2008;53:2140–3.

96. Pasha SF, Sharma VK, Carey EJ, et al. Utility of video capsule endoscopy in the detection of small bowel tumors. A single center experience of 1000 consecutive patients. Proceedings of the 6th International Conference on Capsule Endoscopy 2007 June 8–10. Madrid (Spain); 2007. p. 45. Available at: www.icce.info/en-int/Documents/2007_program_book_madrid.pdf.

97. Ohmiya N, Taguchi A, Shirai, et al. Endoscopic resection of Peutz Jeghers polyps throughout the small intestine at double-balloon enteroscopy without laparotomy. Gastrointest Endosc 2005;61: 140–7.

98. Ross AS, Semrad C, Waxman I, et al. Enteral stent placement by double balloon enteroscopy for palliation of malignant small bowel obstruction. Gastrointest Endosc 2006;64:853–7.

99. Lee B, Choi H, Choi K, et al. Retrieval of a retained capsule endoscope by double balloon enteroscopy. Gastrointest Endosc 2005;62:463–5.

100. Fry LC, Neumann H, Kuester D, et al. Small bowel polyps and tumors: endoscopic detection and treatment by double-balloon enteroscopy. Aliment Pharmacol Ther 2008;29:135–42.

Index

Note: Page numbers of article titles are in **boldface** type.

Radiol Clin N Am 51 (2013) 189–194
http://dx.doi.org/10.1016/S0033-8389(12)00236-9
0033-8389/13/$ – see front matter © 2013 Elsevier Inc. All rights reserved.

Moving?

Make sure your subscription moves with you!

To notify us of your new address, find your **Clinics Account Number** (located on your mailing label above your name), and contact customer service at:

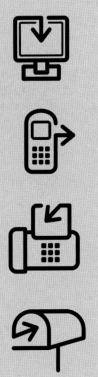

Email: journalscustomerservice-usa@elsevier.com

800-654-2452 (subscribers in the U.S. & Canada)
314-447-8871 (subscribers outside of the U.S. & Canada)

Fax number: 314-447-8029

Elsevier Health Sciences Division
Subscription Customer Service
3251 Riverport Lane
Maryland Heights, MO 63043

*To ensure uninterrupted delivery of your subscription, please notify us at least 4 weeks in advance of move.